multiple lead
ECGs

A Practical Analysis of Arrhythmias

multiple lead

ECGs

A Practical Analysis of Arrhythmias

Kathryn M. Janic Lewis RN PhD

DELMAR
CENGAGE Learning™

Australia • Brazil • Japan • Korea • Mexico • Singapore • Spain • United Kingdom • United States

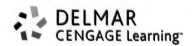

Multiple Lead ECGs: A Practical Analysis of Arrhythmias
Kathryn M. Janic Lewis RN PhD

Vice President, Career and Professional
    Editorial: Dave Garza

Director of Learning Solutions: Sandy Clark

Product Development Manager: Janet Maker

Managing Editor: Larry Main

Associate Project Manager: Meaghan O'Brien

Editorial Assistant: Amy Wetsel

Vice President, Career and Professional
    Marketing: Jennifer Baker

Executive Marketing Manager: Deborah S. Yarnell

Senior Marketing Manager: Erin Coffin

Marketing Coordinator: Shanna Gibbs

Production Director: Wendy Troeger

Production Manager: Mark Bernard

Senior Content Project Manager: Jennifer Hanley

Art Director: Benj Gleeksman

Technology Project Manager: Christopher Catalina

Library of Congress Control Number: 2009927066

ISBN-13: 978-1-4354-4124-8
ISBN-10: 1-4354-4124-9

Delmar
5 Maxwell Drive
Clifton Park, NY 12065-2919
USA

Cengage Learning is a leading provider of customized learning solutions with office locations around the globe, including Singapore, the United Kingdom, Australia, Mexico, Brazil and Japan. Locate your local office at: **international.cengage.com/region**

Cengage Learning products are represented in Canada by Nelson Education, Ltd.

For your lifelong learning solutions, visit **delmar.cengage.com**

Visit our corporate website at **www.cengage.com.**

NOTICE TO THE READER
Publisher does not warrant or guarantee any of the products described herein or perform any independent analysis in connection with any of the product information contained herein. Publisher does not assume, and expressly disclaims, any obligation to obtain and include information other than that provided to it by the manufacturer. The reader is expressly warned to consider and adopt all safety precautions that might be indicated by the activities described herein and to avoid all potential hazards. By following the instructions contained herein, the reader willingly assumes all risks in connection with such instructions. The publisher makes no representations or warranties of any kind, including but not limited to, the warranties of fitness for particular purpose or merchantability, nor are any such representations implied with respect to the material set forth herein, and the publisher takes no responsibility with respect to such material. The publisher shall not be liable for any special, consequential, or exemplary damages resulting, in whole or part, from the readers' use of, or reliance upon, this material.

Printed in the United States of America
1 2 3 4 5 XX 11 10 09

Table of
Contents

PREFACE . . . . **XVII**

CHAPTER 1
Review of Cardiac Anatomy and Function 1

Introduction. 1

Review of Cardiac Function 1

The Heart's Mechanical Structures 3

Cardiac Position and Movement 3

The Cardiac Valves 4

Cardiac Muscle 5

Ventricular Systole 8

Ventricular Diastole 8

Coronary Artery Perfusion 9

Summary 11

Self-Assessment Exercise 11

CHAPTER 2
Electrophysiology of the Heart 13

Introduction. 13

Electrophysiology of the Heart 13

The Phases of the Cardiac Cycle. 14

Properties of Cardiac Muscle 14

The Nervous System Control of the Heart. 16

The Electrical Conduction System 16

Summary 19

Self-Assessment Exercise 19

CHAPTER 3
The ECG and the Multiple Lead System 21

Introduction. 21

The ECG Leads: A Point of View 21

    Limb Leads 22

    Augmented Leads. 23

    The Precordial (Chest) Leads 24

    Monitoring the Posterior Surface of the Heart. 25

    MCL Leads. 26

    Clinical Lead Groups 28

    Hazards of Improper Lead Placement 28

Summary 29

Self-Assessment Exercise 29

CHAPTER 4
Rate, Rhythm, and Wave Forms 31

Introduction. 31

Calculating Rate and Rhythm. 32

Wave Forms, Complexes, and Intervals. 36

    P Waves 37

    PR Interval. 38

    QRS Complex 38

    ST Segment 40

    T Wave 40

    QT Interval 41

    U Wave. 42

Abnormal Wave Forms 43

    Abnormal P Waves. 43

    Abnormal PR Interval 44

    Abnormal QRS Complexes 45

    Abnormal QT Interval. 45

    Abnormal U Waves 46

Alterations of ECG Wave Forms. 47

    Drug-Induced Changes on the ECG 47

    Hyperkalemia 49

    Hypokalemia. 50

    Hypercalcemia 50

    Hypocalcemia 51

    Low-Voltage QRS 51

Pericarditis. 53
Ventricular Aneurysm. 55
Hypertrophic Cardiomyopathy .56
Increased Intracranial Pressure .56
Pulmonary Embolism 56

Summary 58

Self-Assessment Exercise 58

CHAPTER 5
Axis Determination and Implications 63

Introduction. 63

Normal Axis. 63

Axis Deviation. 64
Right Axis Deviation 64
Left Axis Deviation. 64

Calculating Axis 65

Normal and Abnormal Values .69

The Lewis Circle 69

Summary 70

Self-Assessment Exercises 71

CHAPTER 6
The Sinus Mechanisms 77

Introduction. 77

Sinus Rhythm 78

Sinus Tachycardia 79
Causes. 79
Intervention. 80

Sinus Bradycardia 80
Causes. 81
Intervention. 81

Sinus Arrhythmia 82
Causes. 82
Intervention. 83

Sinus Arrest 83
Causes. 84
Intervention. 84

Sinoatrial (SA) Block. 85

    Causes. 85

    Intervention. 86

Summary 86

Self-Assessment Exercise 87

CHAPTER 7
The Junctional Mechanisms. 93

Introduction. 93

The Origin of Junctional Mechanisms. 94

    Causes. 95

Escape Junctional Complex 95

    Causes. 95

    Intervention. 96

Junctional Rhythm 96

    Causes. 97

    Intervention. 97

Accelerated Junctional Rhythm 97

    Causes. 98

    Intervention. 98

Junctional Tachycardia. 98

Premature Junctional Complex. 98

    Causes. 100

    Intervention. 100

Idiojunctional Rhythm. 100

    Summary of Causes of Junctional Mechanisms. 100

Summary 102

Self-Assessment Exercises 102

CHAPTER 8
The Atrial Mechanisms 107

Introduction. 107

Premature Atrial Complex (PAC). 108

    Nonconducted (Blocked) PACs. 110

    Causes. 111

Atrial Bigeminy 112

    Causes. 112

Atrial Tachycardia. 112

PACs with Aberrant Ventricular Conduction. 114

   Intervention. 114

   Multifocal Atrial Tachycardia. 116

   Causes. 116

Paroxysmal Atrial Tachycardia (PAT). 116

   Causes. 117

Supraventricular Tachycardia (SVT). 117

   Causes and Consequences. 120

   Intervention. 121

Atrial Flutter 123

   Causes and Consequences. 125

   Intervention. 126

Atrial Fibrillation 126

   Causes and Consequences. 128

   Suspected Stroke Assessment and Actions 129

   Intervention. 130

   Differentiation of Atrial versus Sinus and Junctional Ectopics 130

Summary 131

Self-Assessment Exercise 132

CHAPTER 9

The Ventricular Mechanisms 141

Introduction. 141

Premature Ventricular Complex (PVC). 142

   Recognizing the PVC. 142

   Characteristics of a Ventricular Ectopic 143

   Narrow Complex PVCs 144

   Variations in PVCs 145

   Intervention. 150

Monomorphic Ventricular Tachycardia. 150

   Intervention. 151

Intermittent Ventricular Tachycardia. 152

   Wide QRS Complex Tachycardia of Uncertain Origin. 152

Polymorphic Ventricular Tachycardia. 154

   Torsades de Pointes (TdP) 154

   The Mechanism of TdP 155

   Intervention. 155

Ventricular Flutter. 156

Ventricular Fibrillation. 156

    Coarse versus Fine Ventricular Fibrillation 157

Ventricular Escape: Idioventricular Rhythm 158

Accelerated Idioventricular Rhythm (AIVR) 159

    Causes. 161

    Intervention. 161

Asystole. 161

    Asystole versus Fine Ventricular Fibrillation .161

    Intervention. 162

Pulseless Electrical Activity. 162

    Causes. 163

    Intervention. 163

Summary 164

Self-Assessment Exercises 164

CHAPTER 10
AV Conduction Defects 173

Introduction. 173

First-Degree AV Block 174

    ECG Characteristics. 175

    Causes. 176

    Intervention. 176

Second-Degree AV Block 176

Second-Degree AV Block Type I (Mobitz I) 176

    ECG Characteristics. 177

    Causes. 178

    Intervention. 178

Second-Degree AV Block Type II (Mobitz II) 178

    ECG Characteristics. 179

    Causes. 180

    Intervention. 180

2:1 Block 180

    ECG Characteristics. 180

Advanced or High-Grade AV Block. 180

    Intervention. 182

Complete AV Block. 184

    ECG Characteristics. 184

Causes. 184

Summary 186

Self-Assessment Exercises 187

CHAPTER 11
Intraventricular Conduction Defects 193

Introduction. 193

The Bundle Branches and Arterial Perfusion 194

Normal Sequence of Ventricular Depolarization
and the QRS Vector 195

ECG Changes in Bundle Branch Block .195

Right Bundle Branch Block. 196
Left Bundle Branch Block 199

Fascicular Blocks. 203

Left Anterior Fascicular Block 203
Left Anterior Fascicular Block and RBBB. 205
Left Anterior Fascicular Block and Myocardial Infarction. 206
Left Posterior Fascicular Block 206

Complete Left Bundle Branch Block 206

Trifascicular Block 208

Summary 209

Self-Assessment Exercise 209

CHAPTER 12
Chamber Enlargement and Hypertrophy 215

Introduction. 215

Right Atrial Enlargement. 215

Left Atrial Enlargement 216

Ventricular Hypertrophy 217

Right Ventricular Hypertrophy 217
Left Ventricular Hypertrophy. 218
Changes in the QRS 219
Ventricular Strain Pattern 223

Summary 225

Self-Assessment Exercise 227

CHAPTER 13

Arrhythmias due to Abnormal Conduction Pathways. . . . 231

Introduction. 231

Preexcitation Defined 232

Physiology of Accessory Pathway (AP) 232

The ECG Wave Forms Affected by Preexcitation 232

    Degrees of Preexcitation 234

    Concealed Accessory Pathway 236

Arrhythmias with Preexcitation 236

Lown-Ganong-Levine (LGL) Syndrome 239

Wolff-Parkinson-White (WPW) Syndrome 240

Summary 242

Self-Assessment Exercise 243

CHAPTER 14

Myocardial Perfusion Deficits and ECG Changes. 247

Introduction. 247

Coronary Artery Perfusion 248

Pathophysiology of Acute Myocardial Infarction. 249

    Consequences of Coronary Artery Occlusion 250

    Reflecting and Reciprocal Leads. 252

Monitoring Myocardial Ischemia, Injury,
and Necrosis on the ECG 254

    Changes in Wave Forms 254

    ECG Indicators of Perfusion Deficits. .261

Inferior Wall (Diaphragmatic) Myocardial Infarction 261

    Clinical Implications 262

Anterior Wall Myocardial Infarction. .264

    Clinical Implications 265

Anteroseptal Wall Myocardial Infarction 265

Anterolateral Wall Myocardial Infarction. 265

    Clinical Implications 266

Lateral Wall Myocardial Infarction 266

    Clinical Implications 267

Posterior Wall Myocardial Infarction .269

    Clinical Implications 269

Right Ventricular Myocardial Infarction............................269
Clinical Implications 272
Non-Q-Wave Myocardial Infarction 272
Pseudo-Infarction Patterns 273
Early Repolarization...274
Nonclassic ECG Presentation of Acute Myocardial Infarction 274
Continuous ST Segment Monitoring...........................274
Brugada Syndrome 276
Cocaine-Induced Chest Pain and Infarction 277
Summary 278
Self-Assessment Exercises 278

CHAPTER 15
Electronic Pacemakers 287

Introduction..287
Pacemaker Codes 288
The Language of Pacemaker Function.........................289
Pacemaker Components..290
Pulse Generator...290
Pacemaker Catheters and Electrodes...........................291
Pacemaker Energy 291
Pacemaker Artifact and Pacer-Induced QRS Complexes.......292
Pacemaker Fusion...292
Temporary and Permanent Pacing.............................293
Classification 293
Hysteresis..295
Atrial Pacemakers...296
Ventricular Pacemakers 296
Ventricular Demand Pacemakers...............................297
Triggered Ventricular Pacemakers..............................297
Rate-Responsive Pacemakers 299
Overdrive Suppression...299
Pacemaker Malfunction...299
Failure to Function..299
Failure to Sense 300
Failure to Capture.. 300

Assessing the Pacemaker ECG 300
    Assessing the Dual-Chamber Pacemaker on ECG 301
Complications of Pacing. 302
    Catheter Dislodgement 302
    Perforation. 302
    Skeletal Muscle Inhibition. 302
Summary 303
Self-Assessment Exercises 304

CHAPTER 16
General Review and Assessment Exercises 311

APPENDIX A
Answers to Self-Assessment Exercises 333

APPENDIX B
Normal Ranges and Variations in the
Adult 12-Lead Electrocardiogram. 423

APPENDIX C
Emergency Cardiac Care Guidelines 425

APPENDIX D
Quick Review of Assessment and
Interventions for Patients with Arrhythmias 437

APPENDIX E
Medication Profiles 443

APPENDIX F
List of Abbreviations 477

GLOSSARY **481**

REFERENCES **489**

INDEX **493**

Foreword

In this day and age, when heart disease is the leading cause of death in the United States, it is imperative that practitioners maintain the skills and knowledge necessary to recognize serious cardiac presentations in a timely fashion and how to best manage them. This situation is even more complex when one factors in the large variety of less serious cardiovascular problems. Our primary goals are to prevent cardiovascular mortality and minimize cardiovascular morbidity. There is rarely room for errors in judgment and decision making.

To meet and exceed the skills required to maintain practice competency, we, as practitioners, require the very best educational resources. In *Multiple Lead ECGs: A Practical Analysis of Arrhythmias*, Kathryn Lewis, RN, BSN, PhD, has created a gold standard textbook designed to be comprehensive from both an educational and practical perspective. In this textbook, Dr. Lewis has synthesized the scientific knowledge regarding the analysis of the multiple lead ECG with evaluating the all-important patient presentation to allow the practitioner to make the most accurate and best patient-care decisions.

The chapters within this text follow an organized progression of education, beginning with cardiac anatomy/function and electrophysiology, progressing through the "anatomy" of the ECG, and on to the analysis of the conduction and chamber mechanisms. With this firm grounding in normal anatomy and physiology, Dr. Lewis then guides the reader through pathophysiology, including conduction defects, arrhythmias, perfusion deficits, and the use of pacemakers. Each problem is approached from both an ECG and clinical presentation perspective. The appropriate management options are clearly and concisely presented with each problem. Finally, Dr. Lewis, ever the educator, has taken the effort to include a general review, based on exercises, and a wonderful collection of appendices, which I will leave to you, the reader, to explore.

Multiple Lead ECGs: A Practical Analysis of Arrhythmias not only represents a labor of love created by a premier educator, it is Dr. Kathryn Lewis's legacy and we are most fortunate to be the beneficiaries.

—*Robert A. Friedman, MD, FAAFP*

Preface

The purpose of this text is to introduce all health care providers to the systematic analysis and interpretation of the electrocardiogram (ECG) as it relates to the heart's function. In this way they will relate the changes, identify the problem, and contribute to and/or help make logical choices in determining patient care. In this text, there is a detailed discussion of cardiac anatomy followed by chapters dealing with specifics of the ECG. Chapters dealing with specific arrhythmias provide clear examples of the ECGs, their characteristics, lists of probable causes, and suggestions for proposed interventions. I have exerted a great deal of diligence and effort to ensure that suggested interventions, medications, and dosages set forth in this text are in accord with current recommendations and practice at the time of this printing.

This text does not replace specific courses detailing cardiac anatomy, physiology, and pathophysiology. Nor does it replace consistent review of updates in procedures, practices, interventions, and medications. The users must also have knowledge of and adhere to the standards and guidelines in their unique work environment.

The key to mastering ECG rhythm analysis and interpretation is consistent application of the steps described in each chapter. You will come to appreciate the ECG as a valuable tool in patient care assessment and intervention. Regardless of your role in the patient care continuum, you are the critical link providing insight and care for the patient in cardiac compromise.

BACKGROUND

The ECG is a powerful tool in the care of any patient. It is critical for any health care professional to know how to interpret the ECG in order to identify patients at high risk for myocardial infarction. The survival of the heart and the patient who houses it depends on early identification of the changes associated with patient presentation and enables the choice of the appropriate interventions in the least amount of time.

Since *time is muscle*, it is becoming increasingly necessary to have 12-lead ECG application and transmission from the prehospital scene to a receiving hospital. Confirmation of myocardial changes within the short "window of opportunity" provides the patient with the best possible opportunity for reperfusion and survival. It is critical that any patient presenting with signs and symptoms of acute coronary syndrome be afforded a multiple lead ECG. The use and interpretation of the 12-lead ECG require the same diligence and effort, and the same organized approach, only adding nine or more leads. Because significant changes may not be seen in some leads, monitoring in just one or two leads is simply wrong.

No matter how sophisticated the technology, the exacting effort and expertise in the hand and eye of the clinician will never be replaced. The clinician has the ultimate responsibility for the interpretation, not the computer.

TEXTBOOK ORGANIZATION

Multiple Lead ECGs: A Practical Analysis of Arrhythmias is organized as follows:

- **Chapter 1, Review of Cardiac Anatomy and Function:** Detailed discussion into the heart's structures and functions as related to its perfusion and the body in which it is housed.

- **Chapter 2, Electrophysiology of the Heart:** Discussion of the properties critical to myocardial electrical activity and the structures of the heart's electrical conduction system.

- **Chapter 3, The ECG and the Multiple Lead System:** Detailed explanation of the differences between unipolar and bipolar leads, the formation of limb leads, and the position of precordial leads. Description of the surface of the heart monitored by each lead and ways to identify the signs of incorrect lead placement.

- **Chapter 4, Rate, Rhythm, and Wave Forms:** Techniques for calculating rate and rhythm; identifying the ECG wave forms, complexes, and their measurements. Discussion on methods of identifying the changes in ECG measurements that may indicate electrolyte imbalance and changes that occur with certain medications and clinical syndromes.

- **Chapter 5, Axis Determination and Implications:** Introduction to the leads used in calculating the direction and flow of the heart's electrical current (axis). Explanations on how to determine normal axis, left and right axis deviation, and the pathology associated with axis deviation.

- **Chapter 6, The Sinus Mechanisms:** Details of sinus rhythm and the mechanisms of the sinus arrhythmias, the probable causes, and proposed interventions.

- **Chapter 7, The Junctional Mechanisms:** Explanations and ECG examples of the junctional mechanisms; differences between ectopy and escape are discussed. Probable causes and proposed interventions are included.

- **Chapter 8, The Atrial Mechanisms:** Descriptions of atrial arrhythmias including ECG examples ranging from single ectopics, to reentry mechanisms within the atria or the AV node and tachycardias whose origins are within the atria. Current efforts to categorize atrial fibrillation are also listed and explained.

- **Chapter 9, The Ventricular Mechanisms:** Details and ECG examples of the ventricular mechanisms; differences between ectopy and escape are discussed. Probable causes and proposed interventions are included. Established methods are provided to assist in dealing with wide QRS complex tachycardias. Identification and confirmation of asystole, the causes, and proposed interventions are discussed. The diagnosis and causes of pulseless electrical activity are presented.

- **Chapter 10, AV Conduction Defects:** Details of anatomical locations and the ECG characteristics of the levels of "the blocks"; the related terminology as well as proposed interventions are clarified and discussed.

- **Chapter 11, Intraventricular Conduction Defects:** ECG recognition of defects within the ventricular conduction system are presented along with probable causes and proposed interventions. The use of axis determination is applied to assist with confirmation of the interpretation.

- **Chapter 12, Chamber Enlargement and Hypertrophy:** The causes, ECG characteristics, and clinical significance of atrial and ventricular enlargement and hypertrophy are discussed. Standardized measurements to assist with confirmation are explained.
- **Chapter 13, Arrhythmias Due to Abnormal Conduction:** The physiology of abnormal and accessory pathways and related syndromes are presented here. Signs and symptoms and proposed interventions are listed.
- **Chapter 14, Myocardial Perfusion Deficits and ECG Changes:** Perfusion deficits and how they are revealed on the ECG. The changes in the wave forms as they "point to" or reflect ischemia, injury, and infarction and related ECG examples are presented.
- **Chapter 15, Electronic Pacemakers:** Discussion of the terminology associated with electronic pacemakers. ECG characteristics as well as signs of pacemaker malfunction are presented.
- **Chapter 16, General Review and Assessment Exercises:** An extensive range of ECG tracings representing the arrhythmias contained in preceding chapters. There is opportunity to systematically assess the ECG, provide an interpretation, and offer proposed interventions.
- **Appendix A, Answers to Chapter Self-Assessment Exercises:** Detailed answers to measurements are provided, patient presentation is explained, and proposed interventions are clarified.
- **Appendix B, Normal Ranges and Variations in Adults on the Multiple Lead ECG:** Normal ranges and variations in the adult 12-lead ECG presented as a table that can serve as a guideline to assess the ECG as it relates to patient conditions.
- **Appendix C, Emergency Cardiac Care Guidelines:** Standard approaches to patient care interventions that have their basis in current guidelines in advanced cardiac care.
- **Appendix D, Quick Review of Assessment and Interventions:** A bulleted approach to patients in situations of compromise with various arrhythmias.
- **Appendix E, Medication Profiles:** A reference for medications; includes dosages, indications, contraindications, and side effects—most dealing with patients who are in cardiac compromise.
- **Appendix F, List of Abbreviations:** A list of common abbreviations used in this text and in clinical practice.
- **Glossary:** A detailed explanation of terminology and phrases in this book and in clinical practice.

FEATURES

The following list describes some of the significant features of this text:

- Clear and concise presentation of concepts and practice skills promotes quicker comprehension and easier application of subject matter.
- Several original ECG tracings with patient presentation are included in the discussion.
- ECG rhythm identification practice sections at the end of each chapter allow readers to test their knowledge.
- Complete chapter focusing on review and assessment exercises helps readers practice everything learned throughout the text.
- Proposed interventions are in accordance with current standards and guidelines.

HOW TO USE THIS TEXT

The text is written in a concise manner and supplemented with detailed ECG tracings, many taken from real-life patient scenarios. There are self-study questions and ECG rhythm identification to allow you, the learner, the opportunity to test baseline knowledge and progress throughout the text. The language of the text provides terminology appropriate to the arrhythmias and related patient care. For the purpose of brevity, the terms *clinician* and *practitioner* include all levels of health care providers. Also, the term *arrhythmia* is used because it is universal and simply describes a deviation from normal—an imperfection or a problem.

The text is designed in a specific format, which, if followed, will help you master the skills necessary for accurate interpretation for each arrhythmia. The introductory chapters provide baseline insight into cardiac anatomy and electrophysiology. Wave forms and timing techniques are explained as they reflect the heart's electrical functions.

Each arrhythmia is introduced; ECG characteristics are detailed and related causes and pathophysiology are listed, described, and explained. As you progress through the chapters and the self-assessment exercises, you may be tempted to study directly from the answer keys—don't do this. The mastery of the sample practice in each chapter builds a stronger foundation.

INSTRUCTOR RESOURCES

Instructor Resources to accompany *Multiple Lead ECGs: A Practical Analysis of Arrhythmias* was developed as a guide to assist instructors in planning and implementing their instructional programs. The CD includes lesson plans, PowerPoint slides highlighting the main topics of each chapter, answers to review questions throughout the book, and additional instructor resources.

ISBN: 1-4354-4125-7

ABOUT THE AUTHOR

Dr. Kathryn M. Lewis is the president of KACEL, Inc. Professional and Community Education. She is also adjunct faculty within the Maricopa County Community College District where she teaches basic and paramedic levels of EMT courses, and is an examiner for the National Registry of EMTs. Dr. Lewis was a critical care nurse and educator for Good Samaritan Medical Center for 20 years. After serving as department chair at Phoenix College since 1986, Dr. Lewis retired in 2005. During that time she was also a member of the Arizona EMS Council (Governor's Appointment), and member of the National EMS Curriculum Development Group. She has worked as a critical care nurse and educator, has authored several articles and contributed to texts on nursing care, education theory and techniques, as well as various cardiovascular topics. Dr. Lewis holds many industry affiliations and credentials, is an active RN and holds a BSN in nursing and a PhD in Education.

ACKNOWLEDGMENTS

The accumulation of knowledge and insight is never a solitary process. I have learned from physicians, nurses, technicians, students, patients, families, and various mentors. Dr. Leonard Caccamo gave my first experiences with ECGs and the patients to whom they belonged. He always reminded me of the humanity the ECG represented and that the ECG should never be considered a stand-alone diagnosis. I am grateful to Dr. Henry Marriott, who gave me the strength to always question "why"; to Drs. Schumacher and Sridahr, who thought out loud no matter the situation.

I will always be indebted to Robert Dotterer, MEd, NREMT-P, who taught the best classes in patient assessment and stressed looking beyond the obvious; and of course for his initial contributions to the medication profiles. Bob was the best street medic in my 30 years in prehospital education.

My thanks to my colleagues and the editorial board who read and reread the manuscripts, listened politely most of the time, oohing and ahhing appropriately, offering simple suggestions, making occasional loud grunts and dramatic eye rolls, and sometimes asking "did you really want to say this?"

Thanks to my students who provided the acid test for each version of this work since its inception in 1977; to those authors who used that work as a foundation for their own publications; and to those past students, now practitioners, who occasionally tell me of a patient encounter and of hearing my voice in their heads: "tell me about the PATIENT."

I am especially grateful to Christian Holdener and the team at S4Carlisle Publishing Services—for patience, firm resolve and boundless knowledge of all aspects of syntax, structure, grammar and all the rules and nuances that translate the author's work into a truly professional text.

Delmar, a part of Cengage Learning, and I would also like to thank the following reviewer not on the editorial board for her valuable suggestions and expertise:

Denise A. Wilfong, PhD(c), NREMT-P
Assistant Professor
Western Carolina University
Cullowhee, North Carolina

Editorial Board

Orlando Alcordo, NREMT-P
Director of Training and Education
PMT Ambulance
Tempe, Arizona

Robert Friedman, MD, FAAFP
Board Certified–Hospice & Palliative Medicine
Medical Director, Vista Care–Austin & San Marcos
Pflugerville, Texas

Eileen Laudermilch, RN, CCRN
Assistant Nurse Manager
Arizona Burn Center
Maricopa Regional Medical Center
Phoenix, Arizona

Krysta Roseberry, RN, CCRN
CCU Staff Nurse; BLS and ACLS Educator
Banner Good Samaritan Regional Medical Center
Phoenix, Arizona

Gary A. Smith, MD
Board Certified Family Physician
Chief Medical Officer: Family Doctors of Arizona
Medical Director: Apache Junction, Gilbert, and Mesa Arizona
    Fire Departments
Mesa, Arizona

Roger D. White, MD
Professor of Anesthesiology
Mayo Clinic College of Medicine
Departments of Anesthesiology and Internal Medicine/Cardiovascular
    Diseases
City of Rochester and Olmsted County Early Defibrillation Program
Co-Medical Director, Gold Cross Ambulance Service
Rochester, Minnesota

Andy Yee RPharm
Senior Staff Pharmacist
Banner Good Samaritan Regional Medical Center
Phoenix, Arizona

Feedback

Delmar and I welcome your feedback. If you have any suggestions that you think others would benefit from, please let us know, and we will try to include them in our next edition.

To send us your questions or feedback, you can contact the publisher at:

Delmar Cengage Learning
Executive Woods
5 Maxwell Drive
Clifton Park, NY 12065
Attn: Emergency Medical Services Team

Dedication

To patients, families, and beloved bystanders past, present, and to come, with all their unique variations. To the students: Remember, just when you thought you knew it all, you will realize you are just beginning. And of course, to the St. Theresa Friday 6:30 AM support group.

Review of Cardiac Anatomy and Function

Premise

To know the heart's mechanical function and purpose is to recognize signs and symptoms of its malfunction.

Objectives

After reading the chapter and completing the Self-Assessment Exercise, the student should be able to

- Describe the position of the heart within the body.
- Identify the structures and functions of the heart and its blood vessels.
- Identify the phases of systole and diastole.

Key Terms

atrial kick	epicardium	pericardium
cardiac output	heart rate	stroke volume
chest pain	myocardium	
endocardium	perfusion	

Introduction

Many students of the electrocardiogram (ECG) are not enchanted with the typical review of cardiac muscle and functions. However, a review is necessary to maintain perspective of cardiac **perfusion**. The ECG will relate problems of ischemia in various surfaces of the heart. The practitioner should be able to read and interpret the ECG, recall the surface of the heart visualized by the various ECG leads and the responsible coronary blood supply that is in jeopardy, and realize the implications in terms of what can happen next with this patient. All this provides a sound basis for patient care decisions.

REVIEW OF CARDIAC FUNCTION

Myocardial contraction and subsequent ejection of blood are a direct result of electrical activation. Electrical activation is complete and accurate if the heart muscle and the conduction system embedded within are well perfused and oxygenated.

In simplest terms, the function of the heart is to pump blood to the lungs for oxygenation and then to pump that blood back into systemic circulation. This process requires blood volume and the timeless, persistent muscular contraction of heart muscle. When there is malperfusion of cardiac muscle, there are problems with electrical function, cardiac output, and systemic circulation.

Cardiac output (the amount of blood ejected from the heart per minute) is the product of heart rate and stroke volume. Variations in cardiac output can be produced by altering the heart rate or the stroke volume. **Heart rate** is the number of contractions, or how fast the heart beats. Heart rate is primarily determined by the integrity of the heart's electrical conduction system and the influence of the body's autonomic nervous system as it tries to identify and respond to changes and needs of the body. **Stroke volume** is the amount of blood ejected with each heartbeat. It is primarily determined by the efficient contraction of cardiac muscle and the blood volume returning to the heart.

Normally, the body compensates for increases and decreases in stroke volume and heart rate, so that as one increases, the other decreases. If the demands of the body's tissues for oxygen are not met due to a decreased cardiac output, the body will display signs and symptoms such as the following:

- Chest pain
- Dizziness
- Altered levels of consciousness
- Syncopal and/or near-syncopal episodes
- Changes in skin temperature and hydration
- Difficulty breathing
- Decreased urinary output

Diminished circulation through the pulmonary system will result in progressive hypoxia, and, if left untreated, the body begins a spiral decline.

For the purposes of this text, **chest pain** is used to describe a range of subjective terms that the patient may use. These terms include:

- Pain
- Discomfort
- Burning
- Pressure
- Tightness
- A constricting band around the chest
- Heaviness
- Diaphoresis (perfuse perspiration)
- Aching
- Fullness
- Hard to breathe
- Cannot take a deep breath
- Heavy weight on the chest
- Sudden anxiety
- Difficulty getting one's breath

When symptoms develop because of a drop in heart rate and the body exhibits the above signs, the patient is said to be symptomatic, that is, hypotensive and hypoperfusing. When the heart muscle is damaged or injured as with infarction, the heart's pumping ability may fail, stroke volume will decrease, and heart rate will increase. Unfortunately, any change in cardiac output requires functioning oxygenated tissue and an increase in myocardial oxygen demand. A poorly perfused myocardium cannot respond to this increased debt, and the problem intensifies.

The Heart's Mechanical Structures

The right atrium and ventricle differ in function and musculature. The right atrium is a low-pressure receptacle, receiving blood from the systemic circulation, and is a thin-walled muscular structure. The right ventricle is thicker than the atrium, to accommodate the pressures necessary to eject blood to the pulmonary circulation. Despite the differences, they act as a single unit to move blood from the great veins to the pulmonary circulation.

The left atrium and ventricle act similarly to move oxygenated blood from the lungs to the high-pressure systemic circulation. The left atrium is a low-pressure receptacle, receiving blood from the pulmonic circulation, and is a thin-walled muscular structure. The left ventricle is thicker than the left atrium and right ventricle because the left ventricle must accommodate the pressures necessary to eject blood to the systemic circulation. Tension in the left ventricular tissue reflects the pressure against which it must pump. Systemic vascular resistance can cause an increase in the size and thickness of the left ventricle. **Figure 1.1** illustrates right and left ventricular structures in relation to their intake and outflow structures and to the lungs.

Cardiac Position and Movement

The terms *right* and *left heart* are not descriptive of their position in the body. The right ventricle is anterior, in front of the left and occupies a position immediately behind the sternum, whereas the left ventricle is rotated so that it faces toward the left side and is more posterior in the thorax.

The heart is suspended and secured in the pericardial cavity by its attachments to the great vessels. The heart is located in the center of the chest, within the mediastinum between the lungs (**Figure 1.2**). Approximately one-third of the heart lies to the right of the midline, and two-thirds of the heart lie to the left of the midline. The heart is superior to the diaphragm, with the apex located to the left of the central portion of the diaphragm. The base of the heart is located superiorly, posteriorly, and to the right of the midline at about the level of the second intercostal space.

The heart is protected anteriorly by the sternum and the rib cage and posteriorly by the vertebral column and the rib cage. The apex is free to move, and in fact, during ventricular contraction, dimensional changes take place within the ventricle, causing the apex to move forward and to strike against the left chest wall in the area of the left intercostal space. This

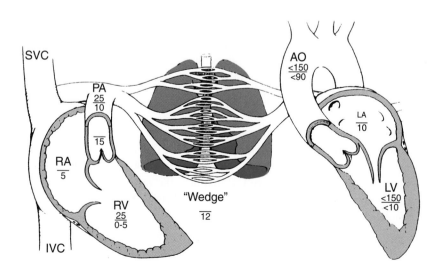

Figure 1.1 Right and left atrial and ventricular structures in relation to their intake and outflow structures and to the lungs. The numbers reflect the normal ranges for each chamber and major artery. "Wedge" (PCWP) pressure provides an indirect estimate of left atrial pressure (LAP). Note the differences in pressures within the right and left ventricles. (SVC = superior vena cava; IVC = inferior vena cava; RA = right atrium; RV = right ventricle; LA = left atrium; LV = left ventricle; PA = pulmonary artery; AO = aorta.)

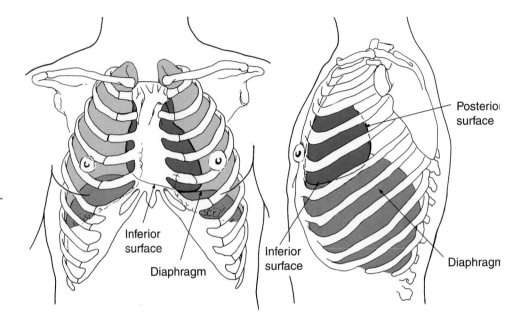

Posterior surface

Inferior surface

Diaphragm

Inferior surface

Diaphragm

Figure 1.2 The position of the heart within the body. The heart is located in the mediastinum, superior to the diaphragm with the bulk of the left ventricle to the left side and posterior.

characteristic thrust is felt by the examiner as the apical pulse. The placement of the heart within the rib cage gives rise to the position of the ECG chest-wall electrodes to best view the heart's surfaces.

The Cardiac Valves

There are four delicate, resilient, but strong valves that guard the entrance and exit of each ventricle (**Figure 1.3**). Even though they function passively, they greatly enhance the movement of blood by preventing backflow. There are no valves between the veins and their entrance into the atria. The heart always must accept the blood that comes to it. Even if the ventricles cannot eject all the blood during systole, blood continues to enter the heart via the atria. This constant flow of blood into the heart will cause the atria to distend and stretch. An abnormal stretch will give rise to various ECG patterns and arrhythmias.

Just at the end of ventricular diastole, in the microsecond prior to ventricular systole, the ventricles tense. It is at this point that the coronary arteries are in greatest jeopardy. They cannot readily perfuse since they are embedded in this tense and rigid muscular structure.

The semilunar valves, so named for their crescent shape, are situated between the ventricles and their respective arteries. The pulmonic (PA) valve is located between the right ventricle and the pulmonary artery; the aortic (AO) valve is located between the left ventricle and the aorta. The aortic and pulmonic valves open completely during ventricular ejection/systole and close completely during ventricular filling/diastole. **Figure 1.3** illustrates the heart's valves during ventricular systole and diastole. Note the apparent bulging of the valves during ventricular systole.

There is a slight enlargement of the aorta and the pulmonary artery in the area of the AO and PA valves. This enlargement provides space behind the open AO valve cusps so that the leaflets do not occlude the openings/orifices of the coronary arteries. This space favors the development of eddy currents (**Figure 1.4**) that hold the valve cusps away from the arterial wall in such a way that they will be easily caught and closed by the backflow of blood at the end of systolic ejection.

The structure of the mitral and tricuspid (AV) valves controls the flow of blood into the ventricles. The valve cusps are extensions of the chordae tendinae, which are, in turn,

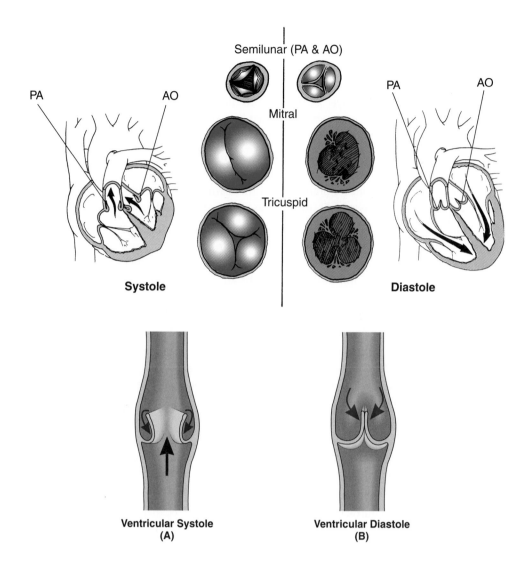

Figure 1.3 A schematic representation of the position of the cardiac valves during ventricular systole and diastole. (PA = pulmonary artery; AO = aorta.)

Figure 1.4 A schematic representation of the eddy currents in the aortic valve during ventricular systole and diastole. The enlargement (A) provides space behind the open aortic (AO) valve cusps so that the leaflets do not occlude the coronary artery orifices in ventricular systole. The eddy currents (B) act to hold the cusps away from the wall of the aorta in ventricular systole and are easily caught and closed at the end of ventricular systole and during ventricular diastole.

extensions of the papillary muscles. Papillary muscles are specialized extensions of the myocardium. Ventricular contraction distorts the valves, which are larger than their openings. This disparity in size allows for complete closure during ventricular systole. Sometimes there is a great disproportion in size, which causes an abnormal movement (called a prolapse) of the valve into the atrium.

The mitral valve has two cusps and is located between the left atrium and ventricle; the tricuspid valve has three cusps and is located between the right atrium and ventricle.

Cardiac Muscle

The wall of the heart is composed of anatomically distinct layers:

1. The pericardium that surrounds the heart and holds the heart in place
2. The *outer* layer or *epi*cardium
3. The middle *muscle* layer or muscular *myo*cardium
4. The *inner* layer or *endo*cardium

The pericardium is a triple-layered sac filled with serous fluid and contains the heart and the roots of the great vessels. The strong outer layer of this sac is called the fibrous pericardium and is composed of dense connective tissue. The fibrous pericardium adheres to the diaphragm inferiorly and is fused to the roots of the great vessels that enter and leave the heart.

The serous pericardium is a closed sac between the fibrous pericardium and the heart. Its outer layer is the parietal layer and adheres to the inner surface of the fibrous pericardium. The parietal layer is continuous with the visceral layer of the serous pericardium or epicardium, which lies on the heart and is considered as part of the wall of the heart.

The **epicardium**, also called the visceral pericardium, is the innermost of the two layers of the pericardium and is continuous with the outer covering of the ventricles. The epicardium contains some small nerve branches and the main coronary blood vessels. Its largest constituent is connective tissue and functions as the heart's protective layer.

The **myocardium** is the muscular middle layer of the wall of the heart. It is composed of spontaneously contracting cardiac muscle fibers that are arranged in elongated, circular and spiral cardiac muscle cells and provide the contractile force. Coordinated contraction of the myocardium propels blood inferiorly through the atria and superiorly from the ventricles to the circulatory system. Cardiac muscle cells, like all tissues in the body, rely on an ample blood supply to deliver oxygen and nutrients and to remove waste products such as carbon dioxide.

The **endocardium** is the innermost layer of tissue that lines the heart and part of the heart valves. It consists of a layer of endothelial cells and an underlying layer of connective tissue. The endocardium contains many nerve fibers and sensory endings that are more abundant in the atria than in the ventricles.

The endocardium is primarily made up of endothelial cells and controls myocardial function. This modulating role is separate from the homeometric and heterometric regulatory mechanisms that control myocardial contractility. The cardiac endothelium (both the endocardial endothelium and the endothelium of the myocardial capillaries) controls the development of the heart in the adult, for example during hypertrophy.

Additionally, the contractility and electrophysiological environment of the cardiac muscle cells are regulated by the cardiac endothelium. The endocardium lines the inner cavities of the heart, covers heart valves, and is continuous with the inner lining of blood vessels.

The Atria. The atria are reservoirs of blood and are very distensible. They are collapsible when partially filled and are usually quite elastic when overfilled. The atrial capacity of the normal adult is 160 milliliters (ml) on the right and about 140 ml on the left. During ventricular systole, forward movement of blood into the ventricles is stopped because of the closed AV valves. At the end of ventricular diastole, the atria contract and blood is added to the already well-filled ventricles. This addition of blood is **atrial kick**. In specific ECG abnormalities, the loss of atrial kick will ensue and the patient will display signs and symptoms of the deficit, such as dizziness, fatigue, and other signs of hypotension and hypoperfusion.

The right atrium has more extensions of the myocardial layer (trabeculae) than the left, perhaps to facilitate the greater pressures from venous flow on the right, that is, superior and inferior venae cavae and the coronary sinus.

The Ventricles. The ventricles are the major force behind perfusion. The more circular left ventricle is designed to support the highly resistant systemic circulation. It is quite effective in developing and maintaining high intracardiac pressures to maintain that circulation. The bellow-shaped right ventricle supports moving blood from the systemic circulation into the low-pressure pulmonary circulation.

The walls of the ventricles are similar in structure to the atria, and for ease of study, the layers are repeated here. There are three anatomically distinct layers:

1.   The outer epicardium
2.   The muscular myocardium
3.   The inner endocardium

The ventricular myocardium is much thicker than that of the atria and is arranged in a much more complicated sequence of layers and bundles. The muscle bundles are trabeculae and are extensions of the myocardium. The dense myocardium is thicker on the left, and the trabecular layer is thicker on the right.

The ventricular septum is the thickest part of the ventricular wall and is common to the right and left ventricular chambers and has trabeculation on both sides.

There are two primary muscle groups, superficial and deep spiral (**Figure 1.5**). The superficial muscles have their origin in the cardiac ring that separates the atria from the ventricles. They wrap around so that they exert a wringing effect during muscular contraction. The deeper spiral muscles are arranged as spirals and coils in clockwise and counterclockwise fashion. The deep bulbospiral muscle in the left ventricle is responsible for the forceful ejection of blood during ventricular systole.

Figure 1.5 illustrates how the fibers leave their origin at the root of the pulmonary artery and the aorta and insert into the papillary muscles and trabeculae. Between the origin and insertion there is a 360-degree path down to the apex and then back onto the inside of the heart at its base.

This is a great simplification of a very complex matrix that supports maximum projection and emptying of blood in ventricular systole and maximum filling of blood in ventricular diastole.

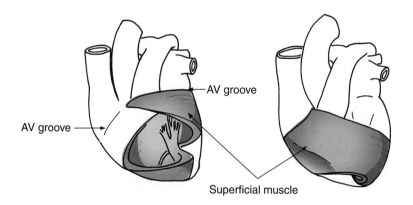

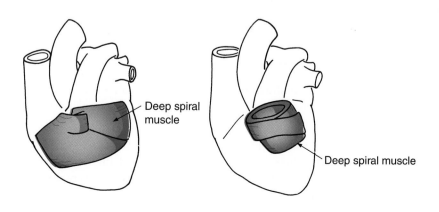

Figure 1.5 Layers of muscles of the right and left ventricles. Two groups of fibers surround the outside of both ventricles and their origin in the atrioventricular (AV) groove. The deep spiral muscle (lower left) also has its origin in the AV groove and encircles both ventricles. The deep spiral muscle (lower right) is specific to the left ventricle.

Knowledge of the muscle groups and their winding configurations will give insight into why, in right inferior myocardial infarction, left ventricular output can be greatly affected.

Ventricular Systole

The spiral arrangement of the ventricular myocardium is adapted to propelling blood flow. During the early stages of ventricular contraction, the inflow tract from atria to apex shortens, and the outflow tract from apex to aorta lengthens, thus making the left ventricle more spheroid. The ventricular septum is activated early on and provides a rigid prop, around which the heart will wring, twist, and thrust in an effort to move the blood out the outflow tract. During this time, the heart rotates somewhat to the right, and the left ventricle is brought forward.

Ventricular contraction (systole) and the associated rapid increase in ventricular pressures promptly close the mitral and tricuspid (AV) valves. The AV valves bulge into the atria, and ventricular pressures rise rapidly as the contraction process begins to squeeze the blood contained inside the ventricle against the closed AV valves. Ventricular pressure continues to increase. As it rises above aortic pressure, the aortic valve cusps are forced open, and the period of rapid ventricular ejection begins.

During the remainder of ventricular systole, ventricular pressure falls below aortic pressure, and a negative pressure gradient develops across the aortic valve. Due to its forward momentum, blood continues to be ejected from the ventricle during this period, in spite of the reversed pressure gradient, but the rate of ejection decreases rapidly.

The fact that blood continues to move forward during this period appears paradoxical, but the total energy of ventricular blood is still higher than the total energy level of the blood in the aorta. About 0.17 second after the onset of the phase of reduced ejection, forward movement of blood out of the ventricles stops, and the flow momentarily reverses as blood attempts to regurgitate into the ventricle. This backflow will catch the aortic valve cusps, and they are promptly closed. It is at this time that the coronary arteries begin to fill.

Ventricular Diastole

Within about 0.06 to 0.08 second after the closure of the aortic valve, ventricular volume is stabilized, and the mitral and tricuspid (AV) valves are still closed. Blood cannot leave or enter the ventricles. This is the period of isovolemic relaxation. During this time, pressure within the ventricles drops rapidly, and relaxation of the ventricular myocardium begins. At the same time, the curve of the AV valves begins to flatten out. When ventricular pressure falls below atrial pressure, the mitral cusps bulge toward the ventricles. At the end of isovolemic relaxation, the ventricular pressures fall below that of the atria. Traction on the valve cusps by the chordae tendinea during diastole plays a role in valve opening.

Opening of the AV valves permits blood that has collected in the atria to rush into the relaxing ventricles; this is the period of rapid ventricular filling early in ventricular diastole. At this point, ventricular pressures are low, and blood is literally sucked into the ventricles. Ventricular filling continues until the atrial and ventricular pressures are similar. After electrical activation, atrial contraction squeezes additional blood into the ventricles. Intraventricular pressures increase, and the process of ventricular depolarization and subsequent contraction begins again.

Figure 1.6 illustrates the phases of ventricular diastole and systole. Note the position of the valves during early and late filling stages and the change in the size of the ventricles. Notice, too, the position of the cardiac valves during the phases ranging from ventricular filling to contraction.

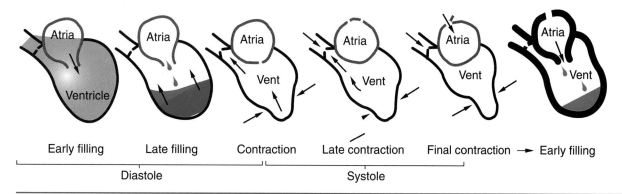

Figure 1.6 Schematic representation of the events in ventricular diastole and systole. During ventricular diastole, the AO and PA valves are closed so that blood enters the ventricles only from the atria. Atrial systole occurs during late ventricular filling (diastole) and contributes to the *boost* of blood volume in the ventricles just prior to ventricular systole (atrial kick).

The right ventricle pumps blood at 25 to 32 millimeters of mercury (mmHg) pressure into the lungs for oxygenation and for release of carbon dioxide. The left atrium receives oxygenated blood from the lungs. The blood then passes into the left ventricle, which pumps at about 120 mmHg pressure into the arterial system. Externally, the anterior and posterior intraventricular sulci contain the coronary blood vessels and a variable amount of fat. The muscular layers of the ventricle are developed so that the muscle mass to the right ventricle is considerably less than that of the left ventricle. This variance in muscle mass is the result of the difference in pressures between the muscular chambers. Although each ventricle pumps essentially the same amount of blood, the major difference in structure reflects the difference in function.

Coronary Artery Perfusion

Like other organ systems, the heart has its own blood supply. However, unlike other organ systems, coronary artery perfusion is occurs during the diastolic phase of the cardiac cycle. Coronary artery perfusion is affected by the unique position at the beginning of the aorta, just behind the aortic cusps. While the right and left sides of the heart receive oxygenated blood from the coronary arteries, the timing for optimal perfusion differs.

For example, the right ventricular myocardium receives a flow of oxygenated blood from the coronary circulation almost continuously throughout the cardiac cycle. Even during ventricular systole, the right ventricle generates lower systolic pressure, which allows for some coronary filling. The left ventricular myocardium receives oxygenated coronary blood flow only during the diastolic phase of the cardiac cycle, probably because the left ventricle exerts systolic pressure equal to or greater than aortic pressure. As a result, intramyocardial tension and pressure hamper blood flow within the myocardium, particularly to the subendocardial layers.

The coronary arteries are also responsible for blood supply to the electrical conduction system. The right coronary artery has its origin behind a cusp of the aortic valve. It proceeds downward and perfuses the right anterior and posterior surfaces of the heart. The posterior descending branch of the right coronary artery also emits septal branches that perfuse the posterior one-third of the ventricular septum and a terminal portion of the inferoposterior division of the left bundle branch, a part of the heart's ventricular electrical conduction system.

The right coronary artery is responsible for about 55 to 60 percent of the blood supply to the sinus node, the major electrical pacemaker of the heart. In about 90 percent of individuals, the posterior descending branch of the right coronary artery perfuses the electrical conduction system at the AV junction: the AV node and the bundle of His. In the remaining

10 percent, dual blood supply from the right posterior descending branch of the right coronary artery and the anterior descending branch of the left coronary artery perfuse the heart's ventricular electrical conduction system.

The common portion of the left coronary artery after its origin from the aorta and before the bifurcation into the left anterior descending (LAD) and circumflex arteries is called the left main trunk (LMT). LAD disease causes loss of a large amount of muscle mass and parts of the electrical conduction system. The LAD is frequently implicated in sudden cardiac death, predominantly in adult males. Clinicians often refer to the LAD as the widow maker because obstruction here predisposes to a high incidence of sudden death. The LAD is usually larger than the circumflex.

The left circumflex branch winds around the left ventricle dividing the left atrium and left ventricle. The extent of perfusion of the left circumflex to the right atrium varies. The left circumflex supplies about 40 percent of perfusion to the sinus node.

Figure 1.7 demonstrates the relative position of each of the major branches of the coronary arteries. Note the large amounts of muscle mass dependent on the LAD.

As blood is perfused through the coronary circulation system, oxygen and nutrients are delivered to myocardial tissue; substrate, carbon dioxide, and metabolic waste products are removed. The deoxygenated blood is collected by smaller cardiac veins that empty into the great cardiac vein, coronary sinus, and finally the right atrium. The venous blood from the posterior aspect is drained into the middle cardiac vein. The remaining blood empties directly into the right ventricle by way of the small Thebesian veins.

Adequate perfusion of the coronary circulation is directly dependent on blood volume and the time in ventricular diastole. The coronary arteries are in jeopardy during ventricular

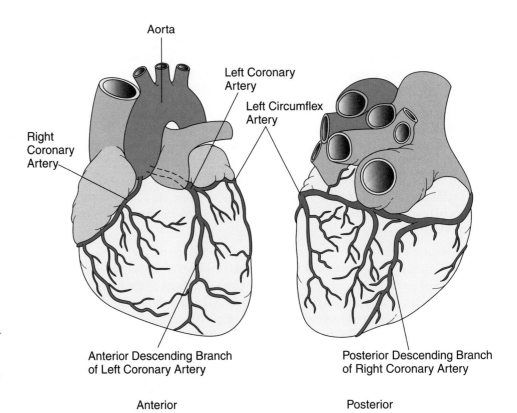

Aorta

Left Coronary Artery

Left Circumflex Artery

Right Coronary Artery

Anterior Descending Branch of Left Coronary Artery

Posterior Descending Branch of Right Coronary Artery

Anterior

Posterior

Figure 1.7 Right and left coronary arteries as they exit from the ascending aorta and perfuse the ventricular myocardium.

systole and must distend and refill during ventricular diastole. Therefore, heart rate and blood volume have an integral part in maintaining coronary artery perfusion. To alter either for a prolonged period of time would hamper myocardial perfusion with great consequence to myocardial function.

SUMMARY

In this chapter, we have come to learn and appreciate the heart's function and purpose, in order to comprehend the magnitude of the signs and symptoms of its malfunction. It is important for us to visualize the landmarks of the surfaces of the heart and the coronary arteries responsible for perfusion to those surfaces.

As practitioners, we will read and interpret the ECG, recall the surface of the heart visualized by the various leads of the ECG, and deduce which coronary blood supply is in jeopardy. From this we should anticipate probable complications and plan patient care decisions. This appreciation and insight will separate practitioners from those who rely solely on an automatic ECG rhythm identification machine for patient care decisions.

Self-Assessment Exercise
Fill in the Blanks

Complete the statements, and then compare your answers with those in Appendix A.

1. The heart consists of right and left sides. The right and left sides of the heart differ in _____ and _____ .

2. The right ventricle delivers unoxygenated blood from _____ circulation to the _____.

3. The left ventricle delivers _____ blood from the _____ to the _____.

4. In comparison, the musculature of the left ventricle is _____ than the right since it is a high-pressure system projecting blood to the _____.

5. The _____ valve lies between the right atrium and the _____ ventricle.

6. The _____ valve lies between the left atrium and the _____ ventricle.

7. Blood exiting the right ventricle passes through the _____ valve to the _____. Blood exiting the left ventricle passes through the _____ valve to the _____.

8. Within the thorax, the heart is _____ and positioned so the right ventricle is more _____. The left ventricle is therefore in a more _____ position.

9. The right coronary artery has its origin behind a cusp of the _____ and proceeds _____ and perfuses the right _____ and _____ surfaces of the heart. The right coronary gives a branch to the AV node at about the same level of the posterior descending branch. The

right coronary perfuses the right atrium and both the _____ and _____ nodes.

10. The posterior descending branch of the right coronary artery also emits branches that perfuse the ventricular septum posteriorly. These are called the _____ branches. These branches supply a portion of the _____, the posterior third of the septum, and a portion of the inferoposterior division of the left bundle branch.

11. The left coronary artery also has its origin behind an aortic cusp. The left coronary divides into two branches, the _____ and the _____.

12. The anterior descending branch perfuses the anterior two-thirds of the ventricular _____, a major portion of the _____, and the anterosuperior division of the _____.

13. The lateral branch, also called the _____, winds around the left ventricle, dividing the left atrium and left ventricle. The extent of perfusion of the left posterior ventricle varies between individuals. The left circumflex also perfuses the _____.

CHAPTER
2

Electrophysiology of the Heart

Premise

There can be electrical activity and no mechanical response, but there can never be mechanical response without electrical activation.

Objectives

After reading the chapter and completing the Self-Assessment Exercise, the student should be able to

- Identify and describe the four properties critical to electrical activity.
- Identify the structures of the heart's electrical conduction system.
- Begin to relate cardiac perfusion deficits to electrical malfunction.

Key Terms

absolute refractory period	contractility	nonrefractory period
action potential	depolarization	refractoriness
automaticity	ectopy	relative refractory period
conductivity	excitability	repolarization
	myocardial cells	specialized cells

Introduction

The electrical activity of the heart precedes mechanical activity (contraction). Electrical activation describes the events that result in the contraction and relaxation of cardiac muscle, thus sustaining perfusion of the body and the heart itself. Chemical reactions cause electrical changes and a chain of events within cardiac muscle that are ultimately displayed on the electrocardiograph, measured, and assessed.

ELECTROPHYSIOLOGY OF THE HEART

Action potential describes the electrolyte exchanges that occur across the cell membrane during depolarization and the four phases of repolarization. **Depolarization** is electrical activation of myocardial cells and a very active process. Unfortunately, ischemia can exist and may not affect the wave forms that reflect depolarization. Unless an ischemic or injury process directly affects an electrical conduction pathway, it will not be visualized in a depolarization wave form.

Depolarization is the process by which the inside of the cell becomes less negative. There are mechanisms by which specific cells depolarize.

- In atrial and ventricular cells there is a rapid influx of sodium into the cell.
- In the His-Purkinje system there is a slow, time-dependent decrease in potassium permeability and an increase in sodium permeability.
- In the sinus node and AV nodes there is a slow, inward flow of calcium.

Repolarization describes *electrical rest and recovery,* the process by which the cells return to the resting level. Repolarization occurs rapidly at first, reaches a plateau, and then accelerates to a longer, more rapid surge until the resting state is reached.

The Phases of the Cardiac Cycle

The phases are described as follows:

Phase 0   Rapid depolarization. As a change in cellular permeability occurs, sodium rushes into the cell, making the cell more positive. This action produces the characteristic upstroke in the action potential.

Phase 1   Initial repolarization. This is the phase in which the rapid influx of chloride inactivates the inward pumping of sodium.

Phase 2   The plateau. During this time, a slow, inward flow of calcium occurs, while the flow of potassium out of the cell is slowed considerably.

Phase 3   Final rapid repolarization. During this phase, there is a sudden acceleration of the rate of repolarization as the slow calcium current is inactivated and the outward flow of potassium is accelerated.

Phase 4   Diastolic depolarization. There is a difference in activities during this phase for working cells and pacemaker cells. In pacemaker cells, there is a time-dependent fall in outward potassium current with a rapid sodium influx, causing depolarization to be self-initiated. The sodium–potassium pump reestablishes the concentration of ions inside the cell.

Diastolic depolarization is very rapid in the cells of the sinus node, less rapid in the bundle of His, and very slow in the terminal fascicles of the bundle branches. Nonpacemaker (working) cells remain in the steady state until their membranes are acted on by another stimulus. **Figure 2.1A** illustrates action potential and electrolyte movement. **Figure 2.1B** illustrates the difference between action potential in pacemaker and working cells.

Properties of Cardiac Muscle

There are two types of cardiac cells. In combination, they are responsible for the mechanical and electrical activity of the heart. **Myocardial cells** make up the bulk of the heart's muscle and are the actual contractile units of the heart. These cells must be able to respond to electrical stimulus.

The other group of cells are **specialized cells** and make up the heart's electrical conduction system. The specialized cells have four specific properties that govern their function: automaticity, excitability, conductivity, and contractility.

Automaticity is the ability of a cell to reach potential and generate an action potential without being stimulated. This property is attributed to the pacemaker cells. In pacemaker

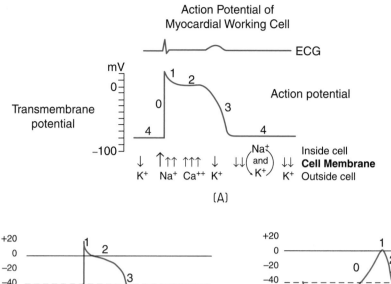

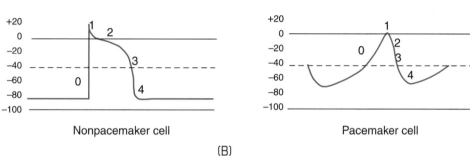

Figure 2.1 (A) Action potential of working myocardial cells; electrolyte exchanges occur across the cell membrane during action potential. (B) Schematic representation comparing action potential of pacemaker and nonpacemaker (working) myocardial cells.

cells, there is a regular, predictable fall in potassium concentration during electrical diastole. The potassium leak and the increased permeability to sodium cause the threshold to be reached and an action potential to occur at regular, usually predictable intervals. The current is then transmitted along all the myocardial cells.

Excitability is the ability of a cell to reach threshold and respond to a stimulus. The smaller the amount of required stimulus, the more excitable the cell. The greater the amount of required stimulus, the less excitable the cell. Cardiac cells become irritable because of the difference in ion concentration. This degree of irritability determines their degree of excitability or responsiveness. Ischemia and hypoxia will enhance excitability and to some extent promote premature, competitive behavior, or **ectopy**.

Conductivity is the transmission or propagation of electrical impulses from cell to cell. Inherent to each cell is the capacity for transmission. There is a difference in the rate of transmission for atrial and ventricular cells.

For instance, from the time the sinus node discharges an impulse, preferential conduction through atrial tissue is roughly 0.08 second, followed by a delay of 0.12 to 0.20 second within the AV node. Subsequent activation of the bundle branch system takes place in only 0.02 second; total ventricular activation is usually 0.10 second or less. These electrical events are translated to the ECG as specific wave forms.

Because of the anatomical interconnection of myocardial muscle fibers, the stimulation of a cardiac cell is facilitated by the many lateral and end-to-end connections within that muscle. Thus, the electrical current can flow from cell to cell and laterally using these interconnections.

Contractility is the ability of cardiac muscle fibers to shorten and contract in response to the electrical stimulation. Contractility is the mechanical response to the other properties just described.

Another property is one of **refractoriness**, which is the ability to reject an impulse or remain unresponsive to a stimulus. It can also be described as the inability of myocardial tissue to accept and transmit an impulse. Refractoriness is divided into three phases:

1. One is the **absolute refractory period**, during which time the cells cannot respond to the stimulus. The term is synonymous with depolarization and is a mechanism that protects the heart from all other ectopic impulses.

2. The **relative refractory period (RRP)** describes the time when only a strong stimulus can cause depolarization. The relative refractory period is when repolarization is almost complete, and some cells can respond, although not entirely in a normal fashion. So some cells may respond normally, some in a bizarre fashion, and some not at all.

    There is a time during the RRP when the cells are most vulnerable. There are enough cells able to respond, although in a disorganized manner. For instance, when an ectopic impulse occurs during this phase, serious, life-threatening arrhythmias can occur.

3. Last is the **nonrefractory period** when all cells are repolarized and ready to respond in a normal fashion.

The length of time for each of the refractory periods can vary between normal individuals and also is affected by medications, recreational drugs, disease, electrolyte imbalance, myocardial ischemia, and myocardial injury.

THE NERVOUS SYSTEM CONTROL OF THE HEART

The autonomic nervous system controls the visceral functions of the body. There are divisions responsible for the heart, smooth muscles, and glands. There are two divisions, the sympathetic and the parasympathetic systems. The sympathetic nerves originate in the spinal cord between the first thoracic and second lumbar vertebrae. They supply both the atria and ventricles, but primarily the ventricles. The chemical mediators of the sympathetic system are the hormones norepinephrine and epinephrine, which have the effect of enhancing excitability and increasing the force of contraction. There is also a modest increase in the rate of discharge in the sinus node. Norepinephrine has a minor effect on the heart; its major effect is on blood vessels.

The parasympathetic nerves leave the central nervous system through the cranial and sacral spinal nerves. The vagus is the parasympathetic nerve controlling the heart, primarily the atria. Stimulation of the vagus causes the release of the hormone acetylcholine. The effects of parasympathetic stimulation are slowing of the rate of discharge of the sinus node, a decrease in atrial and AV nodal conduction, and minimally, a decreased transmission through the Purkinje fibers. **Figure 2.2** illustrates parasympathetic and sympathetic innervations of the heart.

THE ELECTRICAL CONDUCTION SYSTEM

The heart's own electrical conduction system consists of the following structures:

- The sinus node
- Atrial tissue

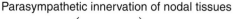

Parasympathetic innervation of nodal tissues

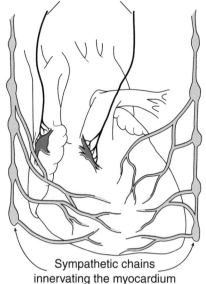

Sympathetic chains
innervating the myocardium

Figure 2.2 Autonomic nervous system innervations of nodal tissue and the myocardium by the parasympathetic (vagus) nerve fibers and the sympathetic chains.

- The AV junction
- The penetrating portions of the bundle branch system
  - The right bundle branch
  - The left bundle branch system
    - Left anterior fascicle
    - Left posterior fascicle
- The Purkinje fibers

Normally the sinus node governs the physiologic heart rate. The sinus node reaches potential more quickly than the rest of the cardiac tissue and is referred to as the pacemaker. A pacemaker is a cell or group of cells that generate an impulse at a predictable rate of speed. There is no recording on conventional ECG that represents SA node depolarization. Such depolarization can be inferred only from subsequent atrial activation that results in a wave form seen on the ECG as a P wave (Chapter 4). Following SA node depolarization, the atrial tissue is activated and is directed inferiorly to the AV node by preferential conduction and from the right atrium to the left atrium via Bachmann's bundle. Preferential conduction also occurs in the left atrium.

The next area to be activated is the AV junction. This area consists of the AV node, which is situated on the floor of the right atrium near the atrial septum, then the bundle of His and continues down to where the His bundle begins to branch (**Figure 2.3**).

The regions that constitute the AV junction are divided according to cell types: atrial-nodal (AN) region, nodal (N) region, and the nodal-His (NH) region. The AV node delays oncoming impulses to afford uniform conduction to the bundle of His and onto the ventricular conduction system. After physiologic delay at the AV node, the impulse is transmitted past the bundle of His and onward through the fascicles of the bundle branch system into the Purkinje fibers (**Figure 2-4**).

The bundle of His has two capabilities: one is simple conduction of the impulse as it comes through from the AV node. An impulse that originates within the bundle of His is conducted through the ventricular bundle branches, resulting in a narrow QRS complex, not unlike a sinus-induced QRS complex. The other capability is generating an impulse

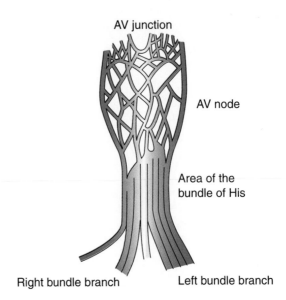

Figure 2.3 Schematic representation of the AV junction, showing the entrance fibers into the AV node, orientation of the AV node to the bundle of His, and the entrance fibers into the intraventricular septum.

forward to the ventricles and retrograde (backward) back up to the atria. For some time it was thought that the AV node functioned as a pacemaker, but the original work of Sherf and James (1968) determined that there are no rapid-sodium channels within the AV node necessary for predictable pacemaker function. The pacing function within AV junctional tissue is referred to by convention as junctional.

During the final stages of myocardial contraction, repolarization is initiated. In normal ventricular tissue, the wave of repolarization starts in the last area to be depolarized and travels in a direction opposite that of depolarization. The forces of repolarization move more slowly, and the magnitude of electrical potential at any given moment is considerably less than the forces of depolarization. Repolarization is a passive process and is greatly affected by ischemic and hypoxic tissue. As a result, recordings of the repolarization are smaller and wider than those of the depolarization wave.

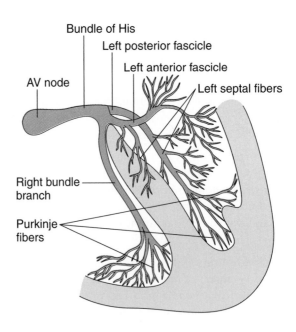

Figure 2.4 Illustration of the conduction system from the AV node through to the His-Purkinje fibers.

SUMMARY

These explanations provide some insight into the processes of depolarization and repolarization. The heart's complex electrical activity can be affected by medications, drugs, and disease. In particular, ischemia of cardiac cells can disrupt the processes to the extent that abnormalities in depolarization and repolarization can lead to lethal consequences.

Self-Assessment Exercise

Fill in the Blanks

Complete the statements, and then compare your answers with those in Appendix A.

1. The heart has both _____ and _____ properties.

2. The ability to spontaneously generate an impulse is called _____.

3. The ability to respond to an impulse is called _____.

4. The ability to transmit an impulse is called _____.

5. The ability to contract is called _____.

6. Finally, without _____, there can be no _____.

The structures of the heart's conduction system are:

7. _____,

8. _____,

9. _____, which consists of two structures,

10. the _____ and the _____.

11. The impulse continues down into the ventricles via the _____, which is thicker and slower in conduction.

12. The impulse also travels down the _____, which divides into the _____ and the _____.

13. Finally, the system terminates in the _____.

The ECG and the Multiple Lead System

Premise

The sensible interpretation of the ECG using the multiple lead system is not difficult if the practitioner:

- Knows the normal ECG wave form configurations.
- Remembers which surfaces of the heart are best "seen" by which leads.
- Associates multiple lead analyses with patient presentation.
- Assesses serial ECG tracings.

Objectives

After reading the chapter and completing the Self-Assessment Exercise, the student should be able to

- Explain the difference between unipolar and bipolar leads.
- Describe the formation of limb leads.
- Identify the position of precordial leads.
- Identify the surface of the heart monitored by each lead.
- Identify the signs of incorrect lead placement.

Key Terms

augmented leads	diphasic	poor R-wave progression
axis	early transition	precordial leads
bipolar leads	frontal plane	R-wave progression
contiguous	horizontal plane	unipolar leads

Introduction

The electrocardiogram (ECG) traces the variation in voltage produced by the heart muscle during depolarization and repolarization. The standard ECG records depolarization and repolarization along designated paths called lead systems. This chapter provides a brief overview of the ECG lead systems and how they visualize the surfaces of the heart.

THE ECG LEADS: A POINT OF VIEW

The word *lead* can be confusing in ECG. Sometimes it refers to the wires that connect the ECG to the patient. Correctly, a lead or lead system is an electrical picture of a heart's surface. We will simply use the term *lead*. Each lead traces the electrical activity between two points called electrodes.

If an electrode faces the advancing wave of depolarization, a positive deflection will be produced. Conversely, if the wave of depolarization recedes away from that electrode, a negative deflection will be produced. The magnitude of the voltage of the wave form depends on the direction of the flow of depolarization.

If the electrodes are parallel to the flow of current, the resulting wave forms will be clearly defined. However, if the electrodes are not directly parallel to the flow of current, the magnitude will be smaller. Electrodes that are perpendicular (at right angles) to the flow of current will show both positive and negative deflections. The resulting wave form is called **diphasic**.

The standard 12-lead ECG system utilizes at least five electrodes: one for each limb, plus a floating electrode on the chest wall. The system is divided into three lead systems: standard limb leads, augmented leads, and precordial (chest) leads.

The initial six leads—I, II, III, aVR, aVL, and aVF—are called the extremity or limb leads because they are derived from electrodes attached to the arms and legs. The precordial leads, V_1 through V_6, are derived from electrodes that are placed across the chest, from front to right or left lateral sites.

Limb Leads

Traditionally in a multiple lead ECG, the limb leads are formed by placing electrodes on the right and left wrists, arms, and ankles, and around the chest (precordial leads). Increasing capabilities of ECG monitoring systems require that for leads I, II, and III the ECG electrodes should be placed above the level of the heart under the clavicle. The left leg electrode should be placed below the heart, preferably inferior to the rib cage, away from bone.

The direction of flow of electrical current as seen in the limb leads lies in the **frontal plane**—a flat plane parallel to the chest. The direct path between two electrodes or between an electrode and the reference point is called the **axis** of that lead.

There are two types of limb leads: bipolar and unipolar. **Bipolar leads** are leads that are composed of one positive and one negative electrode. The bipolar leads record the difference in voltage between two extremities. The bipolar leads are I, II, and III.

Unipolar leads are leads that are composed of one positive electrode and a neutral reference point. The unipolar limb leads are aVR, aVL, and aVF (the augmented leads). The unipolar precordial leads are V_1, V_2, V_3, V_4, V_5, and V_6 and V_{1R}, V_{2R}, V_{3R}, V_{4R}, V_{5R}, and V_{6R}. In some clinical settings, V_7 and V_8, on the right and left sides, are evaluated.

Lead I. In lead I, the ECG designates the left arm as the positive electrode and the right arm as the negative electrode. Lead I records electrical activity from left to right across the chest, providing a view of the left lateral wall of the heart. When the flow of current is to the left, an upright (positive) deflection will be written. Normally, the predominant direction of the flow of depolarization is toward the left; therefore positive deflections are seen in lead I.

If there is an alteration in depolarization so that the direction of flow is to the right, the receding flow of current will be seen as a primarily negative deflection in lead I.

Lead II. In lead II, the negative electrode is on the right arm, and the positive electrode is on the left leg. Lead II provides a view of the inferior surface of the heart. Because the predominant direction of the flow of depolarization is inferior and to the left, positive deflections are generally seen in lead II. If there are deviations in the normal depolarization wave front—that is, superior and to the left—the wave form in lead II will be either diphasic or predominantly negative.

Lead III. In lead III, the positive electrode is on the left leg and the negative electrode is on the left arm. Lead III provides a view of the right inferior surface of the heart. Lead III is usually a positive deflection.

Leads I, II, and III are typically represented by a triangle that depicts the spatial orientation of these leads. If the electrodes are placed correctly and the leads recorded simultaneously, voltage of the wave form in lead II should equal the sum of the voltages in leads I and III. In other words, the amplitude of lead I plus the amplitude of lead III is usually equal to the amplitude of lead II. If the R wave in lead II is not equal to the sum of lead I and lead III, this is a clue that the leads may not placed appropriately.

Augmented Leads

The *a* in leads aVR, aVL, and aVF stands for **augmented** or amplified, so named because these leads are automatically set to increase in size by 50 percent without any change in the configuration of the electrodes by the machine's property.

Lead aVL. In lead aVL (augmented vector left), the electrode on the left arm is positive while the electrode on the right arm and left leg determines the neutral reference point. Lead aVL visualizes the left lateral wall of the heart. Lead aVL is usually positive and sometimes diphasic.

Lead aVF. Lead aVF (augmented vector foot), is the third of the inferior wall leads. In aVF, the electrode on the left leg is positive while the electrode on the right and left arms determines the neutral reference point. Lead aVF is usually positive and sometimes diphasic.

Lead aVR. In lead aVR (augmented vector right), the electrode on the right arm is positive while the electrode on the left arm and left leg determines the neutral reference point. Lead aVR is sometimes called no-man's-land or, northwest, or the orphan lead because it stands alone and does not view any single surface of the heart as directly as other lead systems. The ECG complexes in lead aVR are usually negative because the mean flow of current and depolarization of the heart goes from right to left, superior to inferior. The majority of current flow goes away from the positive electrode in aVR; therefore, the summative wave forms in that lead are predominantly negative.

In most normal ECGs, looking at lead aVR is an easy point of reference to help determine the proper placement of the limb lead electrodes. If the electrodes are placed correctly and the leads recorded simultaneously, the sum of the voltages in aVR, aVL, and aVF should equal 0. In other words, amplitudes in aVR plus aVL plus aVF = 0.

Figure 3.1 shows the position of leads I, II, III, aVR, aVL, and aVF in relation to the heart.

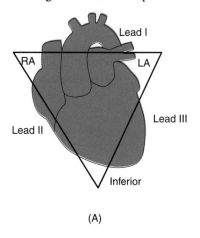

(A)

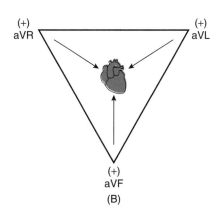

(B)

Figure 3.1 The surfaces of the heart are visualized from the point of view of the positive electrode in a specific lead. In (A), limb leads I, II, and III are superimposed on the heart. (B) shows the augmented leads in relation to the heart's surface; note that leads II, III, and aVF face the inferior surface.

The Precordial (Chest) Leads

The **precordial leads**, also called the chest leads, provide specific views of the heart's electrical activity. These leads are placed directly over the heart and encircle the precordium. The axes of the precordial leads lie in a **horizontal plane** perpendicular to the chest and to the frontal plane of the limb leads. Leads V_1, V_2, V_3, and V_{1R} through V_{6R} are referred to as the right precordial leads. The left precordial leads are V_1 through V_6. All precordial leads are unipolar, and because of their close proximity to the heart, they do not require augmentation. Proper and consistent placement of the precordial leads is essential for obtaining accurate ECG tracings. Serial ECG recordings should be taken to determine the patient's progress, lack of progress, or change in the electrical conduction system. Consistent placement of the electrodes is critical to accurately determine trends in the patient.

Lead V_1. Lead V_1 is placed on the fourth intercostal space at the right sternal border. This lead provides a view of the anterior wall of the heart. V_1 will also display the activity of the intraventricular septum.

Lead V_2. Lead V_2 is placed on the fourth intercostal space at the left sternal border. This lead provides a view of the anterior wall of the heart. V_2 will also display the activity of the intraventricular septum.

Lead V_3. Lead V_3 is placed midway between V_2 and V_4. This lead monitors the activity occurring in the anterior surface of the heart.

Lead V_4. Lead V_4 is placed in the fifth intercostal space at the midclavicular line. This lead monitors the activity occurring on the anterior surface of the heart.

Lead V_5. Lead V_5 is placed on the fifth intercostal space (same level as V_4) at the left anterior axillary line. This lead monitors the left lateral wall of the heart.

Lead V_6. Lead V_6 is placed on the fifth intercostal space (same level as V_4) at the left midaxillary line. This lead monitors the left lateral wall of the heart.

Lead V_{1R}. Lead V_{1R} is placed on the fourth intercostal space at the left sternal border.

Lead V_{2R}. Lead V_{2R} is placed on the fourth intercostal space at the right sternal border.

Lead V_{3R}. Lead V_{3R} is placed midway between V_{2R} and V_{4R}.

Lead V_{4R}. Lead V_{4R} is placed on the fifth intercostal space at the mid clavicular line. This is the most useful of the right chest leads. It is used to assess patients for right ventricular wall involvement who present with inferior wall myocardial infarction.

Lead V_{5R}. Lead V_{5R} is placed on the fifth intercostal space (same level as V_{4R}) at the right anterior axillary line.

Lead V_{6R}. Lead V_{6R} is placed on the fifth intercostal space (same level as V_{4R}) at the right midaxillary line. **Figure 3.2** illustrates the position of the electrodes for the precordial leads.

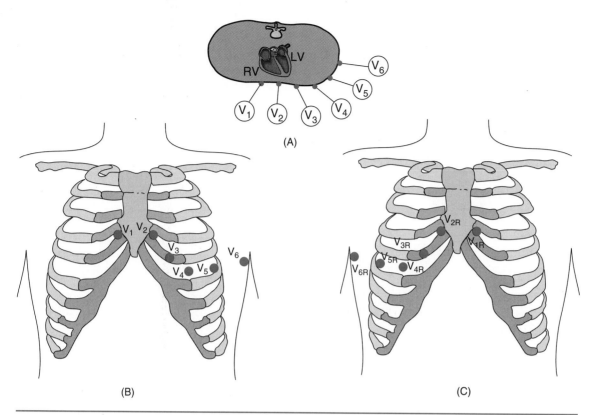

Figure 3.2 The placement of the precordial electrodes. (A) shows the precordial leads as they reflect the surface of the myocardium; (B) is the traditional left-sided placement of electrodes; and (C) is the placement of electrodes on the right side.

When a 12-lead ECG is not available, the monitoring system may be modified so that V_4R can be taken and evaluated. This is critical when the patient presents with signs and symptoms of myocardial ischemia and/or infarction.

Modified V₄R

1. Prepare as for MCL_1:
2. Place one electrode on the right chest in the V_4 position.
3. Place another electrode on the left shoulder.
4. Attach the right chest electrode to the positive lead wire.
5. Attach the left shoulder electrode to the negative lead wire of the same lead pair (in this case, lead I).
6. Turn the ECG recorder to the lead number of the wire pair you used.

Monitoring the Posterior Surface of the Heart

The posterior surface of the left ventricle lies in a plane parallel to the frontal plane. It is hidden from the precordial exploring electrodes by the anterior and septal surfaces. Infarctions of the posterior surface, usually by occlusion of the posterior descending coronary artery, may produce subtle ECG changes. Such damage will be primarily reflected in accentuation of depolarization forces over the anteroseptal surface, in V_1 to V_3, as a mirror image of the posterior surface. **Figure 3.3** shows the position of anterior precordial leads as they mirror the changes in the posterior surface of the heart.

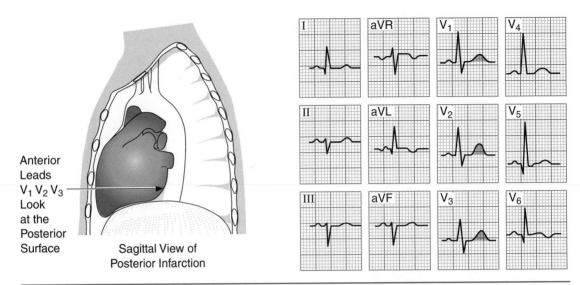

Figure 3.3 The position of the anterior precordial leads as they mirror the posterior surface of the heart. Leads V_1, V_2, and V_3 are more positive as they reflect depolarization away from the posterior surface in this patient with a posterior myocardial infarction.

When assessing the precordial leads, the R waves become taller and the S waves become smaller as we move from right to left across the precordium. This is called **R-wave progression**. The precordial pattern can be summarized as follows:

- V_1 and V_2 depict an rS complex where a small R wave represents depolarization of the septum and right ventricle and the deeper S wave represents activation of the left ventricle. This is called the right ventricular pattern, because these leads lie over the surface of the right ventricle.
- V_3 and V_4 depict an RS complex. In these leads, the complex seems to be equiphasic; that is, the R and S waves are about equal in amplitude. This is called the transition zone.
- V_5 and V_6 depict a qR complex, in which a small q wave represents septal depolarization and the tall R wave represents ventricular activation. This is sometimes called the left ventricular pattern.

When the QRS complex does not become predominantly positive by lead V_4, or the R waves in V_1 and V_3 do not progressively increase in size, and transition is not seen until V_5 or V_6, this is called **poor R-wave progression**.

Early transition occurs when the QRS complex becomes predominantly positive in V_1 or V_2. It can be a manifestation of posterior infarction or ventricular hypertrophy, or it may be simply a normal variant.

Reversed R-wave progression is possible with certain pathology. However, misplacement of the precordial leads can mimic reversed R-wave progression and cause confusion and misdiagnosis. **Figure 3.4** illustrates the QRS complexes showing R-wave progression.

MCL Leads

MCL_1 is a popular bipolar chest lead that simulates V_1. In 1968 Dr. Henry J. Marriott modified the placement of electrodes in the bipolar chest lead. He placed the positive electrode on the chest at the fourth intercostal space and the negative electrode on the left chest under the

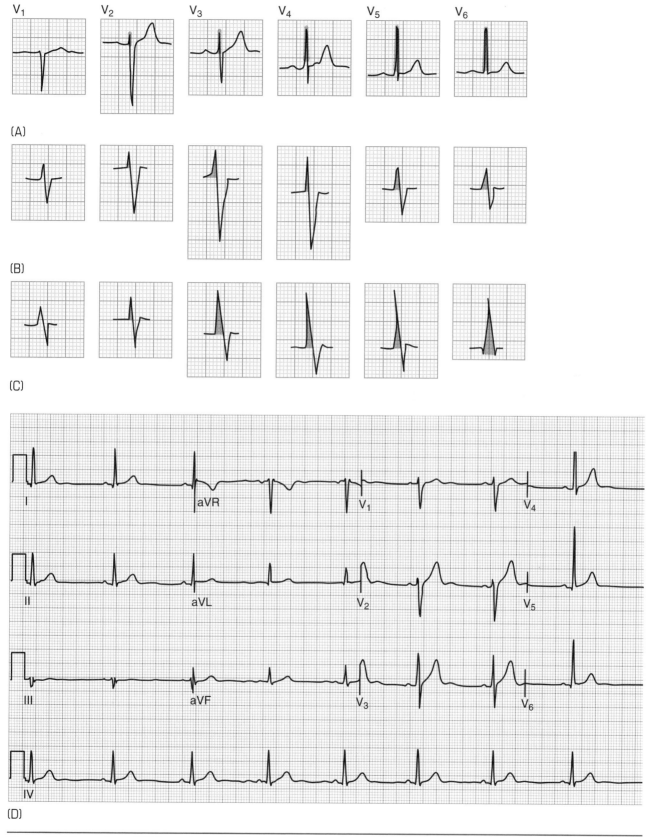

Figure 3.4 Illustrations of QRS complexes with (A) normal R-wave progression; (B) poor R-wave progression, note the transition occurred late in V_5 and V_6; (C) early transition seen in V_1 and V_2; and (D) a 12-lead ECG with normal R-wave progression.

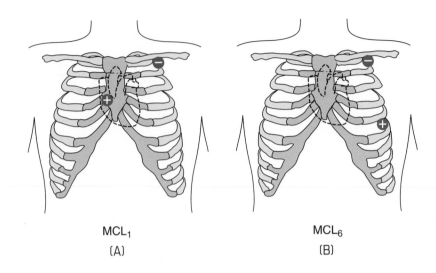

Figure 3.5 The position of the electrodes for the MCL leads. (A) For MCL₁, the negative electrode is under the left clavicle, the positive at the level of V_1. (B) For MCL₆ the placement of the negative electrode is unchanged, and the exploring (+) electrode is in the V_6 position.

left clavicle. The modified chest lead in the V_1 position became known as MCL₁. **Figure 3.5** shows the position of the electrodes for MCL₁.

When using a three-lead ECG, move the left leg wire to the chest lead (fourth intercostal space), and visualize the ECG on lead III.

Another option is to set the ECG on the typical lead II monitoring lead, reverse the arm leads, and then place the left leg wire as the chest lead (fourth intercostal space).

The advantages of monitoring in MCL₁ were helpful in

- Differentiating right from left ventricular ectopics
- Differentiating right from left bundle branch block
- Finding elusive P waves

With the increased portability and the increased knowledge of the multiple lead ECG, most clinicians are not as dependent on MCL₁.

Clinical Lead Groups

There are several leads, each recording the electrical activity of the heart from various perspectives that correlate to a specific surface of the heart. Two leads that look at the same anatomical surface are said to be **contiguous**. Any two precordial leads that are next to one another are also termed contiguous.

- *Inferior* leads II, III, and aVF look at the heart from the perspective of the inferior surface.
- *Lateral* leads I, aVL, V_5, and V_6 look at the heart from the perspective of the lateral wall of the left ventricle.
  - V_5 is closer to the left posterolateral wall.
  - V_6 is actually closer to the left high lateral wall.
- *Septal* leads V_1 and V_2 look at the ventricular septal wall.
- *Anterior* leads V_3 and V_4 look at the anterior surface.

Hazards of Improper Lead Placement

Improper placement of leads can create misleading ECG patterns. The most common error is a switch between right arm and left arm leads. The resulting ECG mimics an anterolateral infarction pattern. Another common mistake is switching right arm and left leg leads.

The hazard here is that the resulting ECG tracing appears as characteristic of inferior wall myocardial infarction. Simply switching right arm and right leg leads creates diffuse, low-voltage wave forms and leads to improper identification and subsequent intervention.

SUMMARY

The standard ECG consists of 12 leads. Six leads—I, II, III, aVR, aVL, and aVF—are the frontal plane leads, also called the limb leads. They provide information about the flow of current as it is directed toward the positive electrode in each lead.

Precordial, or chest leads, are the leads for the horizontal plane and provide information about the flow of current that is right, left, anterior, and posterior. The precordial leads extend from the right chest, at the sternal border from V_1 to the left midaxillary line. A mirror image of these leads on the right chest, from V_1 and extending to the right midaxillary line, is the placement for right precordial leads.

The bipolar leads I, II, and III are common to many monitoring systems. The axes of these limb leads form a triangle about the heart. The axis for the unipolar limb leads—aVR, aVL, and aVF—are from the positive electrode on the limbs, aVR (right arm), aVL (left arm), and aVF (left leg). Some monitoring systems provide lead I or II in combination with a precordial lead, usually V_1.

Proper lead placement is critical to accurate ECG interpretation. Each of the leads offers a perspective of the heart's electrical activity from the point of view of the positive electrode in that lead. No one lead is 100 percent demonstrative of the heart's electrical activity. The clinician must learn the surfaces of the heart as seen by each lead and the groupings that best provide information for analysis, diagnosis, and the planning of appropriate interventions.

Self-Assessment Exercise
Fill in the Blanks

Complete the statements, and then compare your answers with those in Appendix A.

1. Lead I visualizes the _____.
2. Lead II visualizes the _____.
3. Lead III visualizes the _____.
4. Lead V_1 visualizes the _____.
5. Lead V_2 visualizes the _____.
6. Lead V_3 visualizes the _____.
7. Lead V_4 visualizes the _____.
8. Lead V_5 visualizes the _____.
9. Lead V_6 visualizes the _____.
10. Lead V_{4R} visualizes the _____.

Rate, Rhythm, and Wave Forms

Premise

Estimating heart rate and evaluating duration and amplitude of wave forms are critical tasks in assessing the ECG. Clinicians need to understand wave forms as they relate to the cardiac cycle, and be able to identify abnormalities and recognize their implications.

Objectives

After reading the chapter and completing the Self-Assessment Exercise, the student should be able to

- Calculate rate and rhythm.
- Identify the normal ECG wave forms, complexes, and their measurements.
- Identify the changes in ECG measurements that may indicate electrolyte imbalance.
- Identify the changes in the ECG that may occur with specific medications.
- Identify clinical syndromes that cause alterations in the ECG.

Key Terms

anorexia nervosa	J point	QRS complex
bradycardia	low voltage	QT interval
delta wave	nadir T wave	R wave
digitalis effect	P mitrale	RR interval
hypercalcemia	P pulmonale	S wave
hypocalcemia	P wave	ST segment
hyperkalemia	pericardial effusion	T wave
hypokalemia	pericarditis	tachycardia
hypomagnesemia	PR interval	U wave
isoelectric line	Q wave	

Introduction

Depolarization and repolarization are displayed on the ECG as wave forms and complexes that can be measured and assessed. A wave of depolarization that moves toward a positive electrode will record an upright deflection on the ECG, whereas a depolarization moving toward a negative electrode will record a negative deflection. When a wave of depolarization is moving perpendicular to the exploring electrode, a diphasic wave is recorded. The deflection of the wave of repolarization should be similar to that of depolarization. Because the heart is a three-dimensional structure, forces of depolarization must be viewed using multiple exploring electrodes that reconstruct the various dimensions of depolarization. In addition to patient presentation, history, and chief complaint, the knowledge of ECG wave forms and the implications of the changes in those forms combine to provide the basis for many patient care decisions; this is the exciting part of ECG analysis.

CALCULATING RATE AND RHYTHM

ECG monitors run at a standard rate and use paper with standard squares. Each small square is equal to 0.04 second. Each large square is made up of 5 small squares equal to 0.20 second. There are 5 large squares per second and 300 beat(s) per minute (bpm). So, an ECG event that occurs once every large square is occurring at a rate of 300 bpm.

Amplitude, or voltage, is measured on the vertical axis and each of the smallest blocks represents 0.1 millivolt (mV). The same small block measures height, with each block representing 1 millimeter (mm). Diagnostic ECG devices should be standardized so that 1 mV is equal to 10 mm. **Figure 4.1** shows the large ECG square with the minimum units of measurement highlighted: 0.04 second, 1 mm, and 0.1 mV.

Small vertical lines appear on the upper or lower margin of most ECG paper. There are 15 of the larger blocks between these margin lines; therefore, they are placed 3 seconds apart—0.20 × 15 = 3 seconds and 0.20 × 30 = 6 seconds. In **Figure 4.2**, ECG paper shows the markers indicating 3- and 6-second intervals.

Time is measured on the ECG on the horizontal, moving from left to right across the ECG paper. We use the ECG paper as a guide to calculate heart rate. When possible, use a QRS that is on a heavy line. First, count the number of large blocks between 2 consecutive QRS complexes, then divide that number into 300 to calculate the estimated heart rate.

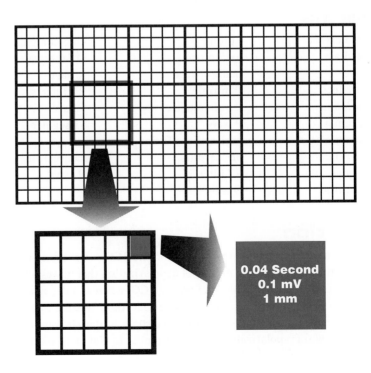

Figure 4.1 ECG monitoring paper with the blocks enlarged to illustrate the minimum units of measurement. The smallest of the blocks has three values: 0.04 second in duration (horizontal measurement), 0.1 mV in amplitude (vertical measurement), and 1 mm in height (also a vertical measurement).

0.04 Second
0.1 mV
1 mm

With very rapid rhythms, count the number of very small blocks and divide into 1,500. This method of calculation is shown in **Figure 4.3** with ECG paper and an ECG rhythm. **Table 4.1** and **Table 4.2** provide an easy reference to these calculations.

Under normal conditions, the sinus node is the pacemaker for the heart. A heart rate that falls below 60 bpm is called sinus **bradycardia**. When heart rate increases to greater than 100 bpm, it is called sinus **tachycardia**.

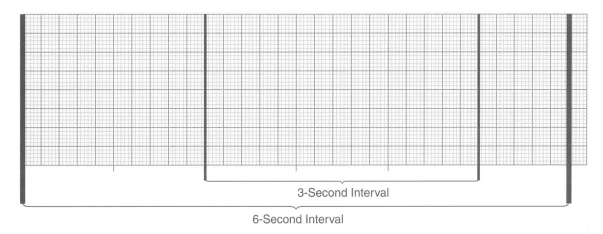

3-Second Interval

6-Second Interval

Figure 4.2 ECG monitoring paper showing markers indicating 3- and 6-second intervals. There are 15 blocks in 3 seconds, and 30 blocks in 6 seconds.

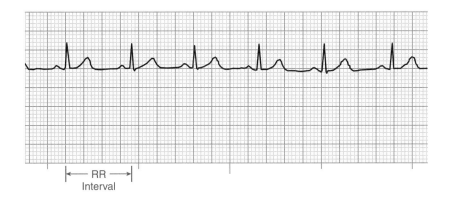

RR
Interval

Figure 4.3 ECG recording with markers denoting the number of large squares (blocks) between the QRS complexes (RR interval). Since there are three such blocks between QRS complexes, dividing 3 into 300 provides the estimated rate of 100 bpm.

Distance between 2 QRS Complexes (No. of Large Boxes)	Estimated Rate per Minute
1	300
1½	200
2	150
2½	125
3	100
3½	86

Table 4.1 Calculating heart rate by counting the numbers of large squares between 2 consecutive QRS complexes and dividing into 300. (Continues)

Distance between 2 QRS Complexes (No. of Large Boxes)	Estimated Rate per Minute
4	75
4½	67
5	60
5½	55
6	50
6½	46
7	43
7½	40
8	37
8½	35
9	33
9½	32
10	30
20	15

Table 4.1 Continued

Distance between 2 QRS Complexes (No. of Small Boxes)	Estimated Rate per Minute
4	375
5	300
6	250
7	214
8	187
9	166
10	150
11	136
12	125
13	115
14	107
15	100
16	94
17	88
18	83
19	79
20	75

Table 4.2 Calculating heart rate by counting the numbers of small squares between 2 consecutive QRS complexes and dividing into 1,500.

Regular rhythms imply regular **RR intervals**—the period of time between two QRS complexes. A regular rhythm doesn't always mean normal sinus rhythm, however. Some arrhythmias may produce a regular rhythm pattern. **Figure 4.4** is an example of various rhythms that have equal RR intervals.

In the case of an irregular rhythm, the rate range should be calculated: first, the widest (slower) of the RR intervals, then the narrowest (faster) of the RR intervals. The calculated rate range is then reported. Many arrhythmias result in an irregular ventricular rhythm. The clinician should avoid the shortcut of calculating the number of like wave forms within 6 seconds and multiplying by 10. This method gives an incomplete description of the arrhythmia, particularly when the range is broad. **Figure 4.5** depicts examples of irregular rhythms.

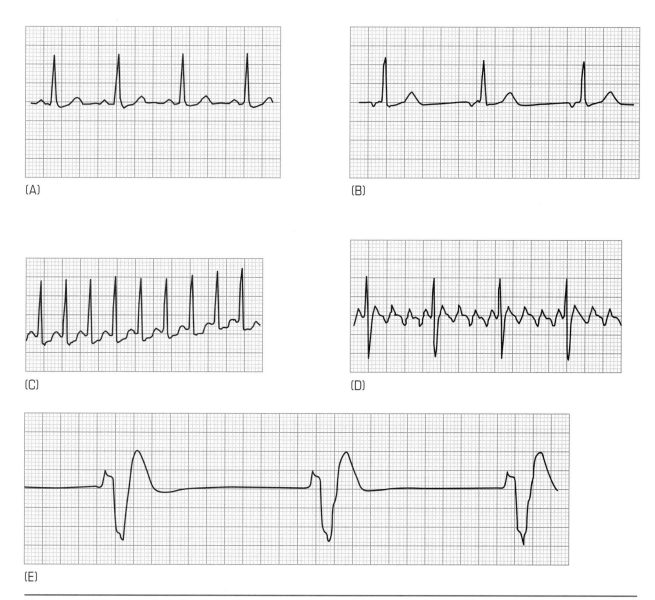

(A)

(B)

(C)

(D)

(E)

Figure 4.4 ECG tracings depicting regular rhythms and their rates: (A) shows the regular RR intervals with a rate of 86 bpm; (B) shows a rate of 55 bpm; (C) shows a rate of 214 bpm; (D) shows a rate of 75 bpm; and (E) shows a rate of 27 bpm.

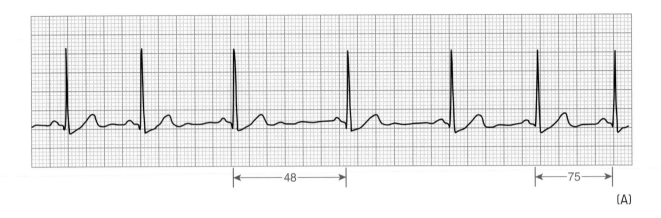

(A)

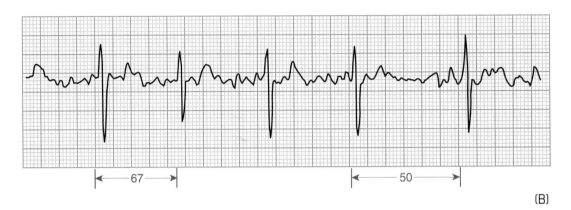

(B)

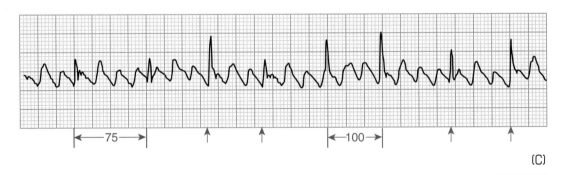

(C)

Figure 4.5 (A) is an example of an irregular QRS rhythm at a rate ranging from 48 to 75 bpm. Calculate the widest and narrowest RR interval for the rate range. (B) shows an irregular QRS rate range of 50–67 bpm. (C) shows an irregular ventricular response of 75–100 bpm.

WAVE FORMS, COMPLEXES, AND INTERVALS

The ECG tracing records the wave forms that represent various stages of myocardial depolarization and repolarization. The association of the wave forms to each other—assessing size, configuration, and duration—is the core of ECG analysis. The following is a brief review of the ECG wave forms and complexes.

P Waves

The **P wave** represents atrial depolarization. When the sinus node is in control, there should be a P wave for each and every QRS complex. The shape, duration, and amplitude of the P waves should be consistent. The P wave usually measures 0.08 second and no more than 0.02 to 0.03 mV in amplitude. Atrial depolarization caused by another source is called a P prime (P′).

Typically, sinus P waves do not plot through an ectopic from atrial tissue, since premature atrial depolarization will reset the sinus cadence. This is called a premature atrial complex (PAC) (Chapter 8). Sinus P waves usually plot through a premature ventricular ectopic complex (PVC) unless there is concealed retrograde atrial conduction (Chapter 9).

Figure 4.6 provides examples of premature complexes and the resulting changes in configuration and rate.

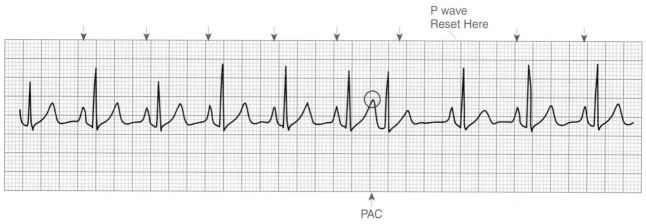

(A)

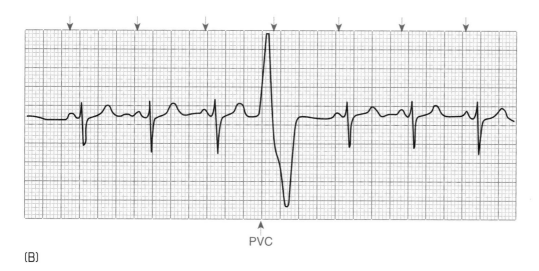

(B)

Figure 4.6 (A) is an example of an ectopic, probably from the atria, and how it alters rhythm (arrow). Plotting P waves through the PAC demonstrates the change in sinus cadence. (B) is an example of an ectopic, probably from within the ventricles (arrow). Plotting P waves through the PVC shows no change in sinus cadence.

PR Interval

The **PR interval** represents the time the impulse initiated by the sinus node travels through the atria to the ventricular conduction system. The PR interval is measured from the beginning of the P wave to the beginning of the QRS complex. A normal PR interval ranges from 0.12 to 0.20 second. The PR interval may vary with heart rate, age, and the patient's physique. There are instances where the PR interval is inversely related to heart rate; in other words, the faster the heart rate, the shorter the PR interval. If a PR interval is greater than 0.20 second, look carefully to determine if there is a distortion to the P wave or if the PR segment is prolonged. **Figure 4.7** provided ECG examples of the PR interval.

QRS Complex

The **QRS complex** represents the ventricular depolarization. It can be comprised of any combination of one, two, or three wave forms.

- The **Q wave** is the first downward, or negative, wave form of the QRS complex.
- The **R wave** is the first positive, or upward, deflection. The R wave can occur with or without a Q wave.
- The next negative wave form is a downward deflection called the **S wave**.

Multiple positive or negative deflections that follow the Q wave are called R prime (R′) or S prime (S′), respectively. Regardless of morphology—that is, whether a QRS, QR, R, RS, or QS is depicted—the complex is referred to as the QRS.

Uppercase letters are usually used to denote a QRS complex. A mix of uppercase and lowercase letters is used to describe the relative size of the wave forms that make up the QRS; for instance, when describing the QRS complex as it is affected by intraventricular conduction defects (Chapter 11).

Larger wave forms are denoted by uppercase letters, and smaller wave forms are denoted by lowercase letters. Therefore, rS means there is a small R wave in relation to the deep (greater than 5 mm) S wave. **Figure 4.8** illustrates the relative size of wave forms and the use of uppercase and lowercase letters.

The normal duration of a QRS complex is about 0.10 second when the speed and direction of depolarization are normal and the voltage (amplitude) generated during ventricular depolarization are normal. Widening of the QRS complex occurs with abnormal activation causing delta waves (Chapter 13) and intraventricular conduction defects (Chapter 11).

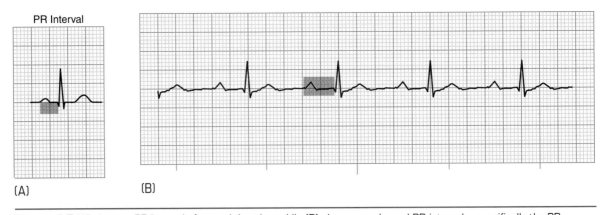

(A)   (B)

Figure 4.7 (A) shows a PR interval of normal duration, while (B) shows a prolonged PR interval—specifically the PR segment. This indicates conduction delay, possibly in the AV node.

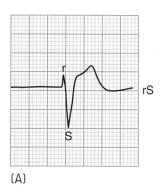

(A)

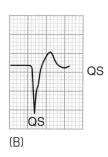

QS

(B)

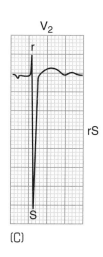

rS

(C)

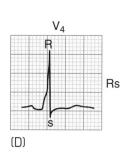

Rs

(D)

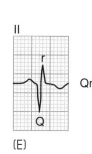

Qr

(E)

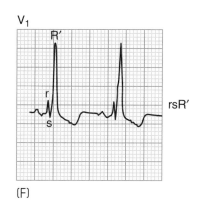

rsR'

(F)

Figure 4.8 Uppercase and lowercase letters are used to describe the variations in sizes of the wave forms in QRS complexes: (A) an rS complex; (B) a QS complex; (C) an rS complex; (D) an Rs complex; (E) a Qr complex; and (F) an rsR' composite of the QRS complex.

There are variations to the amplitude of the QRS, but it generally ranges from 5 mm or the 0.5 mV to 15 mm or 1.5 mV depending on the lead. The duration of the Q wave should not exceed 0.04 second and the depth should be less than 5 mm. Q waves are not normally present in all leads; however, small Q waves can be normal in Leads I, aVL, aVF, V_5, and V_6. Once Q waves are seen, the challenge is to determine how recently they have appeared. If Q waves are new or just evolving in the patient, the clinical presentation and/or patient history will assist in the diagnosis of infarction (Chapter 14).

The height of an R wave is usually proportional to the percentage of the heart's depolarization that occurs toward a given lead. The depth of an S wave represents the portion of depolarization that moves away from the positive electrode in a given lead.

Increased QRS amplitude may be seen in adolescents and those who have a thin chest wall. Intraventricular conduction defects (Chapter 11), ventricular hypertrophy (Chapter 12), and abnormal conduction pathways (Chapter 13) may also generate increased QRS amplitude.

Decreased QRS amplitude can occur in

- Cardiomyopathy
- Hypoparathyroidism
- "Old" myocardial infarction (MI)
- Obesity
- Old age
- Pericardial effusion

ST Segment

The **ST segment** represents the window between ventricular depolarization and repolarization. The ST segment is an extremely sensitive visualization tool. If there are ischemic or injury processes within the heart, they will be seen in the ST segment in the lead facing the affected area.

The ST segment extends from the end of the QRS (the **J point**) to the beginning of the T wave. The ST segment is normally at baseline, that is, at the **isoelectric line**. One way to estimate deviation from the baseline is to draw a line from the PR segment, extending it through the T wave.

The ST segment may be elevated or depressed with myocardial injury, ischemia, ventricular aneurysm, and with some medications. A normal ST segment may be elevated (above the baseline) for 1 to 2 mm; however, elevation greater than 1 mm in a symptomatic patient with chest pain is highly suspicious of hypoxia, ischemia, or injury in the myocardial surface exhibited by the lead facing that surface.

The J point and ST segment may be elevated up to 2 mm in the precordial leads in normal persons. ST segment elevation greater than 4 mm in the lateral precordial leads is rarely considered normal. During exertion a normal person's ST segments will become isoelectric. ST segment elevation seen in normal persons represents early repolarization of a portion of the ventricular myocardium. **Figure 4.9** is an example of ST segments. A straight or horizontal ST segment above or below the baseline is highly suggestive of ischemia. Significant ST segment changes also occur in hypothermia.

T Wave

The **T wave** represents ventricular repolarization. Usually a normal T wave is rather asymmetrical and low in amplitude, not exceeding 5 mm in the limb leads or 10 mm in the precordial leads. Symmetrical T-wave inversion greater than 5 mm is termed a **nadir T wave**,

Ventricular Repolarization
ST Segment

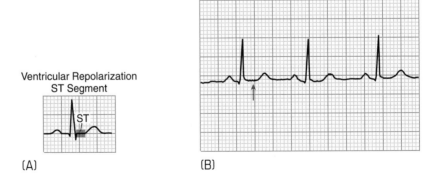

(A) (B)

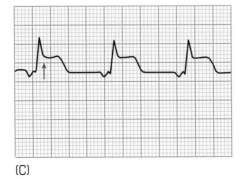
(C)

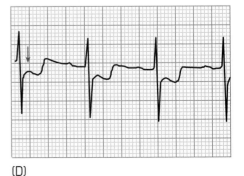
(D)

Figure 4.9 (A) is an ST segment at baseline highlighted within a cardiac cycle. Note the variations in the ST segments in (B), which is normal at baseline; (C), which has a 3 mm ST segment elevation; and (D), which has a 3 mm ST segment depression.

which can be an acute sign often indicating ischemia and/or injury. **Figure 4.10** is an illustration of variations in the T wave.

QT Interval

The **QT interval** indicates the time from ventricular depolarization to repolarization. It is measured from the beginning of the QRS to the end of the T wave and ranges from 0.24 to 0.38 second. The normal QT interval is less than one-half the underlying RR interval; it should not exceed 50 percent of the RR interval. The duration of the QT interval may vary depending on several factors including heart rate, gender, age, disease, obesity, and medications. The Bazette formula for corrected QT (QTc) based on heart rate is:

$$QTc = kQT/\sqrt{RR} \ (k = 0.297 \text{ male}; \ 0.415 \text{ female})$$

The normal QTc related to heart rate is:

60 bpm	0.33–0.43 second
70 bpm	0.31–0.41 second
80 bpm	0.29–0.38 second
90 bpm	0.28–0.36 second
100 bpm	0.27–0.35 second

By convention, the uppermost limit would be considered 0.40 second.

It is sometimes difficult to accurately measure the QT interval where there are low-amplitude T waves. Sometimes T waves will merge with subsequent isoelectric lines or with U waves. Several leads should be compared. The longest clearly visible QT interval should be the measurement reported. The importance of measuring a QT interval is to determine whether it is prolonged. A prolonged QT interval reflects an extended period of ventricular vulnerability to life-threatening arrhythmias. **Figure 4.11** illustrates the measurements of the QT interval.

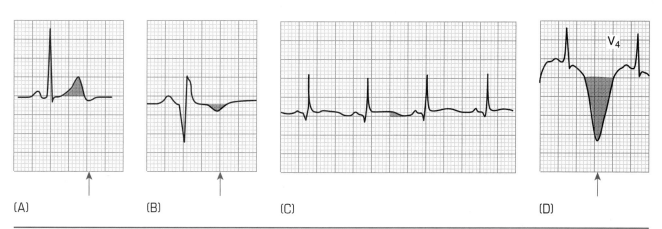

(A) (B) (C) (D)

Figure 4.10 The normal PQRST complex: (A) highlighting the normal T wave; (B) highlighting T-wave inversion; (C) highlighting flattened T waves; and (D) highlighting a nadir T wave.

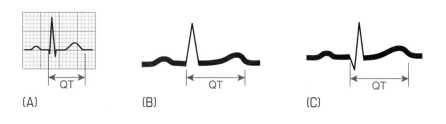

(A) (B) (C)

Figure 4.11 (A) The QT interval highlighted within the cardiac complex; (B) and (C) show the measurement of the QT interval based on the wave forms that make up the QRS complex.

U Wave

There are many theories about the generation and importance of **U waves**. One is that they represent recovery of the Purkinje system or repolarization of papillary muscles. Recent electrophysiologic studies suggest that U waves represent repolarization of a population of subepicardial cells with unique activation properties. Conditions that favor U waves occurring include electrolyte abnormalities, left ventricular hypertrophy, and myocardial ischemia. When visible, U waves are usually easily recognized in leads V_2 and V_3.

It is not necessary to see U waves in all leads. Prominent U waves are frequently seen in patients with hypokalemia, with slow heart rates, and in patients who are taking certain medications including digitalis and beta-blockers. Generally U waves are the same polarity as the preceding T wave. A negative U wave following a positive T wave may be indicative of myocardial ischemia. **Figure 4.12** illustrates the wave forms of the cardiac complex showing P wave, QRS complex, ST segment, and T and U waves. **Table 4.3** provides a summary of the various wave forms and their characteristics.

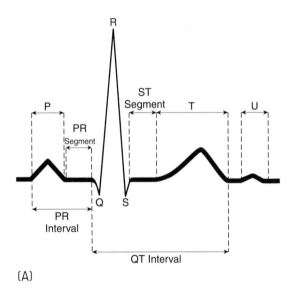

(A)

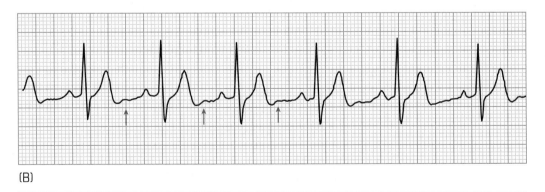

(B)

Figure 4.12 (A) Wave forms showing P wave, QRS complex, ST segment, T and U waves; (B) is an ECG tracing of a sinus rhythm with U waves (arrow).

P Wave

- Represents sinus-induced atrial depolarization.
- Measures 0.08 second and 2 to 3 mm in amplitude.
- Shape is usually symmetrical and upright.
- May be notched in appearance.
- P' (P prime) indicates atrial depolarization from an atrial or junctional source.

PR Interval

- Total supraventricular activity; activation of the His-Purkinje system.
- Measures 0.12 to 0.20 second.
- PR segment represents AV nodal delay and measures about 0.12 second.

QRS Complex

- Represents ventricular depolarization.
- When supraventricular in origin, it is less than or equal to 0.10 second and 1 to 1.5 mV in amplitude.
- When ventricular in origin, it usually measures greater than 0.10 second. and the amplitude is often greater than the normal QRS, and the QRS will be opposite in direction from the T wave.

ST Segment

- Represents early ventricular repolarization.
- Measures less than or equal to 0.12 second and may be angular, depressed, or elevated.
- Deviations may reflect ischemia.

T Wave

- Represents completed ventricular repolarization.
- Measures less than or equal to 0.12 second and 5 to 6 mm.
- May be positive or negative.
- Rarely distorted or notched (atrial repolarization may distort (amplify) the T wave; this additive influence is referred to as aT distortion where *a* denotes the atrial depolarization) and *T* means ventricular repolarization/
- Asymmetrical.

QT Interval

- Total ventricular activity, 0.24 to 0.38 second.
- Affected by ventricular rate and certain medications and electrolytes.

U Wave

- Positive or negative deflection following the QRS.
- Most often flat and unseen.

Table 4.3 Summary of ECG wave forms and measurements.

ABNORMAL WAVE FORMS

Abnormal P Waves

A peaked P wave may indicate right atrial enlargement (RAE). This pattern is sometimes called **P pulmonale** because it is often associated with conditions such as pulmonary stenosis, pulmonary hypertension, hypertensive heart disease, and chronic obstructive pulmonary disease (COPD). P pulmonale is most evident in lead II.

Notching of a P wave in lead II may indicate left atrial enlargement (LAE). This is sometimes referred to as **P mitrale** because it is often associated with disease of the mitral valve such as mitral stenosis. In V_1, notching of the P waves and a negative deflection in the terminal part of the P wave deeper than 1 mm and lasting longer than 0.04 second may indicate LAE. The LAE pattern is particularly common in mitral regurgitation and certain myocardial lesions. LAE is also commonly seen with hypertensive heart disease. **Figure 4.13** illustrates the variation in P waves.

Abnormal PR Interval

A PR interval longer than 0.20 second can be a normal variation or an effect of drugs such as digitalis, certain calcium channel blockers, and some antiarrhythmic medications. It is also commonly associated with aging, and may be the first indicator of underlying conduction system disease.

A shortened PR interval (less than 0.12 second) may be a normal variant or may occur when the electrical complex is promulgated along accessory tracts. Rhythms that originate in the high AV junction will have an inverted P wave prior to the QRS with a PR interval less than 0.12 second. **Figure 4.14** illustrates the variations in the PR interval.

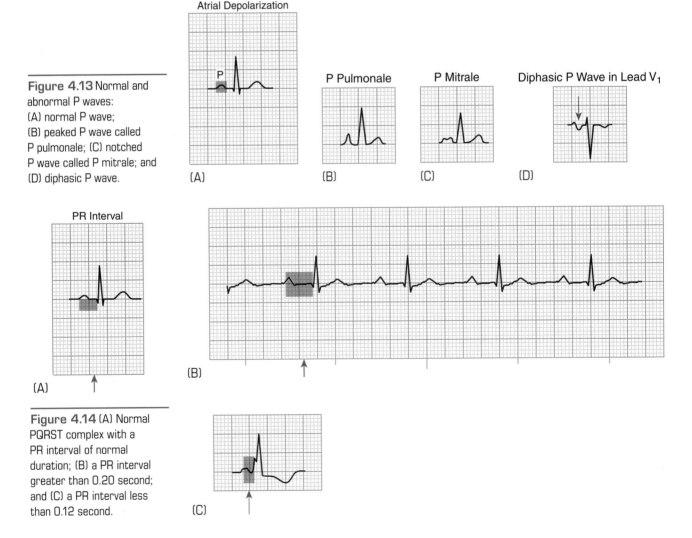

Figure 4.13 Normal and abnormal P waves: (A) normal P wave; (B) peaked P wave called P pulmonale; (C) notched P wave called P mitrale; and (D) diphasic P wave.

Atrial Depolarization

P Pulmonale   P Mitrale   Diphasic P Wave in Lead V_1

(A)   (B)   (C)   (D)

PR Interval

(A)   (B)

Figure 4.14 (A) Normal PQRST complex with a PR interval of normal duration; (B) a PR interval greater than 0.20 second; and (C) a PR interval less than 0.12 second.

(C)

Abnormal QRS Complexes

QRS complexes greater than 0.10 second may indicate abnormal intraventricular conduction. Prolongation itself is not the definitive diagnosis of the defect. Change in the amplitude of the QRS coupled with prolongation of the QRS duration may indicate abnormalities and specific fascicles of the ventricular conduction system. For instance, if the left anterior fascicle is obliterated or delayed, ventricular depolarization will be seen on the ECG as a small R and deep S waves, noted as an rS complex. (These are discussed in detail in Chapter 11.)

When the QRS bulges on the upslope or on the downslope it is said to be slurred. Slurring of the QRS can occur with abnormal ventricular conduction or if there is conduction using an accessory pathway. Notching of the QRS can occur with no evidence of pathology; however, notching is uncharacteristic and therefore suspicious of intraventricular conduction defects when the duration is greater than 0.10 second. Consequently, there are two items to look for: if the QRS is greater than 0.10 second and if the QRS complex has an uncharacteristic jagged look. These two conditions together may indicate a problem with intraventricular conduction. Again, the duration is the first and most important consideration.

Delta waves make the QRS appear slurred. When this occurs, they represent preexcitation of the ventricle using an accessory atrioventricular pathway. The QRS takes on a slurred or sometimes a more rounded upstroke and is usually associated with a short PR interval. A delta wave does not have to be visible in all leads. **Figure 4.15** illustrates the variations of the QRS complex.

Abnormal QT Interval

A prolonged QT interval (greater than 0.38 second) indicates a delay in ventricular repolarization caused by the ST segment and T waves. Prolongation of the QT interval is a predictor of cardiovascular mortality even in the absence of overt heart disease. Prolonged QT intervals may be caused by:

- Anorexia nervosa
- Cerebral hemorrhage
- Congenital
- Hypertrophic cardiomyopathy
- Hypocalcemia
- Hypokalemia
- Hypomagnesemia
- Hypothermia

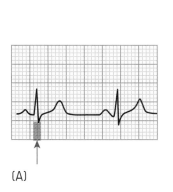

(A)

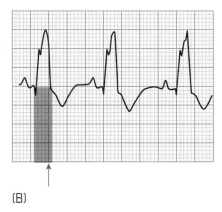

(B)

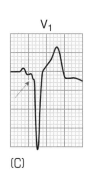

V_1

(C)

Figure 4.15 Variations in the QRS complex: (A) a normal QRS complex; (B) a wide-notched QRS complex; and (C) slurring of the QRS complex, called a delta wave.

- Medications
- Myocardial ischemia or infarction
- Obesity

Prolongation of the QT interval is a potentially dangerous side effect of many antiarrhythmic medications. Antibiotics such as levofloxacin, erythromycin and ketoconazole, the antihistamine agents astemizole and terfenadine, the phenothiazines, and terodiline (a drug used to treat incontinence) have been associated with prolonged QT intervals, torsades de pointes (TdP), and sudden death. Prolongation of the QT interval can occur suddenly. The autonomic dysfunction that occurs commonly in diabetics and alcoholics may show up as prolonged QT intervals. Shortening of the QT interval is caused by hypercalcemia and hyperkalemia. Prolongation of the QT interval is frequently observed in hypomagnesemia and is thought to occur because of the resulting altered potassium transport. The electrolyte imbalances seen with anorexia nervosa and resultant changes in the QT interval are also being studied. **Figure 4.16** illustrates normal and abnormal QT intervals.

Abnormal U Waves

U waves should be the same polarity as the preceding T waves. Negative U waves that follow positive T waves suggest ischemia and/or ventricular hypertrophy. Enlarged U waves (greater than 1 mm in amplitude) may be caused by:

- Hypercalcemia
- Hypokalemia
- Intracranial hemorrhage

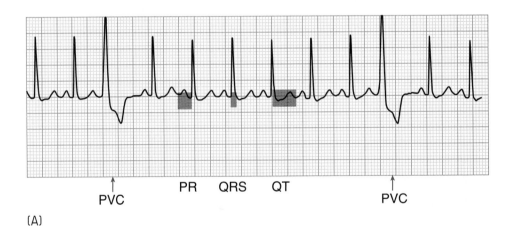

(A)

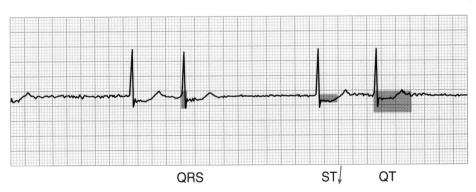

Figure 4.16 (A) shows normal QT interval; (B) shows prolonged QT intervals.

(B)

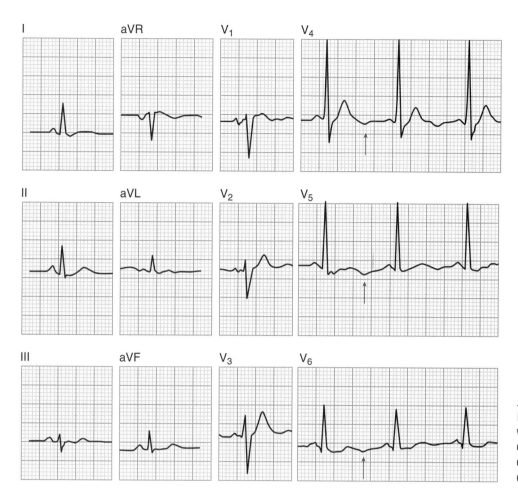

Figure 4.17 A 12-lead ECG where U waves are more obvious in some leads than others. Negative U waves are evident in V$_4$ through V$_6$.

- Left ventricular hypertrophy
- Physical exercise

Figure 4.17 shows a 12-lead ECG depicting U waves.

ALTERATIONS OF ECG WAVE FORMS

Electrolyte imbalance can influence the heart's electrical function, causing changes in duration and amplitude of ECG wave forms, complexes, segments, and intervals. Similarly, ST segment elevation, depression, coving and scooping, and arrhythmias can be induced by medications and certain pathological conditions. The clinician does well to recognize the changes, but clinical correlation is critical. The following section discusses the changes that occur with electrolyte imbalance, cardiac medications, and certain clinical diseases.

Drug-Induced Changes on the ECG

Numerous medications and electrolyte imbalances can influence the heart's electrical function, altering ventricular rate and the duration and amplitude of ECG wave forms. Similarly, ST segment elevation, depression, coving or scooping, and arrhythmias can be induced by medications.

Antiarrhythmic medications used for noncardiac conditions will alter the patient's ECG tracing. Examples include the use of beta-blockers for migraine therapy, timolol eye drops for control of glaucoma, and calcium channel blockers for control of hypertension. To recognize all the possible causes for ECG changes, the clinician should carefully take a medical history to include prescription drugs, over-the-counter (OTC) drugs and supplements, herbal and homeopathic preparations, and illegal chemicals. It is also critical to determine if the patient has borrowed medications. As with any other diagnostic tool, clinical correlation is imperative.

The unexpected effects on the heart by medications given for any reason warrant attention, as do the effects from medications given to treat cardiac problems. Interpretation and anticipation of possible outcomes and knowledge of the adverse effects of specific medications alone or in combination can be critical. Medications alone may produce visible ECG changes including increases in heart rate and prolonged QT intervals.

Although many ECG changes are produced by antiarrhythmic medications, these changes may not be present in all ECG leads and may vary from individual to individual. Many medications are known to prolong the QT interval and, therefore, cause ventricular arrhythmias. Patients, even without underlying heart disease, who take medications that alone or especially in combination with another medication cause prolonged QT intervals can develop life-threatening arrhythmias. Too often patients are prescribed medications by different physicians and may neglect to share with each of their doctors the list of all the medications they are taking.

Patients with congenital prolonged QT intervals can develop ventricular arrhythmias as a result of taking medications that prolong the QT interval. Concomitant use of medications known to prolong the QT interval will increase the risk of an arrhythmia. Included but not limited to this category are certain of the following types of drugs:

- Antiarrhythmics
- Antipsychotics
- Antidepressants
- Antianginal drugs such [as bepridil (Vascor)
- Antifungal medications taken orally or intravenously
- Azole class (Diflucon fluconazole])
- Broad-spectrum antimicrobials such as erythromycin, clarithromycin (Biaxin), and sparfloxacin (Zagam)
- Calcium channel blockers
- Cocaine
- Neuroleptic agents
- Tricyclic antidepressants

The preceding list is not an exhaustive review of all possible medications that can affect the heart's normal conduction and functioning. Treatment modalities dealing with the causative conditions and specific pathologies are beyond the scope of this text.

Digitalis. Digitalis preparations (Lanoxin [digoxin]) are used to treat patients with heart failure and certain arrhythmias. One of the effects of digitalis is to shorten ventricular repolarization. This results in a reduction of the QT interval, specifically the ST segment and T wave.

A more typical change affected by digitalis is the characteristic ST segment change, that is, a negative coving or scooping. This change is sometimes called the **digitalis effect**. This characteristic scooping of the ST segment reflects the digitalis effect and does not imply toxicity. Toxicity must be proven by lab analysis and clinical presentation.

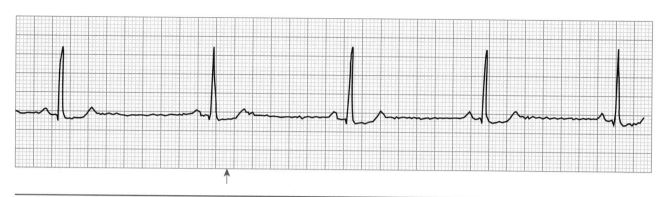

Figure 4.18 ECG tracing showing sinus bradycardia and ST segment depression characteristic of a patient on digitalis.

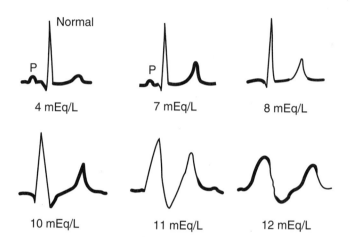

Normal

P   P

4 mEq/L   7 mEq/L   8 mEq/L

10 mEq/L   11 mEq/L   12 mEq/L

Figure 4.19 ECG tracing in a patient with documented hyperkalemia. Note the progressive changes in QRS complex associated with specific serum potassium levels.

When the digitalis effect is seen on the ECG, the ST segment and T wave are often fused so that clear distinction between the two is impossible. **Figure 4.18** provides ECG tracings of changes in ST segments and T waves from patients with the digitalis effect. Note the bradycardia that may be an effect of digitalis.

Hyperkalemia

Hyperkalemia is a condition in which there is an excessive amount of potassium in the blood. An increased serum potassium level greater than 5.2 milliequivalent per liter (mEq/L) is often referred to as clinically mild hyperkalemia, whereas a level reported greater than 6.0 mEq are referred to as severe hyperkalemia. Hyperkalemia can cause a narrowing and peaking of the T wave. There is a characteristic tenting of the T wave as the amplitude increases. Tall tented T waves by themselves may not reflect hyperkalemia. The combination of prolonged PR interval and decreased amplitude of the P waves are better evidence of suspected hyperkalemia.

In clinical persistent hyperkalemia, such as seen with renal failure, the increased QRS complex duration will manifest intraventricular conduction delay. As this change occurs, the QRS becomes distorted and takes on an undulating appearance. **Figure 4.19** is an ECG tracing showing changes in the QRS complex, ST segments, and T waves from a patient with hyperkalemia.

Hypokalemia

Hypokalemia is a condition in which there is decreased concentration of potassium in the blood, that is, serum potassium levels less than 3.5 mEq/L that produce ST segment depression. U waves may also occur. The U waves may merge with the T waves making the QT interval appear prolonged. T waves also may flatten and U waves increase to a size greater than the amplitude of the T waves. The most common cause of hypokalemia is diuretic therapy without concurrent use of potassium supplements. Prolonged bouts of emesis, gastric suctioning, and diarrhea may also produce hypokalemia. **Figure 4.20** provides an ECG tracing showing changes in the QRS complex, ST segments, and T waves in a patient with documented hypokalemia.

Hypercalcemia

Hypercalcemia is a condition in which there is an excessive amount of calcium in the blood. Serum calcium levels greater than 10.3 milligrams per deciliter (mg/dL) or an ionized calcium level greater than 2.46 mEq/L cause decreased ventricular repolarization and subsequent decrease in the QT interval. Hypercalcemia is associated with multiple myeloma and hyperparathyroidism, and may be seen in cancer patients, particularly those with breast and lung cancer. Hypercalcemia can cause seizure, coma, and death in severe cases.

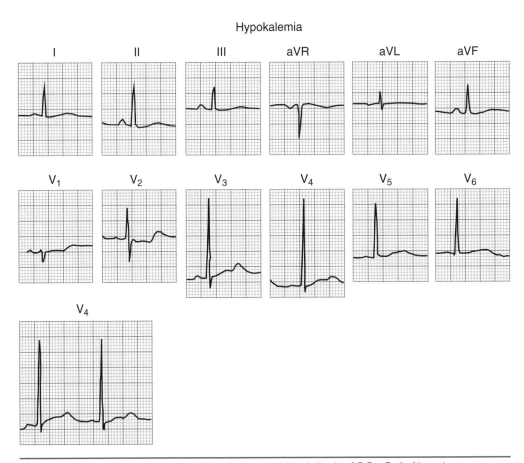

Figure 4.20 ECG tracing in a patient with documented hypokalemia of 2.2 mEq/L. Note the progressive changes in T and U waves. (Adapted from *Clinical Electrocardiography* by Goldberger and Goldberger, 1977, St. Louis: C.V. Mosby.)

Hypocalcemia

Hypocalcemia is a condition in which there is an abnormally low level of calcium in the blood. Serum calcium levels less than 8 mg/dL, or an ionized calcium level less than 2.24 mEq/L, cause prolongation of the QT interval. Common causes of hypocalcemia include pancreatitis, renal failure, hypoparathyroidism, malnutrition, and certain intestinal malabsorption syndromes. **Figure 4.21A** and **Figure 4.21B** provide ECG tracings of changes in the QRS complex, ST segments, and T waves from patients with hypocalcemia and hypercalcemia. **Table 4.4** summarizes changes in ECG wave forms and complexes associated with certain medications and electrolyte imbalance. This is not an exhaustive list. These changes must be correlated with clinical history and serum levels.

Low-Voltage QRS

Low voltage describes the diminished amplitude (less than 5 mm) of the QRS complex in all the extremity leads: I, II, III, aVR, aVL, and aVF. A common ECG sign of pericardial effusion is low-voltage QRS complexes due to the diminished conduction through the fluid surrounding the heart.

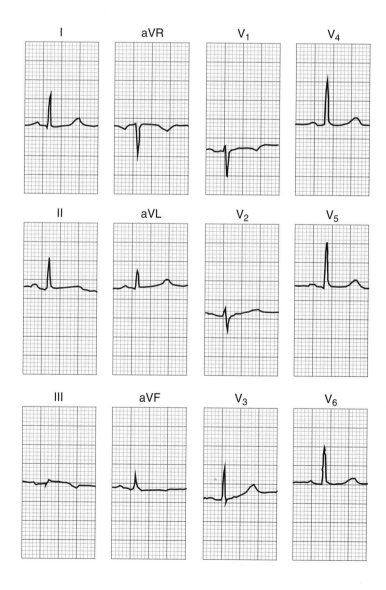

Figure 4.21A An ECG tracing of a patient with documented hypocalcemia; note the long ST segment.

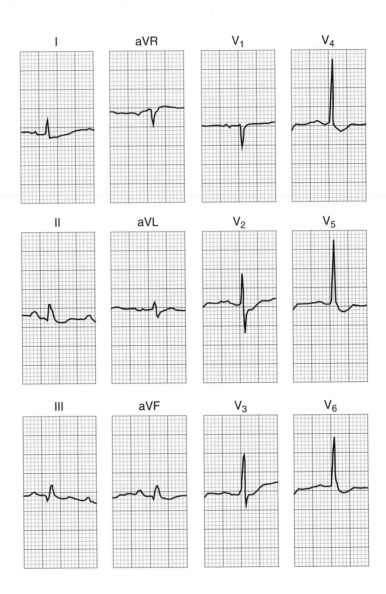

I   aVR   V₁   V₄

II   aVL   V₂   V₅

III   aVF   V₃   V₆

Figure 4.21B An ECG tracing of a patient with documented hypercalcemia; notice the short ST segment.

ECG Wave Forms/Complexes	Medication*	Electrolyte Imbalance
P-wave amplitude↓	Hyperkalemia	
P wave notched	Quinidine	
PR interval >0.20 second	Digitalis Procainamide Quinidine Verapamil	Hyperkalemia
QRS complex >0.10 second	Disopyramide Procainamide Quinidine	Hyperkalemia
ST segment↓	Digitalis Quinidine	Hypokalemia

Table 4.4 Summary of ECG changes induced by some medications and electrolyte imbalance. (Continues)

*The ECG measurements are sensitive to many drugs with antiarrhythmic potential, including medications taken for other reasons; for example, calcium channel blockers for hypertension and beta-blockers for angina. This list is not all-inclusive.

ECG Wave Forms/Complexes	Medication*	Electrolyte Imbalance
T-wave amplitude↓	Digitalis Procainamide	Hypokalemia
T-wave amplitude↑	Quinidine	Hyperkalemia
T wave↓	Digitalis Procainamide	Hypokalemia
U-wave amplitude↑		Hypokalemia Hypomagnesemia
QT interval↓		Hypercalcemia
QT interval↑		Hypocalcemia Hypomagnesemia
(may be a normal variant)		

Table 4.4 Continued

In emphysema, the accumulation of trapped air acts as a deterrent to the flow of current. In pericarditis, low-voltage QRS is seen in the precordial leads. Low-voltage QRS may also be a normal variant. Other conditions that can result in low-voltage QRS are:

- Amyloidosis
- Hypothyroidism
- Heart failure
- Myocardial fibrosis

Pericarditis

Pericarditis is an inflammation of the pericardial sac caused, for example, by viral or bacterial infection, metastasis, infarction, or uremia. Pericarditis of any etiology may show localized ST segment elevations and subsequent T-wave inversion and is easily mistaken for acute myocardial ischemia.

Early in Stage 1 of pericarditis, there is diffuse concave ST elevation in all the leads except for aVR. In aVR the ST segment is depressed and the PR segment is elevated. The term *global* is used to describe when these changes are present in all the leads. Usually, there are no convex ST segments and no reciprocal changes.

ST segment elevation in pericarditis usually represents general involvement of the ventricular subepicardium. Localized involvement of only the subepicardium is rare. If that is the case, ST elevation will occur in only a few leads with reciprocal ST depression. Q waves are not always associated with pericarditis. If Q waves are present they may suggest evolving or causative pathology. T waves are generally upright, while the PR interval is classically depressed except in lead aVR, where it is elevated. The segment between the end of the T wave and beginning of the P wave, the so-called TP segment, is a more accurate baseline for measuring ST segments.

Pseudonormalization occurs in Stage 2. *Pseudonormalization* is a term that describes when the ECG looks normal. ST segments return to baseline and may even be isoelectric; T waves are upright. The PR interval may be depressed, but is usually close to baseline.

In Stage 3 of pericarditis, the T waves change. T-wave inversion is now present in the leads that previously had concave ST segment elevation; the ST segment itself is isoelectric. This pattern may last for days to weeks.

Stage 4 involves resolution. The PQRST complex resumes its original shape. In the early phases, ST segment elevation can be seen due to the inflammation of the epicardium. However, there is never Q-wave formation with pericarditis, and the resolution of the ST segment and T-wave changes takes place over a much longer period of time. The ST segment changes are usually seen in all leads, as opposed to myocardial infarction, where the acute changes of Q waves, ST elevation, and T-wave inversion are seen in the leads facing the localized infarcted myocardial tissue. Remember, there are no reciprocal changes with pericarditis. **Figure 4.22** provides ECG tracings of changes in the ST segments and T waves in patients with pericarditis.

Pericardial Effusion. Pericardial effusion refers to abnormal accumulation of fluid within the pericardial sac. In most cases this is a complication of pericarditis, but can occur with hypothyroidism, uremia, and other systemic pathologies. The clinical significance of pericardial effusion is dependent on the rapidity with which the fluid accumulates. The tension created by the accumulation of fluid can cause progressive decrease in ventricular filling

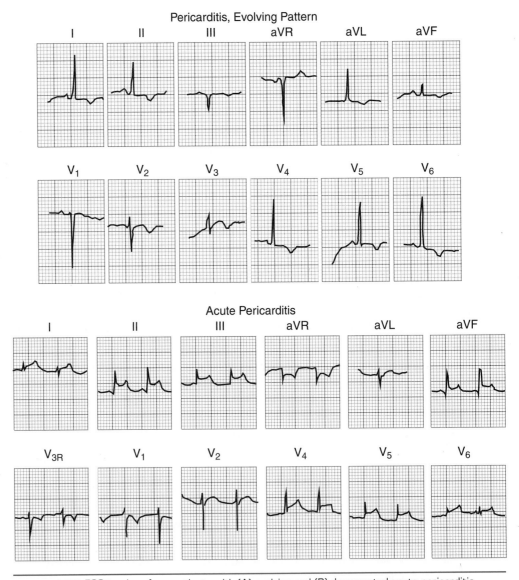

Figure 4.22 ECG tracings from patients with (A) evolving and (B) documented acute pericarditis.

to the point of pericardial tamponade. Fluid collects between the heart muscle and the pericardial sac. The pressure within the sac prevents the heart from expanding fully and filling the ventricles, with the result that a significantly reduced amount of blood circulates within the body. The heart becomes so restricted because of this intrapericardial pressure that, if left unchecked, the condition will result in death. Tamponade usually causes low-voltage ECG wave forms.

Ventricular Aneurysm

Left ventricular aneurysm resulting from extensive infarction may cause persistent ST segment elevation over the damaged muscle. This ST segment elevation may be present for years and may be confused with acute necrosis. Such ST segment elevation and aneurysm formation may hide subsequent ischemic episodes. **Figure 4.23** shows ECG tracings of changes in the ST segments and T waves in a patient with ventricular aneurysm.

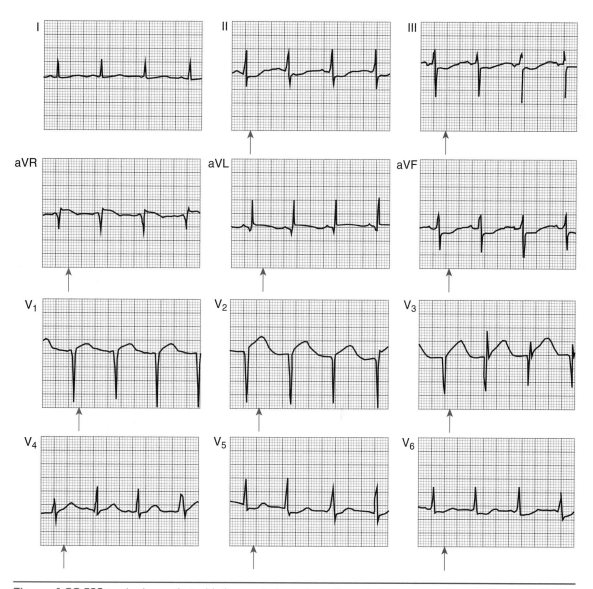

Figure 4.23 ECG tracing in a patient with documented anterior wall ventricular aneurysm. Note the Q waves in V_1, V_2, V_3, and aVL and ST depression in II, III, aVF, V_5, and V_6.

Hypertrophic Cardiomyopathy

Inappropriate myocardial hypertrophy, often with the septum showing more involvement than the free ventricle wall, is common to hypertrophic cardiomyopathy (HCM). Up to 70 percent of HCM cases have familial patterns of occurrence with autosomal dominant inheritance. In children and adolescents, the ECG may be a more sensitive marker of early disease than an echocardiogram.

Patients with HCM often (25 to 50 percent) have significant Q waves on their ECG. Rather than infarction, these Q waves represent hypertrophied asymmetric ventricular muscle with distortion of normal depolarization patterns. Giant negative T waves in mid-precordial leads may be seen. "Voltage criteria" for left ventricular hypertrophy (LVH) in association with repolarization abnormalities is also common, but isolated increases in voltage without ST and T-wave changes are infrequent. A pseudoinfarction pattern should always be suspected when the clinical setting and laboratory data do not correlate with electrocardiographic findings. **Figure 4.24** shows ECG tracings of changes in the ST segments and T waves in a patient with hypertrophic cardiomyopathy.

Increased Intracranial Pressure

In patients with increased intracranial pressure (ICP), QT prolongation may occur along with deep T-wave inversion and sometimes abnormal U waves. This is an almost universal ECG finding in this patient population. With sudden increases in intracranial pressure there may also be dramatic alterations to the T waves and ST segments. These changes do not reflect a primary myocardial problem, but rather changes in repolarization due to enhanced sympathetic nervous system activity. Supraventricular and ventricular arrhythmias, as well as conduction abnormalities, have been well documented in patients with cerebral hemorrhage and increased ICP. Severe life-threatening arrhythmias in patients with subarachnoid hemorrhage include TdP in the setting of marked prolonged QT interval. **Figure 4.25** provides a 12-lead ECG from a patient with increased ICP showing "cerebral" T waves.

Pulmonary Embolism

An embolism can occur and obstruct the pulmonary artery causing a sudden change in the ECG. Acute pulmonary embolism may cause right ventricular dilation and strain which is seen on the ECG as T-wave inversion in the precordial leads V$_1$ through V$_4$; new right axis

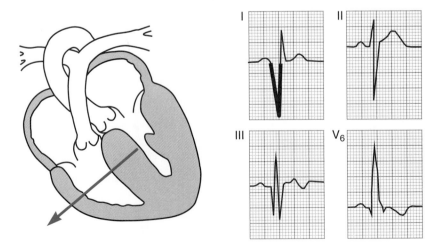

Figure 4.24 (A) Illustration of hypertrophic cardiomyopathy. (B) An ECG tracing in a patient with hypertrophic cardiomyopathy; note the highlighted Q wave in lead I.

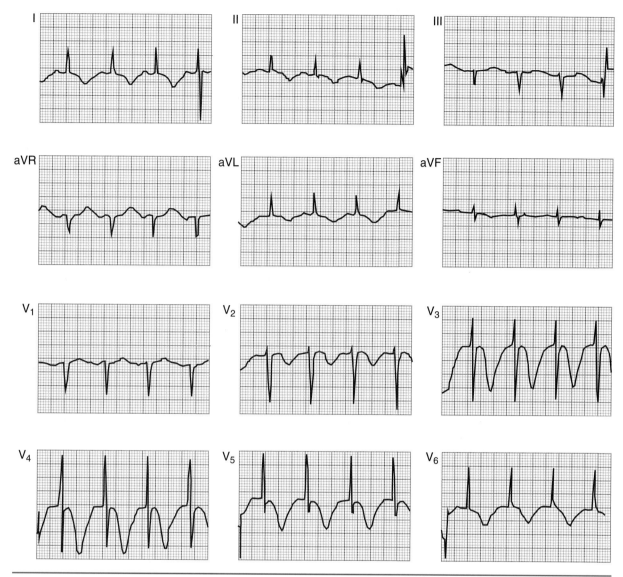

Figure 4.25 A 12-lead ECG from a patient with increased intracranial pressure. Note the QT interval of 0.48 second and the amplitude of the T waves in the precordial leads.

deviation may also be seen. New right bundle branch block could also be the sequelae to a massive pulmonary embolism.

Additionally, S waves in lead I and new Q waves in lead III with T-wave inversion may occur. Referred to as an $S_1Q_3T_3$ pattern, this also is seen with inferior wall myocardial infarction. With pulmonary embolism, there is right axis deviation and the QRS is often greater than 0.10 second and the ventricular rate is often greater than 100 bpm. This is not the case in acute myocardial infarction. **Figure 4.26** provides ECG tracings of changes in the ST segments and T waves from a patient with pulmonary embolism.

Acute Pulmonary Embolism

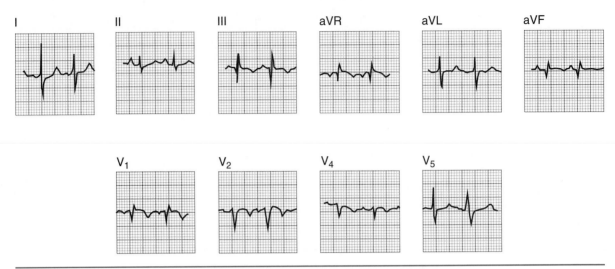

Figure 4.26 ECG tracing from a patient with documented pulmonary embolism.

SUMMARY

In this chapter we have reviewed ECG wave forms and how they relate to the heart's electrical conduction. We have identified some of the causes and resulting changes on the ECG. Deviation in the ECG wave forms could have clinical implications. Variations must be corroborated with clinical presentation and appropriate diagnostic studies.

Self-Assessment Exercise
ECG Rhythm Identification Practice

For the following ECG practice rhythms:

1. Identify the P, Q, R, S, T, and U waves (if evident).
2. Calculate the measurement and rates asked for in each strip.
3. When complete, compare your answers with those in Appendix A.

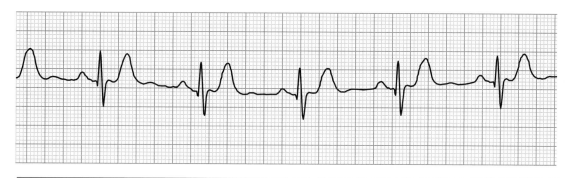

Figure 4.27

1. Can you identify P, Q, R, S, T, and U waves?

2. Look to the left of the QRS and identify each P wave. Is the P wave positive or negative?

   _____

3. QRS (ventricular) rate/rhythm

   _____

4. P (atrial) rate/rhythm

   _____

5. PR interval

   _____

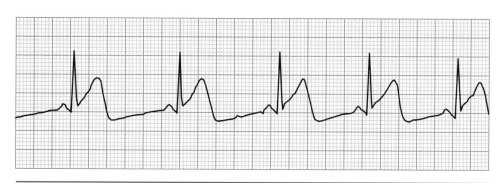

Figure 4.28

1. Can you identify P, Q, R, S, T, and U waves?

2. Look to the left of the QRS and identify each P wave. Are the P waves positive or negative?

   _____

3. QRS (ventricular) rate/rhythm

   _____

4. P (atrial) rate/rhythm

   _____

5. PR interval

   _____

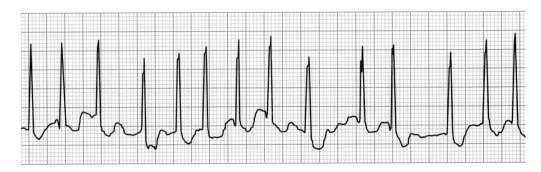

Figure 4.29

1. Can you identify P, Q, R, S, T, and U waves?

2. Look to the left of the QRS and identify each P wave. Is the P wave positive or negative?

   _____

3. QRS (ventricular) rate/rhythm

   _____

4. P (atrial) rate/rhythm

   _____

5. PR interval

   _____

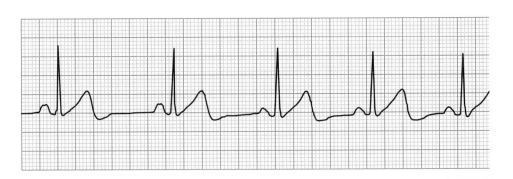

Figure 4.30

1. Can you identify P, Q, R, S, T, and U waves?

2. Look to the left of the QRS and identify each P wave. Are the P waves positive or negative?

   _____

3. QRS (ventricular) rate/rhythm

   _____

4. P (atrial) rate/rhythm

   _____

5. PR interval

   _____

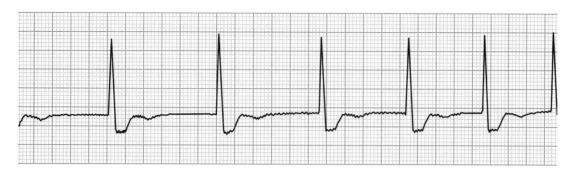

Figure 4.31

1. Can you identify P, Q, R, S, T, and U waves?

2. Look to the left of the QRS and identify each P wave. Is the P wave positive or negative?

    _____

3. QRS (ventricular) rate/rhythm

    _____

4. P (atrial) rate/rhythm

    _____

5. PR interval

    _____

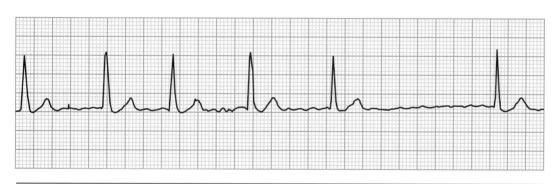

Figure 4.32

1. Can you identify P, Q, R, S, T, and U waves?

2. Look to the left of the QRS and identify each P wave. Is the P wave positive or negative?

    _____

3. QRS (ventricular) rate/rhythm

    _____

4. P (atrial) rate/rhythm

    _____

5. PR interval

    _____

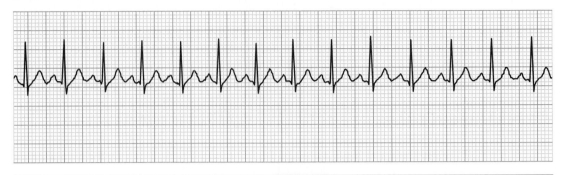

Figure 4.33

1. Can you identify P, Q, R, S, T, and U waves?

2. Look to the left of the QRS and identify each P wave. Is the P wave positive or negative?

   _____

3. QRS (ventricular) rate/rhythm

   _____

4. P (atrial) rate/rhythm

   _____

5. PR interval

   _____

Axis Determination and Implications

Premise

Calculating axis allows clinicians to understand the flow of electrical current as it reflects the heart's electrical conduction system.

Objectives

After reading the chapter and completing the Self-Assessment Exercises, the student should be able to

- Identify the leads used in calculating axis.
- Determine normal axis.
- Determine left and right axis deviation.
- Explain the pathology associated with axis deviation.

Key Terms

cardiac axis   normal axis   vector
left axis deviation   right axis deviation

Introduction

The average direction of the spread of the depolarization wave front through the ventricles as seen in the frontal plane is called the **cardiac axis**, and is useful in deciding whether the wave front is flowing in a normal direction. The axis is derived from the QRS complex as seen in leads I, II, and III, and is sometimes simply called the net area of the QRS. **Figure 5.1** shows examples of the net area of QRS complex and the reciprocal values of leads I and III.

NORMAL AXIS

Normal axis means that the depolarizing wave is spreading toward leads I, II, and III; therefore, the net area of the QRS is seen as primarily positive. Since normal depolarization flows primarily inferior and to the left, the most positive wave form would be lead II. **Figure 5.2** shows the normal axis as seen in leads I, II, and III.

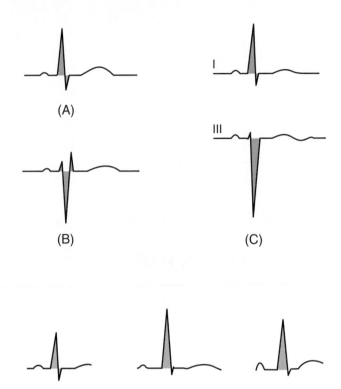

Figure 5.1 (A) is the positive net area of a QRS complex; the shaded area of the QRS above the isoelectric line is more positive than the area below the line. (B) is the negative net area of a QRS complex; the shaded area of the QRS below the isoelectric line is more negative than the area above the line. (C) is the positive net area in lead I and the negative net area in lead III. Lead III is a mirror image of lead I; therefore, the current is directed away from lead III.

Figure 5.2 The net areas of leads I, II, and III are positive, with the greatest positive net area in lead II.

AXIS DEVIATION

Axis deviation may occur as a normal variant, but its presence should alert the clinician to assess for intraventricular conduction defects and ventricular hypertrophy.

Right Axis Deviation

If the flow of depolarization swings toward the right of normal, the QRS deflection in lead I is negative and lead III is positive; this is called **right axis deviation**. **Figure 5.3** compares a negative net area in lead I with positive areas in leads II and III. Note that lead III is more positive than lead II.

Left Axis Deviation

Similarly, when the flow of depolarization swings toward the left of normal, so the QRS deflection is positive in lead I, equiphasic in lead II, and extremely negative in lead III, **left axis deviation** exists. **Figure 5.4** illustrates a net area in lead I that is very positive. In comparison, leads II and III are negative; note that lead III is more negative than lead II.

Figure 5.3 A negative net area in lead I and positive net areas in leads II and III, with lead III showing the greatest positive net area, is characteristic of right axis deviation.

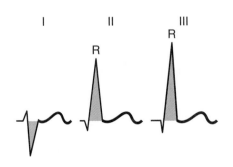

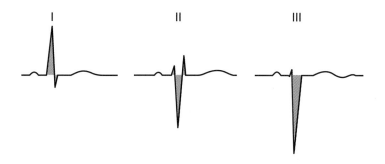

Figure 5.4 A positive net area in lead I and negative net areas in leads II and III, with lead III showing the greatest negative net area, is characteristic of left axis deviation.

CALCULATING AXIS

Calculating the mean axis determines the predominant direction of the flow of electrical current in the heart. This is usually measured during ventricular depolarization (QRS) and uses the morphology of the QRS complexes in the limb leads. Calculating axis is one tool used to determine fascicular block. Calculating the mean flow of current (axis) can be done in several ways. Since not all QRS complexes are clearly different in polarity or configuration, the clinician would do well to learn several methods.

The hexaxial reference system—an intersecting pattern of 6 limb leads—is used to determine the axis of the heart in the frontal plane; in other words, this system refers to the flow of current as it occurs within the heart's conduction system. This is important clinically because deviation from normal can aid in differential diagnosis of many cardiac conditions and pathology within the heart's conduction system.

To apply the hexaxial system, the clinician must first understand the concept of vectors. A **vector** is the direction of force of electrical energy within the heart. The mean cardiac vector is a representation of the flow of electrical current during a cardiac cycle. To understand the hexaxial system, first imagine the triangle formed by leads I, II, and III. As those lines intersect, they create the skeleton for the hexaxial system. Next, add the position for aVR, aVL, and aVF, which also will intersect, producing 3 additional lines of reference. You would now see 12 lines as they visualize the heart's electrical system. **Figure 5.5** illustrates building the hexaxial reference system.

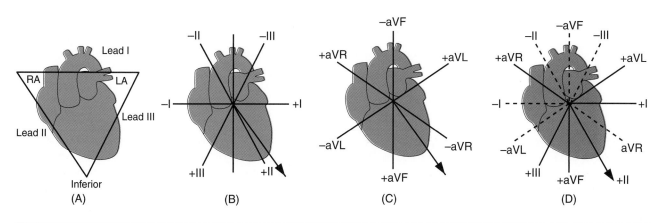

Figure 5.5 In (A), a triangle is formed by leads I, II, and III. (B) shows the intersection of the lines of I, II, and III as they form the skeleton of the hexaxial figure. (C) incorporates the addition of aVR, aVL, and aVF. (D) shows the completed hexaxial system.

Figure 5.6 The mean flow of current in a heart with normal ventricular conduction. When referencing the mean flow current or the mean vector, a heavy arrow is used to indicate the direction of flow.

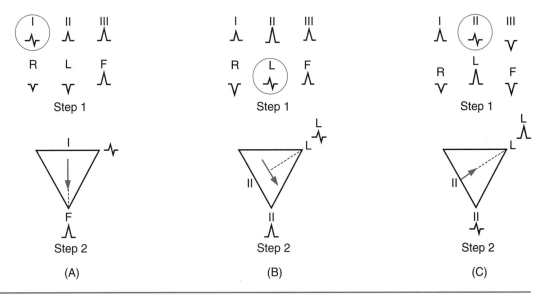

Recall that, in the normal heart, the flow of electrical current usually travels downward from right to left. This generates what is called the normal axis of the heart. **Figure 5.6** illustrates the mean flow of current in a heart with normal conduction.

Calculating the mean flow of current—or axis—can be done in several ways. The common two-step method is as follows:

1. Identify the equiphasic QRS.
2. Identify the lead perpendicular and positive to this lead. (Remember, lead I is at a right angle to aVF, lead II is at a right angle to aVL, and lead III is at a right angle to aVR. The flow of current, or axis, will be parallel to the perpendicular lead.)

Figure 5.7 illustrates the two-step method.

Figure 5.7 In (A), step 1: Look for the equiphasic deflection; in this figure, it is lead I. Step 2: Look for the lead perpendicular (at a right angle) to lead I; in this example, it is lead aVF. Conclusion: The current (axis) is flowing inferior toward the positive electrode of aVF. In (B), step 1: Look for the equiphasic deflection. In this figure, it is lead aVL; therefore, the current flow must be perpendicular to that lead. Step 2: Look at the lead perpendicular to lead aVL; it is lead II. Conclusion: The flow of current is directed inferior toward the positive electrode, lead II. In (C), step 1: Look for the equiphasic deflection. In this figure, it is lead II; therefore, the current flow must be perpendicular to that lead. Step 2: Look at the deflection in the lead perpendicular to lead II; in this example, it is lead aVL. Conclusion: The current is flowing superior toward the positive electrode of aVL. (Adapted with permission from *Understanding Electrocardiography*, 6th ed., by M. B. Conover, 1992, St. Louis: C.V. Mosby.)

Another method used to calculate axis is the quadrant method. This method is useful when there are no equiphasic complexes or when there is more than one lead with equiphasic deflections. The quadrant method is as follows:

1. Look at lead I and determine if the flow of current is to the right or the left; draw an arrow in that direction. Remember that a positive (+) QRS indicates the flow is to the left and a negative (−) QRS indicates the flow is to the right.

2. Look at lead aVF and determine if the flow is superior or inferior; draw an arrow in that direction. Remember that a positive (+) QRS indicates the flow is inferior, toward aVF, and a negative (−) QRS indicates the flow is superior, away from aVF.

3. This creates a quadrant—look for the most positive lead in that quadrant. This will tell you the direction (axis) of current flow for that patient's QRS.

Figure 5.8 illustrates the step-by-step use of the quadrant method.

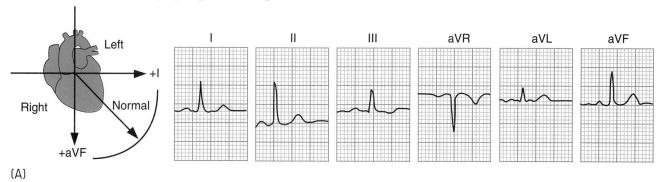

(A)

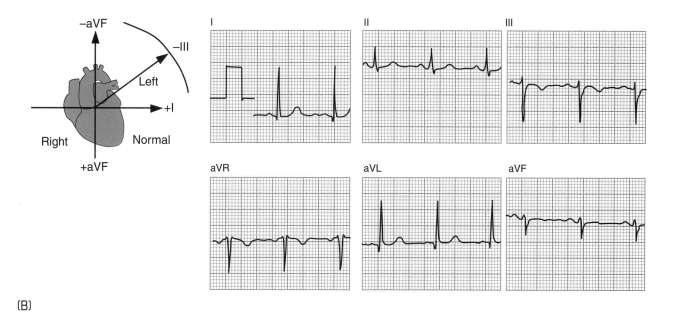

(B)

Figure 5.8 In (A), lead I is positive; the first arrow should be drawn toward the positive electrode in the lead. Next, lead aVF is perpendicular to lead I and the QRS in lead aVF is positive, so draw an arrow toward aVF. You have now localized the flow of current between leads I and aVF. The QRS in lead II is most positive, so the current of flow is directed inferior and to the left, within the normal limits. In (B), lead I is positive; the first arrow should be drawn toward the positive electrode in that lead, Next, lead aVF is perpendicular to lead I and the QRS in lead aVF is negative, so draw an arrow away from the positive electrode in aVF. You have now localized the flow of current between the positive electrode in lead I and the negative electrode in lead aVF. The QRS in lead III is negative, so the current flow is directed superior and to the left, outside the normal limits. This deviation from normal is called left axis deviation. (Adapted from *Understanding Electrocardiography*, 6th ed., by M. B. Conover, 1992, St. Louis: C.V. Mosby.)

It is important to remember that if the QRS in leads I and II are both positive, there is no deviation from normal and no other calculation is necessary. If the QRS in either lead I or II is negative, there is a deviation from normal and further calculation is required.

A flow of current far to the left (superior) is considered a deviation from the normal flow, that is, left axis deviation (LAD). The QRS will be more positive in leads I and aVL than in lead II; leads II and III will be predominantly negative.

A flow of current far to the right (inferior) is considered a deviation from the normal flow, that is, right axis deviation (RAD). The QRS will be more negative in leads I and aVL than in lead II; leads II and III will be predominantly positive, III being the most positive.

Another quick method is to:

1. Look at lead I: if the current flow is toward the right, lead I will be the most negative deflection of the three limb leads.
2. Look at lead III: if the current flow is too far right (inferior), lead III will be very positive and the greatest positive deflection of the three limb leads. This is RAD.

or:

1. Look at lead I: if the current flow is toward the left, lead I will be the most positive deflection of the three limb leads.
2. Look at lead III: if the current flow is too far left (superior), lead III will be very negative and the greatest negative deflection of the three limb leads. This is LAD.

Figure 5.9 illustrates using the net area in leads I and III as a quick reference to determine axis.

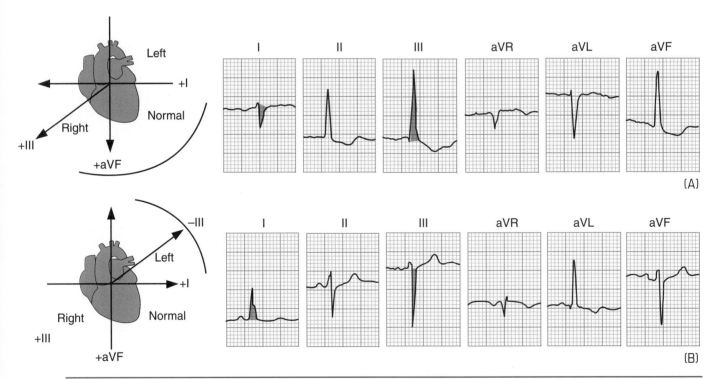

Figure 5.9 (A) shows an ECG tracing of leads I, II, and III highlighting the net QRS complex in leads I and III. Note that in lead I, the net QRS is negative, and in lead III, the net QRS is positive. Note also that the net QRS in lead III is the most positive net QRS seen in the limb leads. (B) shows an ECG tracing of leads I, II, and III highlighting the net QRS complex in leads I and III. Note that in lead I, the net QRS is positive, and in lead III, the net QRS is negative. Note also that the net QRS in lead III is the most negative net QRS seen in the limb leads.

NORMAL AND ABNORMAL VALUES

We have learned that deviation of current to the far left of normal is considered abnormal. This may be caused by a problem with conduction in the left anterior fascicle of the bundle branch system, driving the net current upward and to the left.

Deviation to the far right of normal is also considered abnormal. This may be caused by a problem with conduction in the left posterior fascicle of the bundle branch system, driving the net current to the far right of normal.

Identify the axis by degrees so that each lead has a landmark:

Lead I	=	0 degrees
Lead II	=	+60 degrees
Lead III	=	(+) at +120 degrees (right) or,
		(−) at −60 degrees (left)
Lead aVF	=	(+) at +90 degrees (normal)
		(−) at −90 degrees (superior or far left)

Once calculations are completed, the interpretation would be, for example, "left axis deviation at −60 degrees" or "right axis deviation at +120 degrees." The implications of axis deviation are discussed in Chapter 11.

The principles of assessing mean electrical axis can be applied to P and T waves. For instance, a sinus P wave is directed inferior and to the left and therefore is positive in lead II and negative in lead aVR. The normal P-wave axis is 60 degrees. If the origin of the P wave is from another source, for example from the AV junction, atrial depolarization would be directed toward the right superior surface. Then the P′ wave will be positive in aVR and negative in lead II.

The T-wave axis shift has been reported to represent a general marker of ventricular repolarization abnormalities and a potential indicator of increased risk for cardiovascular mortality.

THE LEWIS CIRCLE

Another quick reference for calculating axis and the related degrees is the Lewis circle. **Figure 5.10** illustrates the heart with the degree values assigned to the limb leads. Note the arrows imposed on the circle to aid in identifying the axis value.

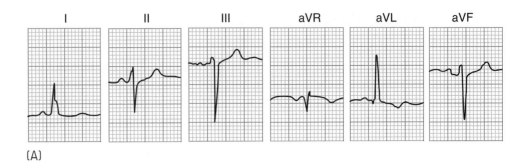

(A)

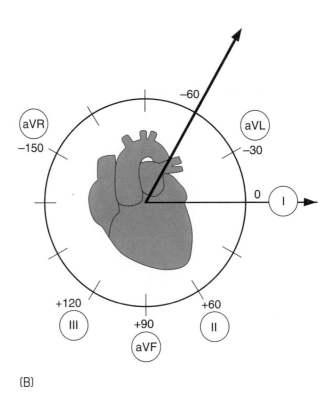

Figure 5.10 (A) is an ECG tracing showing leads I and II being different in polarity; leads I and aVL are positive; lead III has the greatest negative net area. (B) shows the heart with the Lewis circle and degree values assigned to the various leads to provide quick reference and reporting of axis value. Lead I is positive, so an arrow is drawn toward lead I. Lead III is the greatest negative, so an arrow is drawn away from lead III. Lead aVL is also positive, but lead III has the greater value. Conclusion: Axis deviation superior and to the left at −60 degrees.

(B)

SUMMARY

The ECG is a sensitive tool that provides valuable information about the heart's ventricular conduction system, identifying the source of a wide QRS complex tachycardia and the surfaces of the heart affected by ischemia, injury, and necrosis. Once a QRS complex is reported to be greater than 0.10 second, the clinician should assess the polarity of the complex. This involves calculating the QRS axis, for which there are several systems available to the clinician.

Self-Assessment Exercises
Matching

Match the ECG finding in the left column with the definition in the right column, and then compare your answers with those in Appendix A. Definitions may be used more than once.

ECG Finding	Definition
____ 1. rS >0.10 sec in leads II, III, and aVF	A. Left anterior fascicular
____ 2. rS >0.10 sec in leads I and aVL	B. Left posterior fascicular
____ 3. QRS axis at −60 degrees	C. Normal axis
____ 4. QRS axis at +30 degrees	D. Right axis deviation
____ 5. QRS axis at +120 degrees	E. Left axis deviation

ECG Rhythm Identification Practice

Identify the ECG criterion listed below each ECG tracing. Then compare your answers with those in Appendix A.

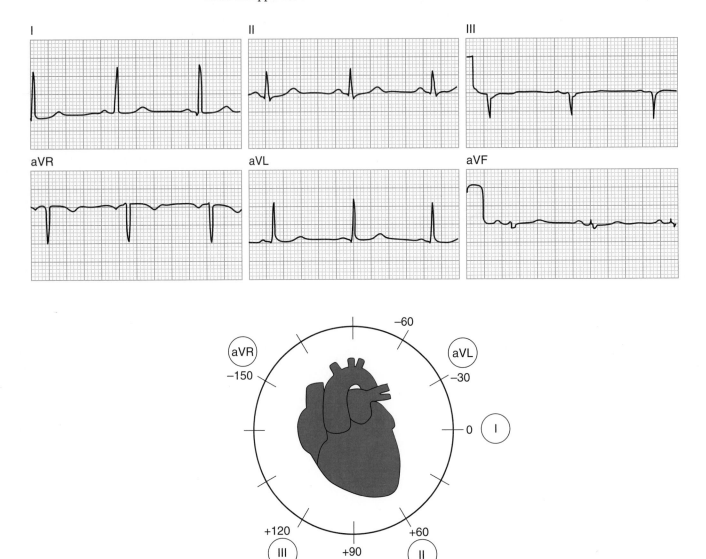

Figure 5.11

1. What is the underlying rhythm? _____
2. What is the axis? _____
    a. Look at leads I and II; are they positive? _____
    b. Are there equiphasic deflections? _____
    c. Draw the arrows on the Lewis circle to verify your calculations.
3. What is your interpretation? _____

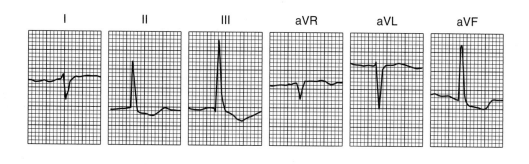

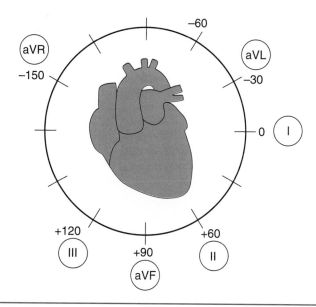

Figure 5.12

1. What is the underlying rhythm? _____
2. What is the axis? _____
    a. Look at leads I and II; are they positive? _____
    b. Are there equiphasic deflections? _____
    c. Draw the arrows on the Lewis circle to verify your calculations.
3. What is your interpretation? _____

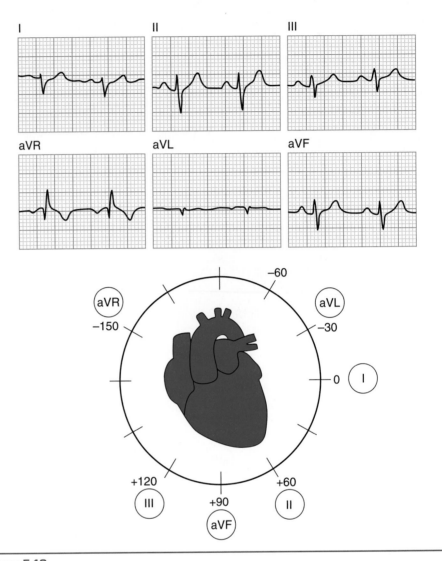

Figure 5.13

1. What is the underlying rhythm? _____
2. What is the axis? _____
    a. Look at leads I and II; are they positive? _____
    b. Are there equiphasic deflections? _____
    c. Draw the arrows on the Lewis circle to verify your calculations.
3. What is your interpretation? _____

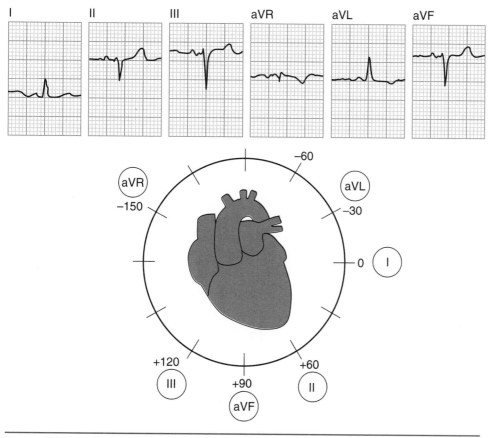

Figure 5.14

1. What is the underlying rhythm? _____

2. What is the axis? _____
   a. Look at leads I and II; are they positive? _____
   b. Are there equiphasic deflections? _____
   c. Draw the arrows on the Lewis circle to verify your calculations.

3. What is your interpretation? _____

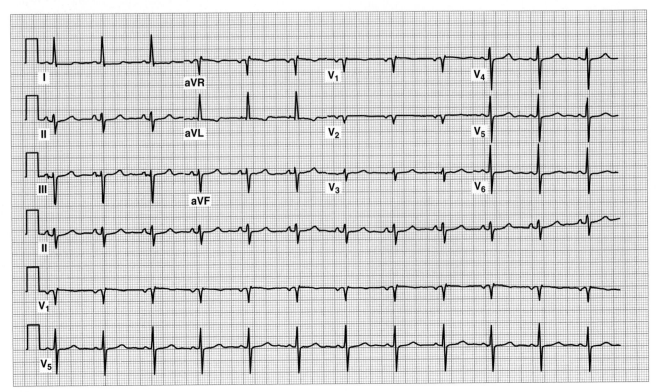

(A)

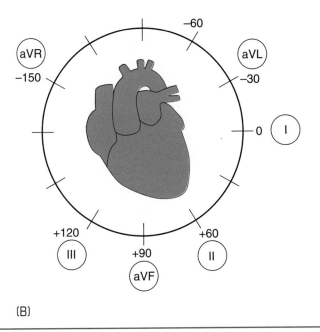

(B)

Figure 5.15

1. What is the underlying rhythm? _____
2. What is the axis? _____
    a. Look at leads I and II; are they positive? _____
    b. Are there equiphasic deflections? _____
    c. Draw the arrows on the Lewis circle to verify your calculations.
3. What is your interpretation? _____

The Sinus Mechanisms

Premise

Abnormalities of heart rhythm are easy to figure out. The key is to find the P wave.

Objectives

After reading the chapter and completing the Self-Assessment Exercises, the student should be able to

- Plot out P waves, calculating rate and rhythm.
- Plot out QRS complexes, calculating rate and rhythm.
- Confirm the association between each P wave and the QRS complex.
- Determine if the rhythm is appropriate to the patient.
- Interpret the configuration and morphology using more than one EGG lead.
- Select the appropriate intervention.

Key Terms

hypoperfusion	sinus rhythm	sinus tachycardia
sinus arrhythmia	sinus (SA) arrest	
sinus bradycardia	sinus (SA) block	

Introduction

Normally, the heart can and will depolarize spontaneously and rhythmically. The rate will be controlled by the pacemaker that depolarizes at the highest rate. The sinus sinoatrial [SA] node normally has the highest frequency of discharge. Subsequent depolarization of atrial tissue will write a P wave on EGG. If the impulse succeeds in traveling through the AV junction and activating the ventricles, a normal QRS complex (0.10 second) will follow. Variations in the sinus mechanisms have to do with rate and rhythm. As long as the sinus fires and atrial tissue responds, the process recurs normally at a given rate of speed. The clue is to look to the left of each QRS and find a single, positive P wave for each normal QRS—that is the sinus mechanism.

To accurately identify the rhythm, specific criteria must be evaluated. In each of the mechanisms, the criteria will be addressed in a consistent manner so the reader can develop a consistent pattern of identification.

All monitors have the capability to look at the heart from various leads. Portable monitors have at least three leads available. When wave forms are not clearly visible on one or more leads, the practitioner should confirm the presence, absence, or abnormality of any wave form in a given set of ECG leads to confirm the absence or abnormality of that wave form.

SINUS RHYTHM

To describe the rhythm of the heart as **sinus rhythm** (the impulse originating in the SA node, the normal pacemaker of the heart) without qualifications, the indicated criteria must be met:

- *P Wave:* The P waves are positive (upright) and uniform in lead II. Every P wave is followed by a QRS complex.
- *PR Interval:* The PR interval (from the beginning of the P wave to the beginning of the QRS complex) is constant and consistently between 0.12 and 0.20 second.
- *QRS Complex:* The QRS complex duration is 0.10 second or less. Every QRS complex is preceded by a single, predictable, positive P wave.
- *QRS Rate:* A normal predictable heart rate is between 60 and 100 beat(s) per minute (bpm) in the adult patient. There is very little variance in rhythm.
- *QRS Rhythm:* The rhythm is regular. Sinus rhythm is the standard against which most arrhythmias are compared, measured, and analyzed.

Figure 6.1 shows a single, positive P wave for each QRS complex, and the PR interval is consistent. The heart rate is between 60 and 100 bpm and rhythmic. **Figure 6.2** consists of two leads from the same patient. In lead II, the P wave is barely visible, but present. When you are not sure that P waves exist, be persistent in your efforts and select a different lead. Comparing leads I, II, and III you will usually see visible P waves more prominently in at least one other lead.

Figure 6.1 An ECG tracing showing one positive P wave to the left of each QRS complex; the PR interval is consistent and the heart rate is between 60 and 100 bpm. These computations represent a sinus mechanism.

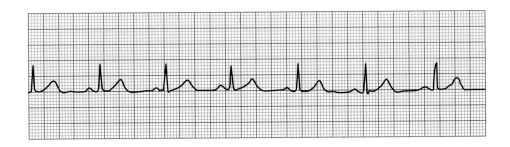

Figure 6.2 An ECG tracing from a patient showing simultaneous leads. Note the difference in the ECG wave forms as depicted in two leads. Note that III depicts the wave forms more clearly. This example illustrates that reliance on only one lead is a disservice to the patient as well as the individual interpreting the ECG tracing.

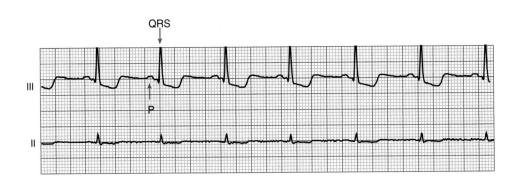

SINUS TACHYCARDIA

Tachycardia means fast (*tachy*) heart (*cardia*), a rate greater than 100 bpm. **Sinus tachycardia** indicates that the origin of the rhythm is the SA node, the normal pacemaker of the heart.

If all the criteria for a sinus mechanism have been fulfilled but the heart rate is greater than 100 bpm, the rhythm is called sinus tachycardia. The range for a sinus tachycardia is usually 100 to 180 bpm. The sinus node rarely exceeds 180 bpm, although rates up to 200 bpm have been seen with exertion. When the ventricular rate exceeds 160 bpm care must be taken to differentiate the source of the tachycardia to determine the source (Chapter 8). EGG characteristics for sinus tachycardia are as follows:

- *P Wave:* The P waves are positive and uniform. Every P wave is followed by a QRS complex.
- *PR Interval:* The PR interval is normal between 0.12 and 0.20 second and is consistent.
- *QRS Complex:* The QRS complex duration is 0.10 second or less. Every QRS complex is preceded by a positive P wave.
- *QRS Rate:* The rate is constant above 100 (100–160) bpm.
- *QRS Rhythm:* The rhythm is regular.

Figure 6.3 shows an EGG of sinus tachycardia.

Causes

Normal body function (physiologic) tachycardia is common for infants at about 120 to 130 bpm. In the adult, sinus tachycardia results from the body's needs for increased perfusion as with exercise and emotions, such as fever, pain, fear, anger, and anxiety,

Sinus tachycardia is a sign of physiologic stress, such as hypovolemia, hyperthyroidism, dehydration, malignant hyperthermia, anemia, pheochromycytoma, sepsis, pulmonary embolism, chronic pulmonary disease, hypoxia, intake of stimulants, or any condition that causes an increased sympathetic stimulation. Other pathologies causing sinus tachycardia are congestive heart failure, cardiogenic shock, valve disease, hypertension, myocardial ischemia, injury, and infarction.

Medications such as atropine and beta adrenergic drugs can cause sinus tachycardia. Drugs that cause vasodilation may have sinus tachycardia as a side effect. These include nitroglycerin, morphine, furosemide (Lasix), and some antihistamines.

Drug abuse and illegal drugs such as methamphetamines cause sinus tachycardia. Opioid intoxication can occur from heroin and cocaine (from cocoa leaves) in various forms and combinations. Other examples are crystal methamphetamine known as crack or rock (smokable cocaine), white crosses (speed) and black beauty, and benzodiazepines (such as flunitrazepam, also known as Rohypnol or "roofies"). Drug abuse includes look-alike drugs made up of mega doses of caffeine such as gamma-hydroxybutyric acid or GHB, also known as "ecstasy"

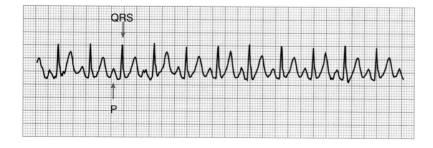

Figure 6.3 An ECG tracing showing one positive P wave to the left of each QRS complex; the PR interval is consistent and the heart rate is greater than 100 bpm. These computations represent a sinus tachycardia.

or the rape drug. All these drugs cause sinus tachycardia, as do marijuana and shurm (marijuana soaked in formaldehyde), PCP (a horse tranquilizer), and MDA (an elephant tranquilizer); PCP and MDA are taken to enhance and create incredible human strength.

If sinus tachycardias persist as a result of any of these conditions, coronary perfusion may be in jeopardy, especially when coronary vessels are narrowed or obstructed, causing myocardial ischemia and injury.

Intervention

When assessing the patient, determine if the circumstances are appropriate to the rhythm/rate presented. Consider how much of a deviation this rate is from the patient's normal physiologic resting rate. Patient care begins with initial assessment, past medical history, focused history, and physical exam in an effort to identify the cause. For patients with chest pain or pressure or with those patients whose clinical presentation indicates they are compromised by the tachycardia, treatment usually begins with high-flow oxygen therapy.

Place the patient on an ECG monitor to determine if the tachycardia is indeed sinus in origin. Assess more than one monitoring lead for signs and symptoms of ischemia and injury. ECG rhythm analysis also should include a 12-lead ECG.

For patients with chest pain or pressure, consider pain relief with nitroglycerin or morphine sulfate according to local protocol. Otherwise, be supportive and continue to identify and treat the underlying cause. Treatment may include appropriate antidotes whenever possible for offending drugs. **Figure 6.4** is an example of sinus tachycardia in an adult allegedly using methamphetamine. **Figure 6.5** shows sinus tachycardia in an exercising adult.

SINUS BRADYCARDIA

Bradycardia means slow (*brady*) heart (*cardia*). If the heart rate is under 60 bpm, but all the criteria for a sinus mechanism have been fulfilled, the rhythm is known as **sinus bradycardia**. The ECG characteristics of sinus bradycardia are as follows:

- *P Wave:* The P waves are positive and uniform in lead II. Every P wave is followed by a QRS complex.
- *PR Interval:* The PR interval is normal between 0.12 and 0.20 second and is constant from beat to beat.

Figure 6.4 An ECG tracing showing sinus tachycardia from an adult allegedly using methamphetamine. Note the wandering baseline caused by rapid respirations and patient movement.

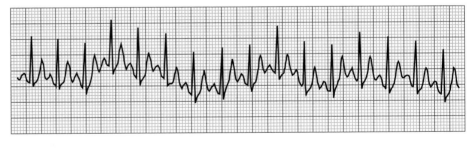

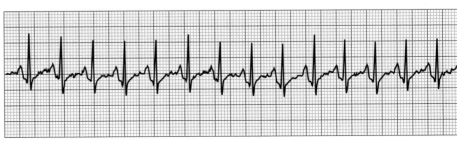

Figure 6.5 An ECG tracing from an exercising adult. Note there is a single positive P wave to the left of each QRS complex; the rate is 150 bpm.

- *QRS Complex:* The QRS complex duration is 0.10 second or less. Every QRS complex is preceded by a P wave.
- *QRS Rate:* The rate is constant below 60 bpm, with little variance.
- *QRS Rhythm:* The rhythm is regular.

Figure 6.6 is an ECG of sinus bradycardia.

Causes

A slow heart rate indeed may be the norm for physically conditioned individuals or may be considered a normal variant. Often, sinus bradycardia is seen with increased vagal tone and not accompanied by hypotension nor **hypoperfusion**. It is also seen in the aging population, in conditioned athletes, and during sleep patterns, and in conditions of hypothermia and some thyroid conditions such as myxedema. When sinus bradycardia is unexpected and is not appropriate for the situation, care should be directed toward assessment and intervention to increase the rate to a level that provides reasonable perfusion. The optimal rate will vary from patient to patient.

Intervention

Patient care begins with initial assessment, which includes past medical history and detailed physical exam. Determine if the rate is physiologic or compromising to the patient. If the patient is symptomatic and hypotensive and has other signs of hypoperfusion, immediate intervention is necessary. The goal is to improve perfusion by increasing heart rate. Two available modalities are medications (atropine) and electronic pacing. There is always the risk that a sudden change in heart rate after atropine may cause an increase in myocardial oxygen debt and further compromise the patient. For any patient with chest pain or pressure, place the patient on an EGG monitor to identify the arrhythmia. Nonphysiologic bradycardia may be the only initial ECG sign that the patient has proximal right coronary artery disease, affecting sinus node function. Assess more than one monitoring lead for signs and symptoms of ischemia and injury. EGG rhythm analysis should also include a 12-lead ECG. **Figure 6.7** shows simultaneous leads of sinus bradycardia in a conditioned adult. **Figure 6.8** illustrates sinus bradycardia in a patient who complained of chest pressure. Note the consistent appearance of the positive P wave to the left of each QRS in all tracings. Note also the ST elevation in lead II indicating possible ischemia and/or injury.

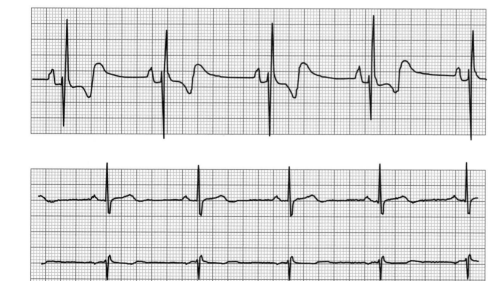

Figure 6.6 An ECG tracing showing one positive P wave to the left of each QRS complex; the PR interval is consistent and the heart rate is less than 60 bpm. These computations represent a sinus bradycardia.

Figure 6.7 An ECG tracing showing sinus bradycardia in two leads from a conditioned adult.

SINUS ARRHYTHMIA

In **sinus arrhythmia**, the impulse has its origin in the sinus node and subsequent conduction is normal. The rhythm of impulse formation, and thus the heart's response, is irregular—irregular (*ar*) rhythm (*rhythmia*). The PR intervals are consistent, but the PP and RR intervals are continually changing. The heart rate varies from about 53 to 58 bpm, about a 10 percent variation. The EGG characteristics of sinus arrhythmia are as follows:

- *P Wave:* The P waves are positive and uniform in lead II. Every P wave is followed by a QRS complex.
- *PR Interval:* The PR interval is normal between 0.12 and 0.20 second and is constant from beat to beat.
- *QRS Complex:* The QRS complex duration is 0.10 second or less. Every QRS complex is preceded by a P wave.
- *QRS Rate:* The rate varies by more than 10 percent.
- *QRS Rhythm:* The rhythm is irregular due to the changing rate.

Figure 6.9 is an EGG showing sinus arrhythmia. Note the gradual increase and decrease of heart rate.

Causes

Sinus arrhythmia is not a disease, nor does it reflect a disease. It is a natural response and meets all the criteria described under sinus rhythm except for the variation in rhythm, naturally associated with the respiratory cycles. It is commonly seen in adolescents.

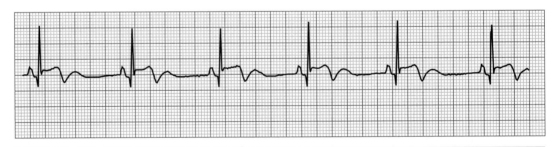

Figure 6.8 An ECG tracing from a patient with chest pressure whose normal heart rate was reported as "usually in the high 70s." Note the ST segment elevation and T-wave inversion indicative of myocardial ischemia/injury. The presence of Q waves in this patient is suspicious. Serial ECGs and comparisons with old ECGs helped differentiate a normal variant from Q waves that represent myocardial infarction.

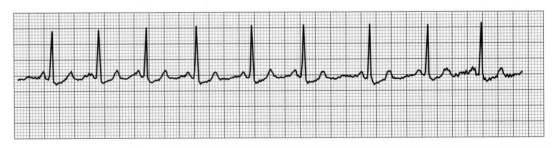

Figure 6.9 An ECG tracing showing one positive P wave to the left of each QRS complex; the PR interval is consistent, but the heart rate varies. These computations and the irregularity represent a sinus arrhythmia. It is helpful to report the rate range. In this patient it is about 66 to 100 bpm.

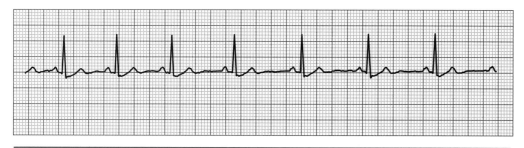

Figure 6.10 An ECG tracing of sinus arrhythmia at 67 to 86 bpm.

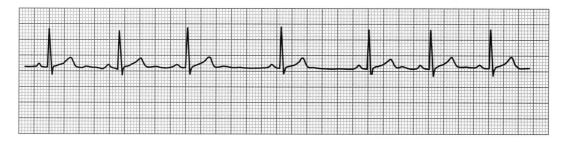

Figure 6.11 An ECG tracing of sinus arrhythmia at 48 to 71 bpm.

Intervention

Unless the arrhythmia is accompanied by a bradycardia that causes hypotension and hypo-perfusion, no intervention is necessary. If such is the case, begin patient care as for sinus bradycardia. **Figure 6.10** and **Figure 6.11** are examples of sinus arrhythmia. Note that despite the irregularity, there is a consistent appearance of the positive P wave to the left of each QRS in all strips.

SINUS ARREST

Sinus (SA) arrest is an event caused by a sudden failure of the SA node to initiate a timely impulse. In sinus arrest, multiples of PQRST complexes are missing, sometimes two, sometimes three or four. There does not have to be a pattern to the frequency of occurrences. In other words, a patient can have periods of SA arrest, missing two or three PQRST complexes. This may not recur for several minutes or hours, and then an episode will recur missing one or several complexes. If the period of arrest is more than one cycle length, physiologically another pacemaker should take over and initiate a new rhythm. In most cases, it is the AV junction. The EGG characteristics of sinus arrest are as follows:

- *P Wave:* Since the SA node has ceased functioning, no sinus P waves are visible.
- *PR Interval:* The PR interval is normal between 0.12 and 0.20 second and is consistent.
- *QRS Complex:* The QRS complex duration is 0.10 second or less. After the arrest, if the escape rhythm is supraventricular, the QRS will remain the same. If the escape rhythm is ventricular, the resulting QRS will be greater than 0.10 second and appear different than the dominant, supraventricular (narrow) QRS.
- *QRS Rate:* Report the overall dominant sinus rate, qualify the length of the arrest (the period of time between QRS complexes containing the arrest period), and report the escape rate.

- *QRS Rhythm:* The underlying rhythm is regular. After the period of arrest, there may be one or more escape beats. If the escape rhythm becomes dominant, its rhythm is usually regular.

Figure 6.12 illustrates an EGG tracing of sinus arrest.

Causes

Sinus arrest reflects a problem within the SA node, usually as a result of proximal right coronary artery disease. If that condition exists, the ability of the AV junctional escape mechanism also may be affected. Sinus arrest also can be seen with sleep apnea as well.

Intervention

Patients are treated based on the degree of hemodynamic compromise. On initial assessment, the patient may complain only of near-syncopal episodes. As with all cases of patient compromise, care begins with documenting patient presentation and past medical history, including medications, and a physical exam.

Begin with high-flow oxygen therapy, and place the patient on a monitor. Include a 12-lead ECG. If SA arrest occurs frequently, an electronic pacemaker may be implanted. Medical direction may recommend the use of atropine as a temporizing measure until a

Figure 6.12 An ECG tracing showing one positive P wave to the left of each QRS complex; the PR interval is consistent, and the heart rate is within normal limits prior to the event of SA arrest. Count the number of large squares between the QRS complexes containing the arrest. Multiply by 0.20 (the value of one large square) for the estimated period of arrest, about 2.76 seconds.

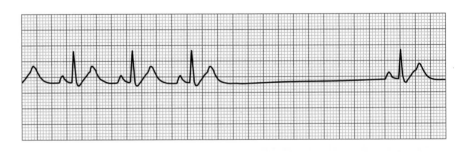

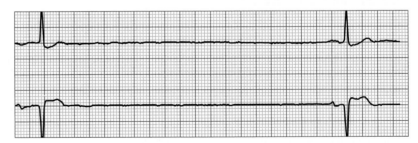

Figure 6.13 An ECG tracing from a 51-year-old patient showing sinus arrest during a sleep apnea episode.

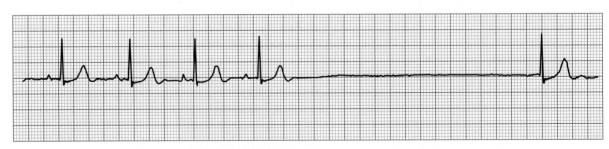

Figure 6.14 An ECG tracing from an 82-year-old patient showing sinus arrest. The patient required insertion of an electronic pacemaker.

pacemaker is implemented. **Figure 6.13** is an example of SA arrest in a 51-year-old male during a sleep apnea episode. **Figure 6.14** shows SA arrest in an 82-year-old male patient who complained of frequent episodes of syncope. The rate was unresponsive to atropine, responded well to transcutaneous pacing (TCP), and eventually had pacemaker implantation.

SINOATRIAL (SA) BLOCK

Sinus (SA) block is also called sinus exit block. SA block is an event and not always reflective of disease within the sinus node. In SA block, the SA node initiates the impulse, but the propagation over atrial tissue is blocked, so the atria are not depolarized. Therefore, there is neither a P wave nor a QRS complex. SA block represents a failure of transmission of the impulse over atrial tissue. The EGG characteristics of SA block are as follows:

- *P Wave:* The P waves are positive and uniform in lead II. However, an entire cycle (P, QRS, and T) is missing. The SA node initiates an impulse, but it is not propagated through the atria; it is blocked, and hence there is no P wave. The pause is a multiple of the regular cycle length.

- *PR Interval:* The PR interval is normal between 0.12 and 0.20 second and is constant from beat to beat except during the pause, when an entire cycle is missing. Also, the PR interval may be slightly shorter following the pause.

- *QRS Complex:* The QRS complex duration is 0.10 second or less except during the pause, when an entire cycle is missing.

- *QRS Rate:* The rate may be constant or varying, according to the number and position of the missing cycles. The RR interval is a multiple of the regular cycle length.

- *QRS Rhythm:* The rhythm may be regular or irregular, according to the number and position of the missing cycles.

Figure 6.15 is an EGG tracing showing SA block. In this example, the sinus P waves plot out. The *X* indicates the missing PQRST complex. The RR interval of the SA block is equal to twice the normal RR interval.

Causes

SA block is most commonly caused by medications, such as quinidine, acetylcholine, and excessive potassium ingestion. Excessive vagal stimulation also may cause SA block; this is episodic and may be documented only if the patient is on a monitor.

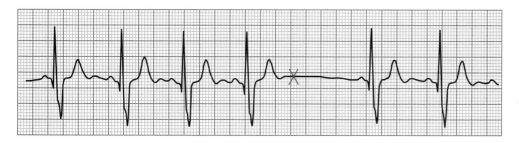

Figure 6.15 An ECG tracing showing one positive P wave to the left of each QRS complex; the PR interval is consistent, and the heart rate is within normal limits prior to the event of SA block. Plot out the P waves and measure the RR interval of the SA block. Note that the long PP interval is equal to two PP intervals. The ECG also shows U waves and broad terminal S waves in the QRS complex.

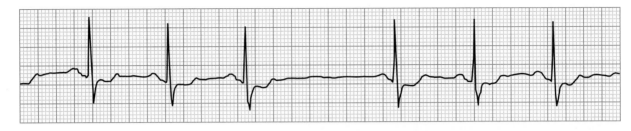

Figure 6.16 An ECG tracing showing SA block. Note that the cadence of sinus P waves plot through the event.

Intervention

Unless the underlying rhythm is slow, intervention is supportive and focused on identifying the cause. This involves performing an initial assessment and completing a focused history with special attention to cardiac conditions and medication ingestion. SA block is rarely life-threatening. **Figure 6.16** is an example of SA block. Note the schematic, which shows how the P waves plot through the event without disturbing the cadence of the sinus rhythm.

SUMMARY

Normally, the sinus node dominates heart rhythm and does so for a lifetime. An arrhythmia is present when the heart rate is too slow, too fast, or irregular, or when depolarization does not propagate over atrial tissue, and, finally, when the SA node fails to produce a stimulus at all. In each of the sinus mechanisms, the visible P wave will be positive and precede each QRS. Where there is no P wave, there is no atrial depolarization.

Most of the sinus arrhythmias are explainable, and the patients tolerate minor deviations. In most instances, identifying and treating the cause remedies the arrhythmias. When the patient situation is complicated with persistent bradycardia and accompanying hypotension and hypoperfusion, treating the patient with a slow rate is appropriate.

Table 6.1 summarizes the ECG configurations of the sinus mechanisms and the proposed treatment.

Sinus	Rhythm	Bradycardia	Tachycardia	Arrhythmia	Exit Block	Arrest
P wave	1 (+) P wave/ QRS	1 (+) P wave/ QRS	1 (+) P wave/ QRS	1 (+) P wave/ QRS	1 (+) P wave/ QRS	1 (+) P wave/ QRS
PR interval	0.12−0.20 sec	0.12−0.20 sec	0.12−0.20 sec	0.12−0.20 sec		
QRS complex	0.10 sec	0.10 sec	0.10 sec	0.10 sec		
QRS rate	60−100 bpm	<60 bpm	>100 bpm	60−100 bpm usually		
QRS rhythm	Regular	Regular	Regular	Irregular	Regular except for the event	Regular except for the event
Event		Gradual onset	Gradual change		Misses one QRS; sinus P plots through; cadence is regular	Misses more than one QRS; sinus P plots through; rhythm after the event may be regular or irregular; perhaps slow

Table 6.1 A summary of the ECG configurations of the sinus mechanisms and the proposed interventions. (Continues)

Sinus	Rhythm	Bradycardia	Tachycardia	Arrhythmia	Exit Block	Arrest
Rx		Consider atropine, fluids, Pace (TCP), pressor for perfusion.	ID and Rx cause such as pain or pressure, fever, anger, anxiety, dehydration, hypovolemia, medications, and/or drug use and/or abuse	Only with bradycardia and patient is hypotensive and hypoperfusing	Only if it persists; increases in frequency and duration; associated with a slow rate; hypotensive and hypoperfusing	Only if it persists; increases in frequency and duration; associated with a slow rate; hypotensive and hypoperfusing

Table 6.1 Continued

Self-Assessment Exercise
Fill in the Blanks

Complete the second and third columns, and then compare your answers with those in Appendix A.

	Sinus Rhythm	Sinus Bradycardia	Sinus Tachycardia
P wave	1 (+) P wave/QRS	1 (+) P wave/QRS	_____
PR interval	0.12–0.20 sec	_____	_____
QRS complex	≤0.10 sec	_____	_____
QRS rate	60–100 bpm	_____	_____
QRS rhythm]	Regular	_____	Regular

Complete the second and third columns, and then compare your answers with those in Appendix A.

	Sinus Rhythm	Sinus Arrhythmia	Sinus Block
P wave	1 (+) P wave Q/RS	1 (+) P wave/QRS	_____
PR interval	0.12–0.20 sec	_____	_____
QRS complex	≤0.10 sec	_____	_____
QRS rate	60–100 bpm	_____	_____
QRS rhythm]	Regular	_____	Regular

ECG Rhythm Identification Practice

For the following rhythms, fill in the blanks and then compare your answers with those in Appendix A.

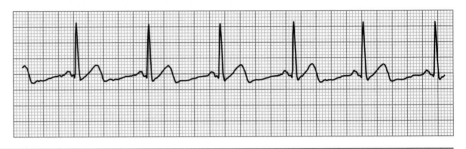

Figure 6.17

1. QRS duration _____
2. QT interval _____
3. Ventricular rate/rhythm _____
4. Atrial rate/rhythm _____

5. PR interval _____
6. Identification _____
7. Symptoms _____
8. Treatment _____

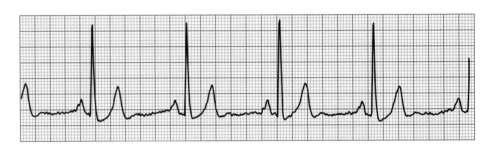

Figure 6.18

1. QRS duration _____
2. QT interval _____
3. Ventricular rate/rhythm _____
4. Atrial rate/rhythm _____

5. PR interval _____
6. Identification _____
7. Symptoms _____
8. Treatment _____

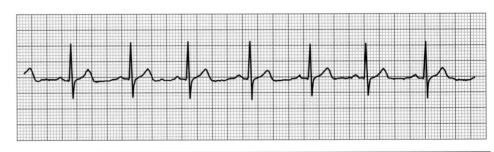

Figure 6.19

1. QRS duration _____
2. QT interval _____
3. Ventricular rate/rhythm _____
4. Atrial rate/rhythm _____

5. PR interval _____
6. Identification _____
7. Symptoms _____
8. Treatment _____

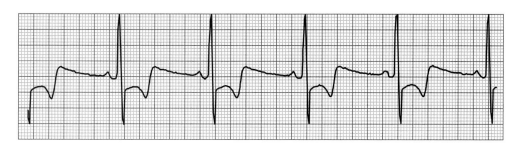

Figure 6.20

1. QRS duration _____
2. QT interval _____
3. Ventricular rate/rhythm _____
4. Atrial rate/rhythm _____
5. PR interval _____
6. Identification _____
7. Symptoms _____
8. Treatment _____

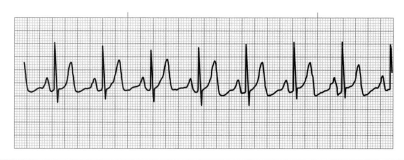

Figure 6.21

1. QRS duration _____
2. QT interval _____
3. Ventricular rate/rhythm _____
4. Atrial rate/rhythm _____
5. PR interval _____
6. Identification _____
7. Symptoms _____
8. Treatment _____

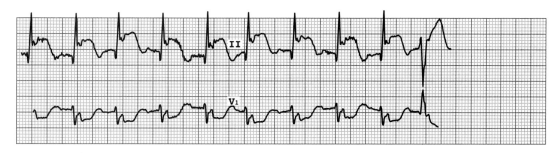

Figure 6.22

1. QRS duration _____
2. QT interval _____
3. Ventricular rate/rhythm _____
4. Atrial rate/rhythm _____
5. PR interval _____
6. Identification _____
7. Symptoms _____
8. Treatment _____

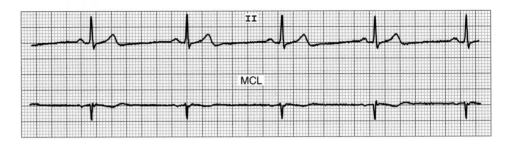

Figure 6.23

1. QRS duration _____
2. QT interval _____
3. Ventricular rate/rhythm _____
4. Atrial rate/rhythm _____

5. PR interval _____
6. Identification _____
7. Symptoms _____
8. Treatment _____

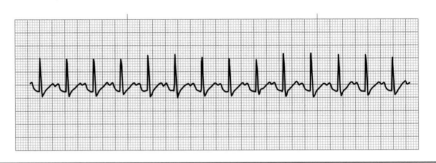

Figure 6.23

1. QRS duration _____
2. QT interval _____
3. Ventricular rate/rhythm _____
4. Atrial rate/rhythm _____

5. PR interval _____
6. Identification _____
7. Symptoms _____
8. Treatment _____

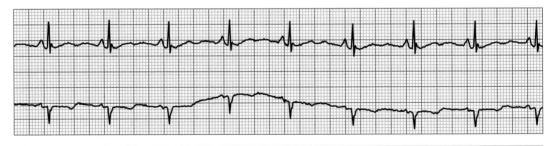

Figure 6.25

1. QRS duration _____
2. QT interval _____
3. Ventricular rate/rhythm _____
4. Atrial rate/rhythm _____

5. PR interval _____
6. Identification _____
7. Symptoms _____
8. Treatment _____

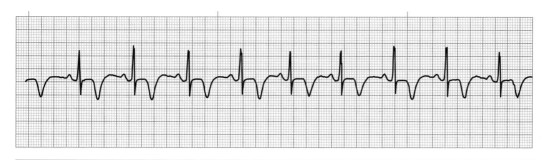

Figure 6.26

1. QRS duration _____
2. QT interval _____
3. Ventricular rate/rhythm _____
4. Atrial rate/rhythm _____

5. PR interval _____
6. Identification _____
7. Symptoms _____
8. Treatment _____

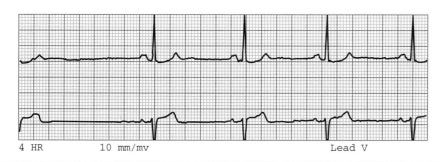

4 HR   10 mm/mv   Lead V

Figure 6.27

1. QRS duration _____
2. QT interval _____
3. Ventricular rate/rhythm _____
4. Atrial rate/rhythm _____

5. PR interval _____
6. Identification _____
7. Symptoms _____
8. Treatment _____

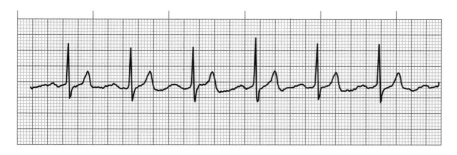

Figure 6.28

1. QRS duration _____
2. QT interval _____
3. Ventricular rate/rhythm _____
4. Atrial rate/rhythm _____

5. PR interval _____
6. Identification _____
7. Symptoms _____
8. Treatment _____

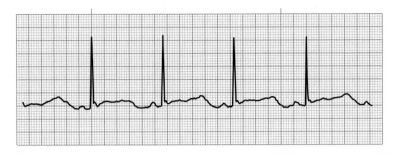

Figure 6.29

1. QRS duration _____
2. QT interval _____
3. Ventricular rate/rhythm _____
4. Atrial rate/rhythm _____

5. PR interval _____
6. Identification _____
7. Symptoms _____
8. Treatment _____

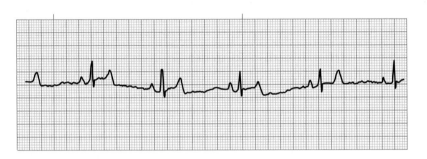

Figure 6.29

1. QRS duration _____
2. QT interval _____
3. Ventricular rate/rhythm _____
4. Atrial rate/rhythm _____

5. PR interval _____
6. Identification _____
7. Symptoms _____
8. Treatment _____

The Junctional Mechanisms

Premise
The difference in ECG recognition between sinus and junctional rhythms is the shape and direction of the P wave.

Objectives
After reading the chapter and completing the Self-Assessment Exercises, the student should be able to

- Recognize the change in direction of the P wave.
- Differentiate between sinus- and junctional-induced P waves.
- Differentiate between ectopic and escape junctional beats.
- Identify the causes for the junctional arrhythmias.

Key Terms

accelerated junctional
  rhythm
AV dissociation
idiojunctional rhythm
junctional (AV)
  tachycardia

junctional escape beat
junctional rhythm
P prime (P′)
premature junctional
  complex (PJC)

retrograde atrial
  depolarization

Introduction
When the sinus node fires, a single positive predictable P wave is created and precedes each QRS with a consistent PR interval. While there are variations in rate and rhythm, the relationship of P wave, PR interval, and the QRS complex remain consistent.

When the sinus node fails to function, the next most likely pacemaker to respond lies within the AV junction. The conduction into the ventricles is usually without problem, and the resulting QRS shows little or no difference from a sinus-induced QRS.

However, if the atria are depolarized by the junctional impulse, they are depolarized in a manner opposite to that of normal. This is known as **retrograde atrial depolarization**, and can occur only if the inferior-superior pathway is capable of conduction. This retrograde atrial depolarization is reflected on the ECG by a negative (downward, inverted) P′ wave in leads II, III, and aVF. The differential interpretation between sinus and junctional-induced QRSs is largely dependent on the analysis of the P wave.

THE ORIGIN OF JUNCTIONAL MECHANISMS

The AV junction consists of the AV node and the bundle of His down to the beginnings of the bundle branches. The regions of the AV junction are divided according to their cell types—that is, the atrionodal (AN), nodal (N) and nodal-His (NH), and the His bundle. The AV junction provides the only electrical connection between the atria and the ventricles.

In the AN region there are two AV nodal pathways: the anterior and superior, fast pathway and the posterior and inferior, slow pathway. Retrograde conduction using one of these pathways to the atria results in a retrograde or negative P wave. These pathways are also responsible for the AV nodal reentry mechanisms causing paroxysmal tachycardia (see Chapter 8).

The N region of the AV node is responsible for rate-related conduction delay. For some time, it was thought that the AN and N cells functioned as pacemaker cells. In 1968 Drs. T.N. James and L. Sherf determined that there are no rapid-sodium channels within the AV node known to be necessary for predictable pacemaker function.

In the NH region the merging of fibers from the lower part of the AV node with those of the His bundle. Most investigators have defined this area as the source for junctional escape rhythms.

An impulse that originates within the NH region of the bundle of His is conducted through the ventricular bundle branches and results in a narrow QRS complex, not unlike a sinus-induced QRS complex. By convention, the pacing function within AV junctional tissue is referred to as junctional. Any P wave that is other than from the sinus node is referred to as **P prime (P′)**. **Figure 7.1** is a graphic illustration of the position of the P′ in three variations of a junctional mechanism.

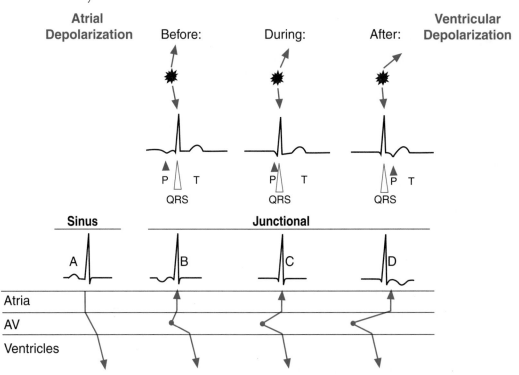

Figure 7.1 Sinus- and junctional-induced QRS complexes. Note the positive P to the left of the QRS in a sinus mechanism. (A) shows a negative P′ wave to the left of each QRS complex. (B) indicates a junctional mechanism. (C) shows a QRS complex without a visible P wave, and (D) shows a negative P′ buried within the ST segment. The schematic above and below the ECG depicts the retrograde depolarization of the atria from the junctional site.

Causes

The junction rarely functions in competition with the sinus node because its primary role is that of a backup pacemaker since it is normally depolarized with each sinus beat. When the sinus fails, or when the sinus impulse is blocked within the AV node, or when there is prolonged AV node conduction time, junction may reach potential and generate an impulse and conduct through to the ventricles. This is termed a **junctional escape beat**. If the rhythm is sustained as the role of pacemaker it is termed an escape junctional rhythm, or simply a **junctional rhythm**.

ESCAPE JUNCTIONAL COMPLEX

A junctional escape beat is one that comes after a delay in the cardiac cycle. There is a pause, as with SA block or SA arrest or a premature atrial complex and at the conclusion of the delay there is a narrow QRS with a retrograde P′ that can occur before, during, or after the QRS, or the P′ may not be visible at all. Wherever the junction P′ occurs in relation to the QRS complex, it is usually consistent for that patient.

Again, the escape junctional beat occurs because the sinus has failed to maintain control and the junction, not having been stimulated by a sinus-induced wave front, reaches its potential and discharges. If the condition persists, the escape beat can take over the pacemaking function. This is the junctional rhythm previously described.

The P′ wave may be completely or partially hidden within the preceding T wave or enhance or diminish the amplitude and distort the preceding T wave. The P′ waves can be seen before, during, or after the QRS complexes and are inverted (negative) in leads II, III, and aVF.

The position of the P′ wave depends on the following:

- The atria are depolarized before the ventricles. The P′ wave is inverted in leads II, III and aVF with a consistent but short (0.12 second or less) P′R interval.
- The atria and the ventricles are depolarized nearly simultaneously; the P′ wave is then hidden within the QRS complex and not clearly visible on the ECG.
  - The atria are depolarized after the ventricles. The P′ wave is then inverted following the QRS complex in leads II, III, and aVF.
- When no P′ waves are visible, a fourth possibility exists: the atria are not depolarized because retrograde conduction is blocked. The QRS complex is 0.10 second or less, with normal ventricular depolarization.

Figure 7.2A and **Figure 7.2B** are ECG tracings showing two examples of sinus mechanisms, each with an escape junctional complex. Note in each example the long pause, ending with a narrow QRS that is similar to the sinus QRSs. However, in each example, there is no sinus-induced P wave prior to the escape junctional QRS complexes. In each example, the QRS complexes do not vary in configuration or size despite the difference in point of origin. Recall that impulses that have an origin above the ventricles typically conduct normally with a narrow QRS as a result.

Causes

Remember, the role of the AV junction is that of a backup when the sinus fails. This may also occur after a premature atrial ectopic has paralyzed the atria.

Figure 7.2 Two ECG tracings showing (A) one positive P wave to the left of each QRS complex; the PR interval is consistent, and the heart rate is within normal limits. The heart rate visibly slows until a long pause of about 1.6 seconds. The next complex is a QRS without the visible sinus P wave to the left. *This is the junctional escape beat.* (B) shows a positive P plus a QRS (a sinus beat), a pause, a QRS with no visible P wave *(the junctional escape beat)*, and a return to a sinus bradycardia. In each example, note that the configuration and measurement of the QRS complex do not vary despite the difference in origin.

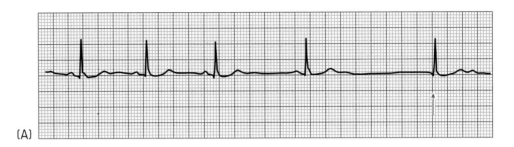

(A)

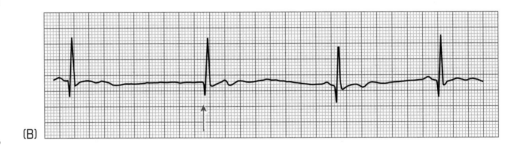

(B)

Intervention

There is no reason to interfere with a junctional escape mechanism. The practitioner must be suspicious as to why the junction took over as a pacer. There is always concern for underlying proximal right coronary artery disease that often results in sinus arrest. Assess for medication-induced prolonged AV conduction time as with digitalis preparations.

JUNCTIONAL RHYTHM

When sinus rate is slow, delayed, or blocked, or an instance of SA arrest occurs, the junctional cells are capable of reaching potential and discharging an impulse. Unless the sinus accelerates, the junction will maintain the rhythm and respond (accelerate) depending on the body's needs.

The AV junction is capable of providing a consistent and predictable heart rate. The inherent rate is 40 to 60 beat(s) per minute (bpm). When the junction becomes the dominant pacemaker, the single impulse originating in the junction can travel in two directions, superior to the atria and inferior activating the ventricles. Retrograde atrial depolarization can occur only if the inferior-superior pathway is capable of conduction.

Again, the ventricles are usually depolarized normally, since the impulse spreads through the bundle of His to the bundle branches and then through to the Purkinje network, leading to ventricular depolarization, Therefore, the QRS complexes are normal in duration, 0.10 second or less.

To describe a rhythm as junctional in origin, the following criteria must be met:

- *P′ Wave:* The P′ that is junctional in origin is negative and visible in front of, within, or after the QRS. Whichever occurs, the position is consistent.
- *P′R Interval:* When the inverted negative P′ waves are visible before the QRS complexes, PR interval is relatively short, about 0.12 second and consistent.
- *QRS Complex:* The QRS complex duration is 0.10 second or less.
- *QRS Rate:* The inherent rate is constant and ranges between 40 and 60 bpm.
- *QRS Rhythm:* Junctional rhythm is regular at any rate range.

Causes

Again, the role of the junctional pacer is that of a backup when the sinus fails, or the sinus-induced wave forms fail to conduct through AV junctional tissue. If an atrial ectopic has suppressed the sinus node this may allow the junction to reach potential and take over pacing the heart. Junctional escape rhythms are common in children and in athletes, and are seen during periods of increased vagal tone, such as during sleep.

Intervention

A junctional rhythm is usually considered a protective mechanism and no intervention is required. It is critical, though, to assess why the mechanism occurred. Look for previous instances of SA block or SA arrest or a premature atrial complex (Chapter 8) and identify the cause of those arrhythmias.

Figure 7.3 shows an ECG of a junctional rhythm. Note that there are no P waves associated with any of the QRS complexes.

ACCELERATED JUNCTIONAL RHYTHM

Accelerated junctional rhythm is the term used when the junctional rate is between 60 and 100 bpm. The rate may be "tachy" for the junction but by convention, the term is reserved for heart rate greater than 100 bpm. The ECG characteristics are as follows:

- *P′ Wave:* The P′ that is junctional in origin is negative and visible in front of, within, or after the QRS. Whichever occurs, the position is consistent.
- *P′R Interval:* When the inverted negative P′ waves are visible before the QRS complexes, PR interval is relatively short, about 0.12 second.
- *QRS Complex:* The QRS complex duration is 0.10 second or less.
- *QRS Rate:* When the junctional rate accelerates to greater than 60 bpm, it is identified as accelerated junctional rhythm.
- *QRS Rhythm:* Junctional rhythm is regular at any rate range.

Figure 7.4 is an example of an accelerated junctional rhythm. Note that the heart rate is faster than 60 bpm and yet very regular; this is the hallmark of a junctional pacemaker.

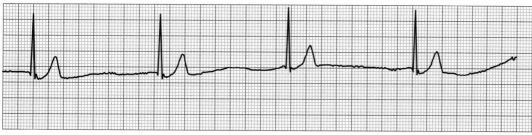

60 yom 40 Dizziness/Near Syncope

Figure 7.3 An ECG tracing showing narrow QRS complexes but no preceding P waves. This indicates a junctional rhythm.

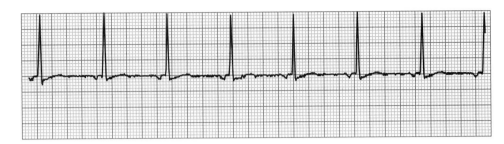

Figure 7.4 An ECG tracing showing a regular, narrow QRS with a negative P′ to the left of each QRS. The QRS rate is 67 bpm. The ECG interpretation would be accelerated junctional rhythm at about 67 bpm.

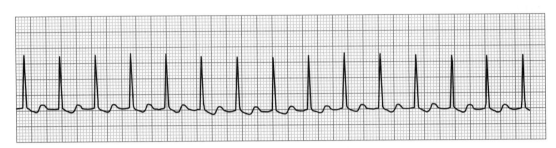

Figure 7.5 An ECG tracing showing narrow QRS with no identifiable P wave to the left of the QRS. The QRS rate is 125 bpm. This is probably junctional tachycardia at 125 bpm.

Causes

The junction can accelerate for the same reasons as the sinus such as with vagal blocking or exercise. Accelerated junctional rhythm may occur in patients with myocarditis, coronary artery disease, digitalis toxicity and following cardiac surgery involving valve replacement. It can also be a normal variant. The junction is able to respond normally to exercise.

Intervention

It is rarely necessary to intervene, except to document signs, symptoms, and patient medical and medication history, and identify and treat the cause.

JUNCTIONAL TACHYCARDIA

The ECG characteristics for junctional tachycardia are similar to those of a junctional rhythm and accelerated junction rhythm, with the exception of rate. In **junctional (AV) tachycardia**, the rate is 101 to 140 bpm. There is a gradual onset and termination occurs when the sinus recurs and again dominates the rhythm. **Figure 7.5** is an ECG showing junctional tachycardia. The rate is rapid at 125 bpm, and the rhythm is very regular. If this were sinus tachycardia, the rate would not be so fast that a positive sinus P wave could be seen easily preceding the QRS.

PREMATURE JUNCTIONAL COMPLEX

A **premature junctional complex (PJC)** originates within the NH region of the AV junction. The PJC depolarizes before the next expected sinus impulse, travels through the His bundle, and activates the ventricles as would a sinus-conducted beat. Thus the sinus and junctional QRS complexes are similar. If there is retrograde conduction through the atria, the P′ wave may be completely or partially hidden within the preceding QRS complex or the T wave. The P′ may also greatly enhance or diminish the amplitude, thus distorting the preceding T wave. The P′ waves that can be seen before, during, or after the QRS complexes are inverted (negative) in leads II, III, and aVF. Retrograde atrial depolarization can occur only if the inferior-superior pathway is capable of conduction. The following is a summary of the ECG characteristics of junctional escape beats and PJCs.

- *P′ Wave:* The P′ that is junctional in origin is negative and visible in front of, within, or after the QRS. Whichever occurs, the position is consistent.
- *P′R Interval:* When the P′ occurs prior to the QRS, the P′R interval differs from the PR interval of the dominant rhythm and is usually less than 0.12 second.
- *QRS Complex:* The QRS complex duration is 0.10 second or less, most of the time. If the resulting QRS changes configuration and is greater than 0.10, this reflects the degree of refractoriness of the conduction tissue.
- *QRS Rate:* The inherent sinus rate is constant.
- *QRS Rhythm:* In the case of the PJC, the regularity of the basic rhythm is disturbed. In the case of an escape beat, there is a long pause that ends with the escape junctional beat.

Three examples of sinus mechanisms with PJCs are shown. In **Figure 7.6** the premature QRS is similar in configuration to the sinus-induced QRSs, but there is no preceding P wave. **Figure 7.7** is an example of the P′ prior to the premature QRS; **Figure 7.8** has no visible P before the premature QRS but a P′ is visible within the ST segment of the ectopic QRS. In each of the examples, the sinus P wave does not plot through the events, indicating a disruption in normal, predictable sinoatrial activity.

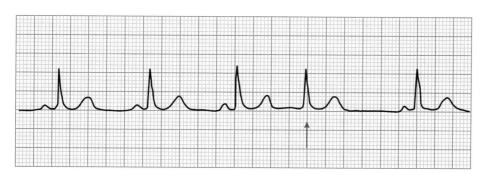

Figure 7.6 An ECG tracing showing one positive wave to the left of each of three sinus complexes. The fourth QRS complex is similar to the sinus QRSs so it is supraventricular in origin, but it is early (premature). There is no positive P wave preceding the premature complex. The sinus P waves do not plot through the event. The interpretation is sinus rhythm at 75 bpm with a PJC.

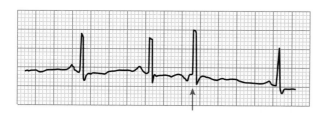

Figure 7.7 An ECG tracing showing one positive P wave to the left of each of the first two sinus beats. The third QRS complex is similar to the sinus QRSs so it is supraventricular in origin, but is early (premature). There is a negative P′ preceding it. The sinus P waves do not plot through the event. The interpretation is sinus rhythm at 77 bpm with a PJC.

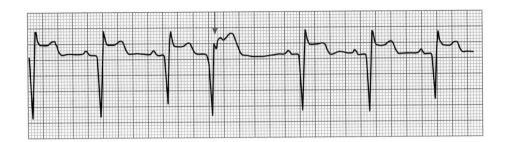

Figure 7.8 An ECG tracing showing a positive P wave for each of two clearly visible QRS complexes, indicating a sinus mechanism. The fourth QRS is similar in appearance, but clearly premature, and there is no positive P prior to the QRS. There is a negative deflection within the ST segment of the premature complex, which may indicate the retrograde conduction from the AV junction. The sinus P waves do not plot through the event, but resume cadence afterward. There is 3 to 4 mm ST segment elevation and deep Q waves 14 to 18 mm and 0.06 second, (which may indicate proximal right coronary artery disease with ischemia, injury, and necrosis). The ECG interpretation would be sinus rhythm at 67 bpm with a PJC, 3 to 4 mm ST segment elevation, and Q waves at 18 mm and 0.06 second.

Causes

PJCs may be idiopathic or symptomatic of digitalis excess. Excessive sympathetic stimulation may also cause PJCs.

Intervention

PJCs are considered symptomatic rather than pathologic. Extensive insight into medication history, particularly digitalis, may be all that is warranted.

IDIOJUNCTIONAL RHYTHM

Idiojunctional rhythm is the term used when atrial and ventricular rhythms are independent (AV dissociation). The term *AV dissociation* is a condition, not a diagnosis. The atria are under the control of either sinus or atrial foci, and the junction (or a site in the ventricles) is the escape pacer for the ventricles. When there is AV dissociation and the junction is in control of the ventricles, the ventricular rate is between 40 and 60 bpm. The ECG characteristics are as follows:

- *P Wave:* A positive P wave that is sinus in origin will plot through the rhythm usually at a regular rate, but independent of the ventricular rhythm.
- *PR Interval:* No PR interval occurs since the sinus does not conduct through to the ventricles.
- *Atrial Flutter or Fibrillation:* Flutter or fib waves can be seen between QRS complexes (see Chapter 8).
- *QRS Complex:* The QRS complex duration is 0.10 second or less.
- *QRS Rate:* The rate is 40 to 60 bpm. When the junctional rate accelerates to greater than 60 bpm, it is identified as accelerated idiojunctional rhythm.
- *QRS Rhythm:* Junctional rhythm is regular at any rate range.

Figure 7.9 is an example of an idiojunctional escape rhythm. The example stresses the need to assess the overall rhythm and each of the PR intervals.

Summary of Causes of Junctional Mechanisms

Junctional escape beats and junctional rhythms are passive escape mechanisms that take control when sinus rate is too slow, during excessive vagal stimulation, acute myocardial infarction, medication-induced delay, or episodes of SA block or SA arrest. Junctional escape beats, single occurrences of a junctional-induced QRS, are often seen after pauses that occur following premature atrial complexes (PACs) or premature ventricular complexes (PVCs).

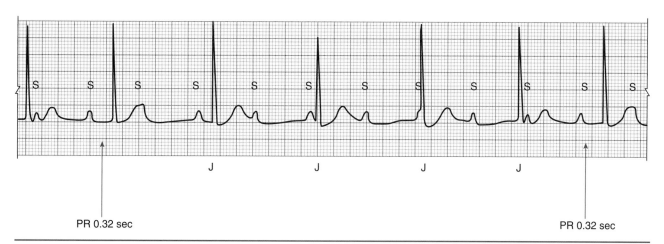

PR 0.32 sec   PR 0.32 sec

Figure 7.9 Sinus rhythm at 96 bpm with an idiojunctional escape rhythm. The overall ventricular rhythm is irregular. The sinus P wave plots out at 96 bpm. The first and last PR intervals are the same at 0.36 second. Then there is AV dissociation with capture—a regular junctional escape rhythm for four beats. Sinus capture claims the last QRS complex.

A junctional escape rhythm can occur when there is no conduction through the AV node (complete AV block), most commonly when the source of the block is at the level of the AV node. This can occur with acute myocardial infarction and with right coronary artery occlusion or spasm.

Enhanced automaticity in the AV junction causes PJCs. *Accelerated junctional rhythm* is the term that describes an AV junction rhythm faster than 60 and less than 100 bpm. *Junctional tachycardia* is the termed used when the junctional rate is greater than 100 bpm and rarely exceeds 140 bpm. Episodes of junctional tachycardia also may occur after open heart surgery. Enhanced automaticity within the AV junction is usually the result of digitalis toxicity but may occur with metabolic disturbances or after cardiac valve surgery.

Digitalis toxicity has catastrophic consequences. Sadly, the signs of toxicity can go unnoticed or attributed to other maladies, even in the face of therapeutic blood levels. AV junctional ectopics and junctional rhythms of increasing rates are some of the ECG signs of toxicity. While the patient's heart rate is within normal limits, the patient has a myriad of signs and symptoms often attributed to long-standing chronic complaints. These include gastrointestinal (GI) disturbances and visual complaints. Psychiatric symptoms range from agitation to feeling listless and apathetic. Nervousness, loss of memory, nightmares, feelings of paranoia, weakness, and fatigue are common complaints, uncorrected with other therapies or interventions.

Most patients tolerate a junctional escape rhythm. However, the situation should not be taken for granted. If the patient is compromised by the slow ventricular rate, for instance, decreased levels of perfusion, or the occurrence of PVCs, consider the use of medications to accelerate the sinus rate. The AV junction can respond to vagal blocking and may accelerate to a more satisfactory rate, or the sinus node will accelerate and regain control.

The initial assessment and history should focus on medication history and compliance. Of interest too is whether or not the patient borrowed medication, such as digitalis preparations. This does occur, and the patient does not perceive this as a wrong thing to do. The presence of a PJC may be the first indication of the enhanced automaticity provoked by digitalis toxicity.

When the heart rate is within normal limits, there is no reason to intervene, other than cataloging signs and symptoms for further study by the responsible physician. When the heart rate is slow, and the patient is symptomatic, hypotensive, and hypoperfusing, the tendency is to treat with medications to increase heart rate.

If digitalis is a suspected cause for the bradycardia, the accelerated junctional rhythm, and/or the junctional ectopics, supportive therapy until the patient can be treated for the digitalis toxicity is in order. This would include preparing for transcutaneous or transvenous pacing.

Vagal maneuvers can help differentiate the narrow QRS tachycardias, if the patient's symptoms warrant. Medications may be useful, but when the patient is considered hemodynamically compromised, synchronized cardioversion should be considered.

SUMMARY

When the sinus node falters or fails, the AV junction can function as a backup pacemaker or be ectopic, challenging the sinus node by generating an impulse and taking control of heart rate from 60 to 140 bpm. The difference between junctional and sinus mechanisms is the polarity of the P waves.

Care of the patient includes detailed physical exam and a medical history focusing on medications, specifically digitalis preparations. Clinical intervention solely to treat a bradycardia in a patient who is not compromised is rare. If the patient is compromised, an electronic pacemaker may be required.

Table 7.1 summarizes the ECG configurations of junctional mechanisms.

	Junctional Escape Beat	Junctional Rhythm	Accelerated Junctional Rhythm	Junctional Tachycardia	Premature Junctional Complex (PJC)
P waves	(−) or none	(−) or none	(−) or none	(−) or none	(−) or none
PR interval	≤0.12 sec	≤0.12 sec	≤0.12 sec	≤0.12 sec	≤0.12 sec
QRS complex	≤0.10 sec	≤10 sec	≤0.10 sec	≤0.10 sec	≤0.10 sec
QRS rate		40–60 bpm	60–100 bpm	>100 bpm	
QRS rhythm		Regular	Regular	Regular	
Intervention	? Med Hx* ? Digitalis	If the patient is symptomatic with the slow rate, consider: atropine, fluids, TCP and/or vasopressor for perfusion	? Med Hx ? Digitalis	? Med Hx ? Digitalis	? Med Hx ? Digitalis

*Hx = history.

Table 7.1 Summary of ECG configurations of junctional mechanisms.

Self-Assessment Exercises
Matching

Match the phrase in the left column with the lettered word or phrase in the right column, and then compare your answers with those in Appendix A.

____1. 0.10 second   A. P wave

____2. 0.08 second   B. QRS complex

____3. 0.12–0.20 second   C. PR interval

____4. 0.36–0.44 second   D. QT interval

Fill in the Blanks

Complete the third column, and then compare your answers with those in Appendix A.

	Sinus Rhythm	Sinus Bradycardia	Junctional Rhythm
P wave	1 (+) P wave/QRS	1 (+) P wave/QRS	_____
PR interval	0.12–0.20 sec	0.12–0.20 sec	_____
QR complex	≤0.10 sec	≤0.10 sec	_____
QRS rate	60–100 bpm	<60 bpm	_____
QRS rhythm	Regular	Regular	_____

ECG Rhythm Identification Practice

For the following rhythms, fill in the blanks and then compare your answers with those in Appendix A.

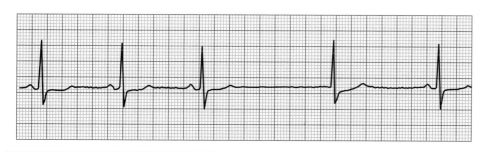

Figure 7.10

1. QRS duration _____
2. QT interval _____
3. Ventricular rate/rhythm
   _____
4. Atrial rate/rhythm _____

5. PR interval _____
6. Identification _____
7. Symptoms _____
8. Treatment _____

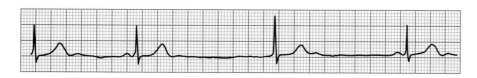

Figure 7.11

1. QRS duration _____
2. QT interval _____
3. Ventricular rate/rhythm
   _____
4. Atrial rate/rhythm _____

5. PR interval _____
6. Identification _____
7. Symptoms _____
8. Treatment _____

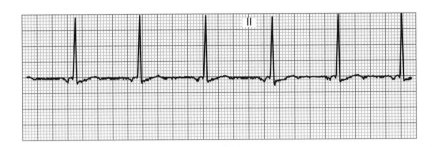

Figure 7.12

1. QRS duration _____
2. QT interval _____
3. Ventricular rate/rhythm
   _____
4. Atrial rate/rhythm _____

5. PR interval _____
6. Identification _____
7. Symptoms _____
8. Treatment _____

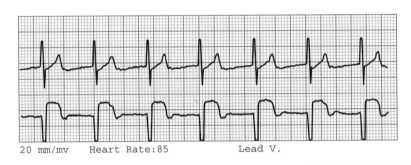

20 mm/mv   Heart Rate:85   Lead V.

Figure 7.13

1. QRS duration _____
2. QT interval _____
3. Ventricular rate/rhythm
   _____
4. Atrial rate/rhythm _____

5. PR interval _____
6. Identification _____
7. Symptoms _____
8. Treatment _____

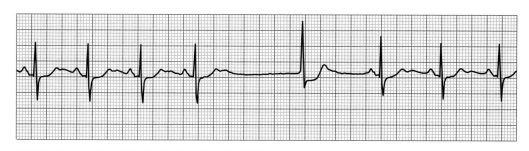

Figure 7.14

1. QRS duration _____
2. QT interval _____
3. Ventricular rate/rhythm

   _____
4. Atrial rate/rhythm _____

5. PR interval _____
6. Identification _____
7. Symptoms _____
8. Treatment _____

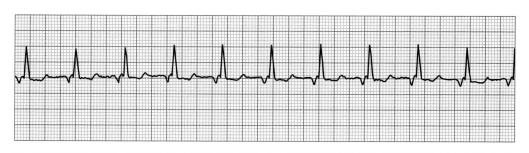

Figure 7.15

1. QRS duration _____
2. QT interval _____
3. Ventricular rate/rhythm

   _____
4. Atrial rate/rhythm _____

5. PR interval _____
6. Identification _____
7. Symptoms _____
8. Treatment _____

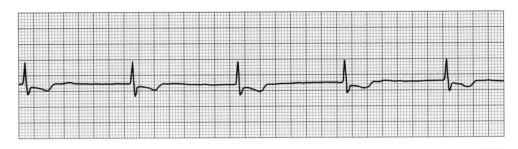

Figure 7.16

1. QRS duration _____
2. QT interval _____
3. Ventricular rate/rhythm
   _____
4. Atrial rate/rhythm _____

5. PR interval _____
6. Identification _____
7. Symptoms _____
8. Treatment _____

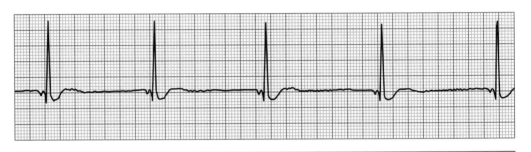

Figure 7.17

1. QRS duration _____
2. QT interval _____
3. Ventricular rate/rhythm
   _____
4. Atrial rate/rhythm _____

5. PR interval _____
6. Identification _____
7. Symptoms _____
8. Treatment _____

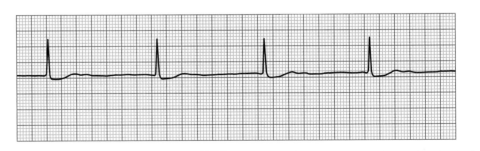

Figure 7.18

1. QRS duration _____
2. QT interval _____
3. Ventricular rate/rhythm
   _____
4. Atrial rate/rhythm _____

5. PR interval _____
6. Identification _____
7. Symptoms _____
8. Treatment _____

The Atrial Mechanisms

Premise

The key to recognizing an atrial ectopic is to remember a few concepts:

- A sinus impulse cannot occur prematurely.
- Atrial ectopics by definition occur in a premature fashion.
- Sinus P waves plot through as regular rhythms unless disturbed by atrial ectopics.
- Always begin by plotting out the sinus P waves.

Objectives

After reading the chapter and completing the Self-Assessment Exercise, the student should be able to

- Identify the ECG characteristics of the atrial mechanisms.
- Differentiate atrial from junctional ectopics.
- Identify and describe the mechanisms for PACs, atrial tachycardias, atrial flutter, and fibrillation.
- List the significant clinical findings in the unstable patient.
- Identify and describe the mechanical, pharmacologic, and electrical interventions used in the atrial arrhythmias.

Key Terms

aberrant
atrial flutter
atrial fibrillation
bigeminy
ectopic
focal atrial tachycardia
idiopathic
multifocal atrial
tachycardia (MAT)

paroxysmal atrial
fibrillation
paroxysmal atrial
tachycardia (PAT)
permanent atrial
fibrillation
persistent atrial
fibrillation

reentrant atrial
tachycardia
reentry
supraventricular
sustained atrial
tachycardia
triggered activity

Introduction

The QRS complex provides information about the origin of the impulse responsible for the ventricular complex. The origin may be from a supraventricular source or from within the ventricles. The term **supraventricular** means the source is from above the ventricles—that is, from the sinus node, the AV junction, or an ectopic within atrial tissue. Analysis of the P wave and calculation of atrial rate and rhythm provide the information for the differential diagnosis of the supraventricular arrhythmias.

The atrial arrhythmias are manifestations of abnormal electrical activity in the atria. Atrial stretch, hypoxia, drugs, medications, and chemical imbalance are factors that contribute to enhanced or triggered automaticity, resulting in an atrial **ectopic**.

A clinical concern is the grave potential for debilitating tachycardias and the formation of mural emboli.

PREMATURE ATRIAL COMPLEX (PAC)

A sinus-induced QRS presents with a single positive predictable P wave preceding each and every QRS with a consistent PR interval. A junction-induced QRS may present with negative P waves preceding or following the QRS or buried within the QRS complex. A premature atrial-induced complex will usually present with a positive P′ and the intrinsic sinus rhythm will be disturbed. The sinus P waves will not plot through rhythmically; the QRS complex remains unchanged and is usually 0.10 second or less if the impulse is conducted normally through the ventricles. When the P′ is superimposed on the previous T wave, the height of that T wave will be a combination of P′- and T-wave amplitudes and may be referred to as aT distortion (P′ + T = aT).

Premature atrial complexes (PACs) occur when an ectopic atrial pacemaker propagates an impulse before the next normal sinus discharge. The ectopic atrial beat is usually easily identified when the atrial ectopic is far outside the sinus node. When the ectopic occurs close to the area of the sinus node, the P′ may be similar to a sinus P wave, but it occurs prematurely. Remember, the sinus node does not suddenly change its rate of automaticity; thus it is said it cannot be a premature occurrence. Premature depolarization of the atria may have a depressant effect on sinus node automaticity, and if that is present, the effects are usually minimal. Once recovered, sinus node activity resumes. The morphology of the QRS complex will be narrow and relatively unchanged. The preceding P′

- Will be early (premature)
- Usually varies in size and configuration from the sinus P waves

The source of the PAC can be from anywhere in the atria.

- If the ectopic focus is inferior and close to the atrial septum, the P′ will be negative in the limb leads II, III, and aVF. This is because the flow of current is directed away from the positive electrode in those leads.
- If the ectopic focus is from the atrial right free wall, then the P′ will be positive in limb leads I and aVL because the flow of current is directed toward the positive electrode in those leads.
- If an ectopic focus arises from the left atrial appendage, the flow of current will be away from the positive electrode of limb lead I and will appear as a negative P′ in that lead.

Finally, PACs disrupt the regularity of the sinus rhythm. The sinus P waves will not plot through the premature event since the premature depolarization will affect sinus activity. When the sinus node regains control, the rhythm and regularity will be restored. The ECG characteristics of PACs are as follows:

- *P′ Wave:* The configuration of the P wave of the PAC differs from that of the dominant rhythm. If the PAC is early, the P′ wave may be completely or partially hidden within the preceding T wave. Often the P' will enhance the amplitude and distort the preceding T wave.

- **P'R Interval:** The P'R interval may be normal or prolonged and often differs from the PR interval of the dominant rhythm. Repeated PACs may not have consistent P'R intervals as compared to each other.

- **QRS Complex:** The QRS complex duration is 0.10 second or less, most of the time, if the resulting QRS changes configuration, is greater than 0.10, and reflects a degree of refractoriness of the ventricular conduction pathways.

- **QRS Rate:** The underlying sinus rate is calculated first, then a reference is made to the number and/or frequency of the PACs.

- **QRS Rhythm:** The regularity of the sinus rhythm is disturbed by the PAC. It may be quite irregular when there are many PACs. Most of the time, the observer can plot through the P waves and determine that sinus rhythm (regularity) is disturbed.

Table 8.1 describes a way of differentiating the supraventricular mechanisms. To differentiate atrial from junctional ectopic, use an area to the left of your ECG tracing, and, by process of elimination, identify the source of the ectopic.

Figure 8.1 is an ECG tracing illustrating a sinus rhythm with frequent PACs. To differentiate atrial from junctional ectopic, use the guidelines in **Table 8.1** and, by process of elimination, identify the PACs.

A guideline for assessing the source of a narrow QRS complex by assessing the P waves.	
Sinus	1 (+) P wave to the left of each QRS complex
Junctional	1 (−) P' wave in front of or behind or buried within the QRS complex, or no P wave at all
Atrial	Premature (+) P' wave in front of the QRS complex

Table 8.1 Use the area to the left of your ECG tracing, and write the letters *S, J,* and *A*. Then, by process of elimination, identify the source of the ectopic. If there are consistent positive P waves, circle the *S*. If there is a premature P' that interrupts sinus cadence, cross out the *S* because you know the sinus cannot give itself an extra beat; cross out the *J* since junctional P waves are negative or you don't see them at all. The P' is atrial in origin.

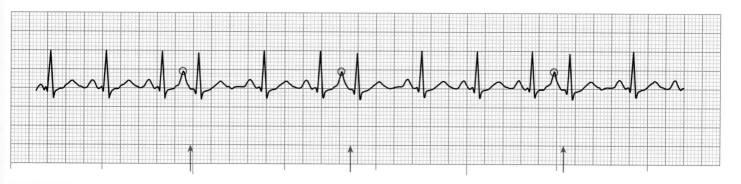

Figure 8.1 An ECG tracing showing one positive P wave to the left of each of the first three sinus beats, a sinus rhythm at 96 beat(s) per minute (bpm). The next QRS complex is similar to the sinus QRSs but is premature and has a positive P' superimposed on the previous T wave and the amplitude of that T wave is equal to the combined amplitudes of a sinus P and normal T wave. The sinus P waves do not plot through the event. The PACs recur (arrows), and each time disturb the sinus rhythm. There is 1 mm of ST depression. The ECG interpretation would be sinus rhythm at 96 bpm with frequent PACs and 1 mm ST↓.

Nonconducted (Blocked) PACs

An atrial ectopic may or may not successfully conduct into the ventricles. The ability to conduct is a matter of timing and opportunity. The AV node has a short absolute refractory period and a longer relative refractory period. So the shorter the distance of the normal QRS to the P′ (RP′ interval), the more refractory the AV node will be and the P′ will not be able to conduct.

- If the atrial ectopic conducts through to the ventricles without any delay, the QRS will be similar to those of the sinus.

- If the atrial ectopic conducts through to the ventricles but one or more of the conducting fascicles is partially refractory, the QRS will conduct abnormally and appear distorted, wider than the sinus-induced QRSs. This is called abnormal or *aberrant* ventricular conduction.

- If the atrial ectopic finds the AV node or the His bundle refractory, the impulse will not conduct through to the ventricles. The term for this is a *nonconducted* or *blocked* PAC.

The position of the atrial P′ may be hidden within the ST segment or T wave and usually can be recognized when there is an alteration of T-wave morphology. For instance, when the amplitude of the T wave changes suddenly, or appears notched, and there is a sudden pause in the cadence of the sinus rhythm, the cause may be a premature P′ superimposed on that T wave.

Figure 8.2 shows an ECG tracing of a sinus rhythm with two nonconducted PACs. Note the increased amplitude of the T waves just prior to the pause in the rhythm (arrow). The P′ created an additive influence on that T wave. The P′ did not conduct into the ventricles; therefore, there was no QRS, and this absence of conduction created the pause seen in the tracing.

Figure 8.3 is an ECG tracing of a sinus rhythm with a nonconducted PAC, causing a sudden pause in the cadence of the sinus rhythm. The pause is followed by junctional escape beats. In this tracing, the P′ is visible in the ST segment (arrow). The PAC did not conduct into the ventricles, and this created the pause seen in the tracing. There is a junctional escape mechanism for two beats, which is not uncommon following atrial ectopics. Sinus P waves seem to be surfacing, and perhaps as the sinus accelerates, it will capture and conduct as it did earlier in the tracing.

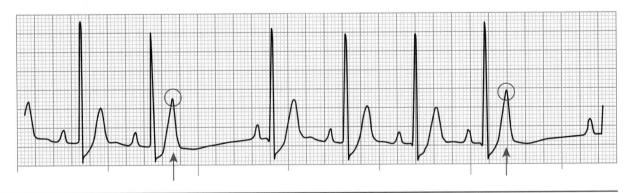

Figure 8.2 An ECG tracing showing one positive P wave to the left of each of the first two sinus beats, a sinus rhythm. There is a sudden pause in the cadence of the sinus mechanism. Look back at the last T wave and note the increased amplitude. The height of the T wave is a combination of the P′- and T-wave amplitudes and may be referred to as aT distortion (P′ + T = aT). The sinus P waves do not plot through the event, and the cadence of the sinus rhythm resumes at about 75 bpm. The ECG interpretation would be sinus rhythm at 75 bpm with frequent, nonconducted PACs.

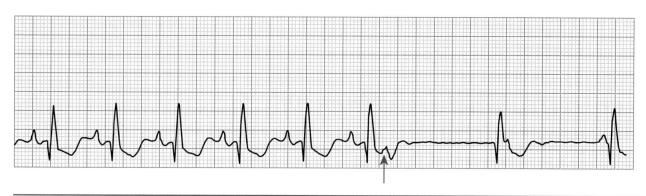

Figure 8.3 An ECG tracing showing one positive P wave to the left of each of the first six sinus beats, a sinus rhythm. There is a sudden pause in the cadence of the sinus mechanism. Look back at the ST segment and note the appearance of the P′. The sinus P waves do not plot through the event. An escape junctional rhythm is the source of the last two QRS complexes; at that point there is AV dissociation. The ECG interpretation would be sinus rhythm at 86 bpm with a nonconducted PAC, followed by a junctional escape rhythm at 50 bpm.

Points to remember:

- The most common cause of the unexpected change in sinus rhythm is a PAC.
- The most common cause of the unexpected pause in sinus rhythm is a nonconducted PAC.
- The most common cause of sudden distortion (usually increased amplitude) of a T wave is the superimposed P′ of the PAC.

Causes

In patients with no significant heart disease, PACs may result from stress, anxiety, or catecholamine surge. Nicotine, caffeine, alcohol ingestion, and various illegal drugs may also cause PACs. And finally, they may be **idiopathic**.

Other significant causes for PACs are structural heart disease such as atrial septal defect or mitral stenosis, atrial distention as with heart failure, ischemia resulting from proximal right coronary artery disease, digitalis excess, sepsis, and pericarditis. Hypoxia and electrolyte imbalance, particularly hypokalemia and hypomagnesemia, may also precipitate PACs. Other causes of atrial stretch include conditions such as chronic lung disease, which results in increased pulmonary vascular resistance.

Atrial ectopy also can occur in the third trimester of pregnancy. At this time, the mother's blood volume has increased by 50 percent. In addition, the perfusion of the fetus and placenta results in increased peripheral vascular resistance. The increased workload can cause an increase in heart size, distention, and ventricular hypertrophy. It is not unusual for the atria to stretch to accommodate the increased workload that has occurred over a rather short period of time. Atrial stretch promotes excitability and enhances automaticity.

Once the infant and placenta are delivered, accompanied by blood loss, there is a significant, sudden decrease in blood volume and peripheral resistance. The sudden diminished volume can leave behind boggy atria, which gives rise to the atrial ectopic. Until the mother's heart size, blood volume, and peripheral resistance return to normal, the potential for atrial arrhythmias exists.

Patients may or may not be aware of PACs, and some may complain of feeling a random flip feeling or the proverbial "skipped beat." If the PACs are not conducted and the rate changes or becomes slow, the clinician should assess for history of syncopal or near-syncopal episodes with the resultant bradycardia.

There is no intervention specifically for PACs. The patient should be advised to minimize intake of offending stimulants.

ATRIAL BIGEMINY

Bigeminy is when every other beat is an ectopic beat—when a PAC follows every sinus beat. The pattern is sinus→PAC→sinus→PAC, and so on. This is called atrial bigeminy, as noted in **Figure 8.4**.

It is possible to have bigeminal nonconducted PACs and misdiagnose the rhythm as sinus bradycardia. Remember, the sinus rarely does anything suddenly except to arrest. When there is a sudden change to a bradycardia, take care to assess the T waves. There may be a distortion of the ST segment or the T waves just prior to the bradycardia, indicating the P′ occurred. The distortion may not be seen in a single monitoring lead, therefore assessing the multiple lead ECG is in order. Remember, the most common cause of the unexpected pause is a nonconducted PAC.

Causes

Atrial bigeminy is not common and may occur in patients as the first sign of congestive heart failure. Assess the patient for signs and symptoms of peripheral edema, sudden weight gain, shortness of breath, and adventitious lung sounds.

ATRIAL TACHYCARDIA

Atrial tachycardia can be classified according to the anatomical location of the atrial ectopic, or by the physiologic mechanism. **Focal atrial tachycardia** is said to originate from a *localized area* such as at the crista terminalis, pulmonary veins, ostium of the coronary sinus, or the atrial septum. The origin of atrial tachycardias can also be from the right or left atrium, the orifices of the vena cava, or the pulmonary veins. Focal atrial tachycardia that originates from the pulmonary veins is thought to trigger atrial fibrillation.

Reentrant atrial tachycardias have a macroreentrant or microreentrant circuit and are typically paroxysmal; that is, they occur suddenly, terminate just as suddenly, and they are rigidly regular. They are seen in patients with structural heart disease or as a result of open-heart surgery. Atrial flutter is one example of reentry within the atria.

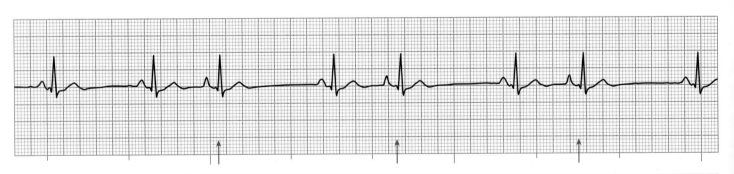

Figure 8.4 An ECG tracing showing a sinus mechanism with one positive P for each QRS. There are also premature QRS complexes that are supraventricular in origin. There is a positive P′ to the left of each premature QRS complex. When every other beat is an atrial ectopic, it is called *atrial bigeminy*. Thus, the ECG interpretation would be sinus rhythm at 55 bpm followed by atrial bigeminy.

Triggered activity is due to delayed afterdepolarizations, which are low-amplitude oscillations occurring at the end of the action potential. These oscillations are triggered by the preceding action potential and are the result of calcium ion influxes into the myocardium. When these oscillations are of sufficient amplitude to reach the threshold potential, depolarization occurs again and a spontaneous action potential is generated. If single, this is recognized as an atrial ectopic. If it recurs and spontaneous depolarization continues, a sustained tachycardia may result.

- *P′ Wave:* Begins abruptly. A visible P′ may be seen and differs in configuration from the sinus P wave. At more rapid rates, however, the P′ is hidden in the preceding T wave and may not be seen as a separate entity.

- *P′R Interval:* While the sinus PR interval is between 0.12 and 0.20 second and is constant from beat to beat, the P′R interval of the atrial tachycardia will be different than sinus but consistent. At rapid rates, the P′R interval is difficult to measure.

- *QRS Complex:* The QRS complex duration is 0.10 second or less. Every sinus QRS complex is preceded by a P wave. The QRS of the atrial tachycardia may be normally or abnormally conducted, depending on the degree of ventricular refractoriness.

- *QRS Rate:* In atrial tachycardia the rate range is 130 to 250 bpm.

- *QRS Rhythm:* Atrial tachycardia is very regular.

Figure 8.5 and **Figure 8.6** are examples of episodes of atrial tachycardia. Note the P′ wave just before the sudden onset of the tachycardia.

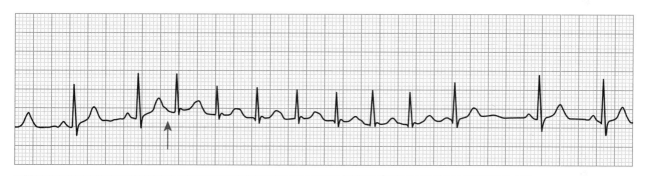

Figure 8.5 An ECG tracing showing a narrow QRS complex of similar configuration throughout. Plotting out the P waves, the sinus rate is 86 bpm for the first two complexes. Then the rate changes suddenly. The sinus P waves do not plot through this event. Note the PAC (arrow) at the beginning of the tachycardia. The rate here is 136 bpm, and T waves are distorted and lumpy indicating the atrial ectopics buried within. The rate changes again, there is a pause and then the sinus rhythm resumes. The identification is sinus at 86 bpm → atrial tachycardia at 136 bpm → sinus at 86 bpm. We see the sudden start and stop, which is the *paroxysm*. The rhythm is then called **paroxysmal atrial tachycardia (PAT)**. Whenever possible it is necessary to define the rhythm and rate before and after the PAT.

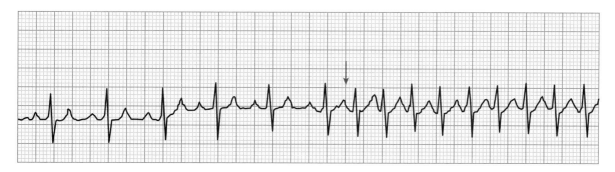

Figure 8.6 An example of the onset of atrial tachycardia. In the beginning, the tracing shows a sinus rhythm at 100 bpm. A PAC (arrow) begins the sudden change in rate at 188 bpm.

PACS WITH ABERRANT VENTRICULAR CONDUCTION

Abnormal ventricular activation will occur if one or more of the bundle branches are partially refractory at the time of the next electrical stimulation. The term is usually applied when a PAC occurs and when there is a transient AV conduction defect or, more commonly, a right bundle branch block. Thus the PAC conducts abnormally through the ventricles, which is in an **aberrant** fashion.

Some PACs have deviated from the normal conduction pathways and produce changing QRS complexes that appear ventricular in origin. Therefore, it is important for the examiner to look for the premature P′ that may be hidden in the previous ST segment or T wave.

Another way to recognize the PAC with aberrant ventricular conduction is to carefully plot out the sinus-conducted P waves. Remember, in a regularly occurring sinus rhythm, the sinus P waves will plot through, usually undisturbed by a PVC, but be reset by the PAC.

Remember, too, PVCs are different from sinus-conducted beats; the QRS is usually opposite from the T wave, and PVCs are usually greater than 0.12 second in duration. However, there are PVCs that are fascicular in origin, and while the QRS complexes are different, they are not broad and bizarre and may be wrongly interpreted as PACs. Again, plot out the sinus P waves; they should march through most ventricular ectopics occur without disturbing the cadence of the sinus rhythm.

In most hearts, the right bundle branch has the longest refractory period. Therefore, aberrantly conducted PACs usually find the right bundle still refractory and may conduct with a right bundle branch block pattern, that is, rSR′. The PAC with aberrant ventricular conduction may present with its T wave in the same direction. Again, plot out the sinus P waves; they should march through the PVC but the sinus cadence will be altered if the abnormal complex is atrial in origin.

Although PACs are the source of most aberrantly conducted complexes, PJCs can conduct abnormally. These complexes are difficult to differentiate from PVCs. Once again, if these abnormal QRSs occur in a sinus rhythm, the sinus rate will not be disturbed provided there is no retrograde conduction from the AV junction to the atria. QRS complexes that are different from the underlying rhythm should be considered ventricular in origin, until confirmed by multiple lead ECG analysis. **Figure 8.7** shows examples of sinus with PACs and aberrant ventricular conduction.

Intervention

Whenever possible, a multiple lead ECG should be performed to determine if the wide QRS complex is ventricular or atrial in origin. A patient who presents with chest pain or other signs of acute coronary syndrome and episodes of wide QRS complex tachycardia is usually treated as though the tachycardia was ventricular in origin until proven otherwise. Treatment of a patient with a reasonable ventricular rate would include assessment and intervention for the chest pain and consideration given to the use of ventricular antiarrhythmic therapy.

Intervention in a patient with an underlying slow sinus rate would be initiated if the bradycardia was thought to cause hypotension and hypoperfusion.

The following is a summary for differentiation of PVC and PAC with aberrancy:

- Look for the sinus P waves and plot them through the event. Sinus-conducted P waves usually plot out independently of the event. The chances of the event being a PVC are better than 12:1 (Conover 2003; Wellens and Conover 2006).

- If the sinus-conducted P waves are disturbed in their cadence and the rhythm is not sinus arrhythmia, look to the left of the event and search for a P′ in the preceding ST segment or T wave.
- Look for other PACs and PVCs in the same patient. If you see conducted or blocked PACs elsewhere in the tracing, the event in question is probably a PAC with aberrant ventricular conduction.

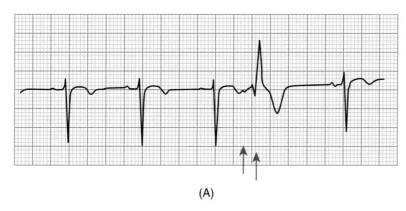

(A)

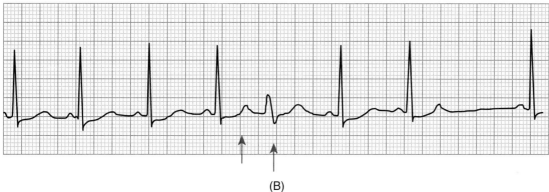

(B)

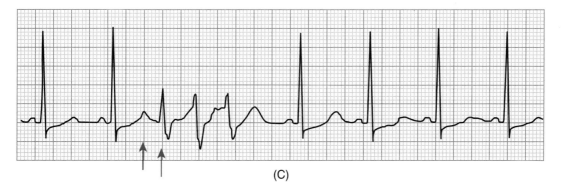

(C)

Figure 8.7 Three ECG tracings illustrating aberrant ventricular conduction. Note in (A) there is a PAC in the previous ST segment. The ECG interpretation for (A) would be sinus at 75 bpm with a PAC and aberrant ventricular conduction. Note that the sinus P waves do not plot through the event. In (B) and (C), the T-wave amplitude prior to the aberrant QRSs is increased. The increased amplitude of the T wave is additive, that is, the combined amplitude of the P′ superimposed on the preceding T wave. The ECG interpretation for (B) would be sinus at 75 bpm with a PAC with aberrant ventricular conduction and a nonconducted PAC. Here, too, the sinus P waves do not plot through. (C) would be interpreted as sinus at 75 bpm, 1 to 2 mm ST segment depression, a PAC with aberrant conduction, and a 3-beat run of atrial tachycardia. Note the sinus P waves do not plot through the event. Notice also that the T wave just prior to the tachycardia is increased in amplitude. That amplitude is additive and measures as the total of the T wave plus the P wave of complexes prior to the event. PACs that occur this early in the cardiac cycle often find the tissue partially refractory, and thus the impulse conducts abnormally or aberrantly.

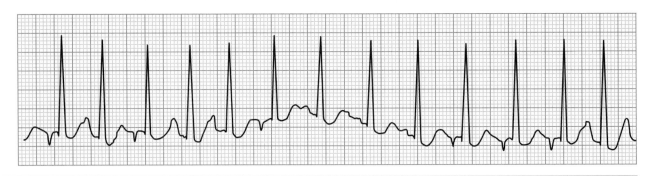

Figure 8.8 An ECG tracing of an example of MAT with P′ waves that are both negative and positive, each with its own P′-R intervals. MAT is easily confused with atrial fibrillation.

- If you are dealing with a tachycardia, look at its onset. A PAC will begin an atrial tachycardia and a PVC will begin the ventricular tachycardia. Look at the underlying rhythm and assess the QRS complexes that are present before the event.
- Treat the patient clinically. Be aware of drug history if at all possible. If you suspect ventricular tachycardia, then treat the patient accordingly.

Multifocal Atrial Tachycardia

There may be multiple, different atrial foci that depolarize the atria at different and rapid rates. The difference is an arrhythmia characterized by atrial tachycardia, with a variation in both P′ contour and the rate of atrial depolarization, **multifocal atrial tachycardia (MAT)**. The atria are discharging at very rapid rates, 150 to 250 bpm. The ventricular rate will be slower and irregular.

At first glance, it may be difficult to differentiate MAT from atrial fibrillation. In MAT, whereas morphology of the P′ waves changes, they recur in a pattern and are often both negative and positive in configuration.

Causes

Multifocal atrial tachycardia is seen in adults with chronic lung disease, sepsis, congestive heart failure, lung cancer, and pulmonary embolism. MAT is also seen in patients with high doses of theophylline. Patients may complain of tightness in the chest, light-headedness, sudden feelings of palpitations, and syncope or near-syncopal episodes. Often patients do not display MAT during examination and the physician may suggest monitoring at home using a portable monitor. Interventions are focused on treating the causative disorder. **Figure 8.8** is an example of MAT.

PAROXYSMAL ATRIAL TACHYCARDIA (PAT)

As we have discussed, an atrial ectopic may develop a rapid rate of depolarization, thus creating a persistent tachycardia. The hallmark is the sudden onset and sudden stop, that is, it appears *and* disappears suddenly. As mentioned, the arrhythmia is referred to as paroxysmal atrial tachycardia (PAT). If the AV node supports the rhythm, every atrial impulse will be conducted through to the ventricles. The paroxysm may recur at a similar, slower, or faster rate. If the arrhythmia persists and is constant with no let-up, it is referred to as **sustained atrial tachycardia**.

- *P′ Wave:* Begins abruptly, at rates of 150 to 160 bpm; a visible P′ may be seen and differs in configuration from the sinus P wave. At more rapid rates, however, the P′ is hidden in the preceding T wave and may not be seen as a separate entity.

- *P′R Interval:* While the sinus PR interval is between 0.12 and 0.20 second and is constant from beat to beat, the P′R interval of the atrial tachycardia will be different than sinus but consistent. At rapid rates, the P′R interval is difficult to measure.

- *QRS Complex:* The QRS complex duration is 0.10 second or less. Every sinus QRS complex is preceded by a P wave. The QRS of the atrial tachycardia may be normally or abnormally conducted, depending on the degree of ventricular refractoriness.

- *QRS Rate:* The rate is 130 to 250 and in some cases up to 300 bpm.

- *QRS Rhythm:* Atrial tachycardia is precisely regular.

Causes

Atrial tachycardias may be idiopathic or occur because of structural or congenital heart diseases. Atrial tachycardia can be precipitated by sympathetic stimulation, as with anxiety, ingestion of caffeine or cocaine, excessive and/or long-term smoking, or excessive alcohol intake. Medication-induced atrial tachycardia has been known to occur with albuteral and theophylline. The patient "feels" the sudden start of an atrial tachycardia, whereas the increase in heart rate in sinus tachycardia often goes unnoticed.

Young adults sometimes have attacks of atrial tachycardia that break spontaneously. The tachycardia also can occur with adults in early stages of menopause or male climacteric.

Patients may present with dyspnea, dizziness, chest pressure, or pain. There is a decline in tolerance for the episodes, and signs and symptoms of heart failure may become manifest. The faster the heart rate, the more likely the patient will feel the onset and become lightheaded. Some patients report syncope or near-syncopal episodes. Hypotension may occur in those patients who present with syncope.

Atrial tachycardia may persist despite vagal maneuvers. Episodes may occur with greater frequency and last longer with each incident. Persistent episodes requires electrophysiolgic investigation to rule out microreentry circuits or structural problems, assess for cardiac dilation, congestive heart failure, and digitalis toxicity.

SUPRAVENTRICULAR TACHYCARDIA (SVT)

The term *supraventricular* has several connotations. First is the category of rhythm—that is, the origin is above (*supra*) the ventricles (*ventricular*), hence the term. Supraventricular (SVT) also denotes the condition where an atrial ectopic has taken control over the atria, and the AV node unwittingly supports the tachycardia. The ventricular rate is very fast and the rhythm is very regular. When the SVT is constant it is referred to as *sustained* SVT.

The three most common mechanisms supporting a sustained SVT are:

1. AV nodal reentry: A retrograde P wave coincidental with abnormal, narrow QRS (most common).

2. Concealed bypass tract: No evidence of heart disease, a younger, healthy patient, but QRSs are wide—no clinical evidence of preexistent bundle branch block (BBB).

3. SA nodal/atrial reentry: Presence of P′ waves before the narrow QRS—and in the presence of organic disease.

Reentry is defined as the ability of an impulse to reexcite some region of the atria through which it has already passed. Reentry usually occurs when an impulse deviates into a circular conduction pathway, forming a loop.

There are dual pathways in the AV node of differing conduction rates and refractory levels, which when activated separately support a reentrant tachycardia. These independent AV pathways are parallel and are capable of bidirectional conduction. The beta pathway is characterized by faster conduction but a longer period of refractoriness. The alpha pathway is characterized by slower conduction but a faster period of refractoriness, as shown in **Figure 8.9**. The PAC enters the AV node and is blocked in the fast (beta) pathway but passes in an antegrade fashion down the slow pathway into the ventricles *and* in a retrograde fashion back up into the atria using the rapid pathway. The return of the current to the atria produces an atrial echo beat, and if this circuit is sustained, the ventricles will respond in a reciprocal fashion.

Like atrial tachycardia, SVT with AV nodal reentry begins abruptly. At the onset, the tachycardia is preceded by a prolonged P′R interval. This mechanism establishes the reentry circuit. The P′ waves may distort the QRS. However, there should be no alteration of the QRS amplitude (QRS alternans).

Two AV nodal reentrant tachycardias can result: one impulse accessing the fast path downward and the slow path in a retrograde fashion (fast-slow) often seen in children; and the other impulse accessing the slow path downward and the rapid path in a retrograde fashion (slow-fast). Since it uses the slow pathway for return to the atria, the RP′ is longer than the P′R interval. The slow-fast is almost always triggered by a PAC associated with a prolonged P′R interval preceding it. Often the P′ is lost or blended into the narrow QRS and impossible to see.

Many small potential circuits (microcircuits) normally exist within a conduction system, such as the AV node and atrial and ventricular tissue where the terminal Purkinje fibers attach to cardiac muscle.

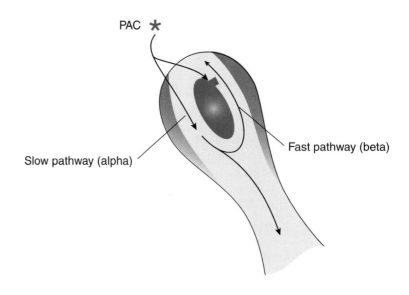

Figure 8.9 The AV node and the dual pathways, alpha and beta. A PAC enters the AV node, proceeding down the alpha pathway to the ventricles. During this time, the impulse crosses over, activates, and conducts back up into the atria.

PAC

Fast pathway (beta)

Slow pathway (alpha)

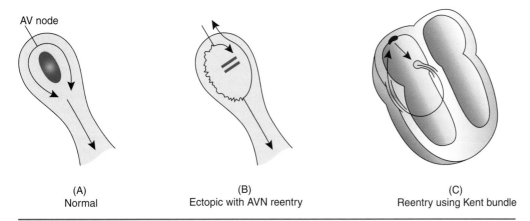

(A)
Normal

(B)
Ectopic with AVN reentry

(C)
Reentry using Kent bundle

Figure 8.10 Three examples of AV conduction: (A) normal AV conduction, (B) a PAC and AV nodal reentry, and (C) a reentry circuit using the accessory Kent bundle.

Macrocircuits or larger circular pathways also may form. These circuits are at least partially composed of cardiac conduction tissue. An example of this phenomenon would be a circuit formed by a congenital accessory pathway or by AV node microcircuits, which are functionally grouped together into two major pathways. **Figure 8.10** is composed of three sketches. The first is the AV node showing normal conduction. The second shows an atrial ectopic with AV nodal reentry. The third shows the Kent bundle as a potential pathway for conduction.

Normally, the impulse travels through the conduction fibers in an even and synchronous manner and collides with itself in the potential circuits. However, conditions of ischemia can affect selected portions of these conduction fibers, altering their speed of conduction. These cells recover slowly from previous impulses and may not conduct new approaching impulses. When the block occurs, there is an abrupt stop to the tachycardia.

An altered circuit may be partially or totally refractory. If the circuit is partially refractory in only one direction, the impulse will be blocked from transmitting in that direction.

When the impulse is blocked in one direction through a pathway, it is a unidirectional block. When an impulse encounters refractory tissue, the impulse detours away from that area, deviating around the conduction pathway and forms a loop. Impulse transmission then becomes asynchronous.

The impulse enters the ischemic area in a retrograde direction and is conducted through ischemic tissue slowly. Remember that ischemic cells are slow cells and have prolonged refractory periods. If tissue surrounding the previously blocked area has recovered sufficiently to be excitable, the emerging impulse will reenter the adjacent tissue. As a result, an original impulse will now reexcite or depolarize the area through which it has just passed. **Figure 8.11** illustrates the concept of unidirectional block and subsequent reentry.

If the reentrant impulse exits early in repolarization, when the disparity in recovery is still pronounced, the impulse may recycle within the circuit, producing a chain-reaction response. The response often disintegrates into chaotic activity.

The ECG characteristics of SVT with AV nodal reentry are as follows:

- *P Wave:* P waves, because of the overall rate, cannot be clearly delineated to establish the diagnosis as sinus, atrial, or junctional.
- *P′R Interval:* P waves are not easily seen; therefore, there is no measurable P′R interval.

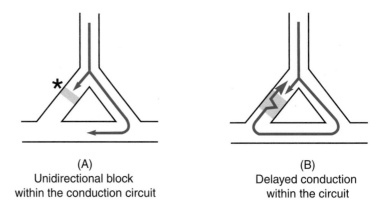

Figure 8.11 (A) Reentry with unidirectional block, and (B) delayed conduction of the reentry circuit.

(A)
Unidirectional block
within the conduction circuit

(B)
Delayed conduction
within the circuit

- *QRS Complex:* The QRS complex duration is 0.10 second or less.
- *QRS Rate:* The rate is greater than 150 bpm.
- *QRS Rhythm:* The rhythm is rigidly regular.

Figure 8.12 is an example of SVT with probable AV nodal reentry. Note the sudden onset, the narrow QRS, and the rapid rate.

Causes and Consequences

SVTs can be seen in patients with organic heart disease of any type, and chronic lung and liver diseases. "Drug abuse" as described in sinus tachycardia can precipitate the tachycardias. SVT and PAT in patients with limited cardiac reserve may precipitate angina pectoris or congestive heart failure. SVT and PAT may also occur in the presence of little or no structural heart disease.

Patient history and chief complaints include sudden onset, feelings of breathlessness, a full feeling in the neck and ringing in the ears, palpitations, dizziness, and hypotension. The observer should expect a change in vital signs. A sudden increase in pulse rate sometimes to 188 bpm or more can understandably cause a decrease in cardiac output. The degree of drop will vary between patients. The patient's tolerance to the arrhythmia and drop in blood pressure will provide a sense of urgency in choosing an intervention.

The patient's level of consciousness is an excellent indicator of the patient's ability to tolerate the arrhythmia. While the sudden onset causes anxiety and apprehension, the patient is usually responsive and alert. Any deviation where the patient is slow to respond or has any altered level of consciousness (LOC) is unstable and is cause for immediate electrical intervention known as synchronized cardioversion.

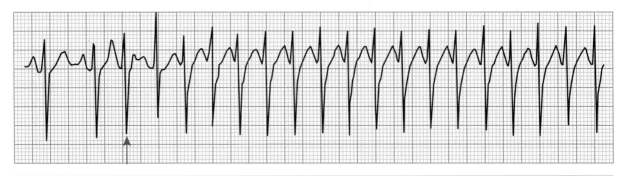

Figure 8.12 An ECG tracing showing a sinus tachycardia, a PAC progressing to a narrow-complex tachycardia at 214 bpm.

Intervention

Ectopic impulses generated as a result of reentry are usually precipitated by fast rates, and recovery time is limited. Many times, the tachycardia will resolve spontaneously or after sedation. When it does not, increasing vagal tone will exert a braking effect on the conduction velocity through the AV junction. Recall that the vagus is part of the parasympathetic nervous system, and the mediator is acetylcholine. The AV node is richly supplied with autonomic nerves and is especially sensitive to acetylcholine. Stimulating the vagus causes acetylcholine release, which delays conduction and increases refractoriness in the AV node.

There are several ways of increasing vagal tone. For example, the patient can be encouraged to try Valsalva's maneuver, which is straining or bearing down as long as possible as if having a bowel movement; or direct the patient to place a hand against the mouth and blow down on the hand as hard as possible for as long as possible. It is critical to document the ECG during the maneuver. The tachycardia may slow down and the clinician can see if the rhythm continues despite the maneuver, or slows down, so the clinician can document the underlying rhythm. If the maneuver results in stopping the tachycardia, the clinician must be vigilant since the tachycardia can resume without warning. **Figure 8.13** is an ECG from a patient responding to vagal maneuver. Note the sudden change in ventricular response.

In uncompromised patients, provoking gagging by placing a finger or catheter down the throat increases vagal tone. However, emesis may result and compromise the airway. Similarly, caution should be used when simulating a dive reflex. This can be done by placing a cold, wet towel over the center portion of the face. This maneuver also increases vagal stimulation.

Deep, profound coughing is another maneuver, but it must be very deep and hard. Pressure on the eyeball is not an acceptable maneuver. It is rarely effective, and may cause retinal detachment. If it did work, it was probably because the patient gasped in fear of enucleation.

Carotid sinus massage (CSM) may be employed by the physician as a method of terminating the arrhythmia. Prior to this maneuver, the physician should assess for carotid bruit, although absence of bruit is not a foolproof method for ruling out plaque formation or stenosis. Any history of dizziness or transient ischemic attacks (TIAs), syncope and the presence of carotid bruit on either side are contraindications for CSM.

CSM should never be applied for longer than 5 seconds and is used with great care in patients over 65 years. CSM can provoke SA arrest, and may result in either an abrupt temporary slowing (not gradual as with sinus tachycardia) or no effect at all.

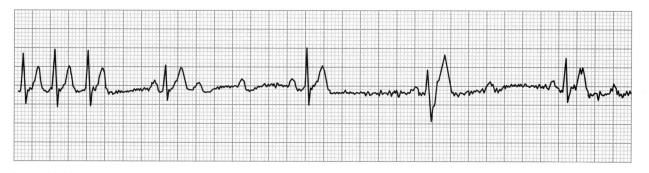

Figure 8.13 An ECG tracing showing atrial tachycardia and the sudden slowing of ventricular rates during a documented vagal maneuver.

Several medications can be used to treat atrial tachycardias. If an offending drug is the cause, using the appropriate antidote while efficiently managing the airway is the treatment of choice.

If the diagnosis is a reentrant tachycardia, use of drugs that decrease conduction velocity and increase refractoriness of AV node is in order.

For any patient who is hemodynamically compromised and in whom rate control drugs are ineffective or contraindicated, synchronized cardioversion should be considered. Some atrial tachycardias cannot be cardioverted. Some atrial tachycardias and MATs may not always respond to electrical cardioversion.

Atrial tachycardia due to digitalis intoxication often manifests with AV conduction defects and/or ventricular ectopics and arrhythmias. Interventions here include discontinuing the drug and correcting any electrolyte disturbances. The administration of antidigoxin antibodies is usually indicated in patients with conduction block, severe bradycardia, ventricular arrhythmias, and congestive heart failure. Electrical cardioversion is contraindicated because it may cause ventricular arrhythmias.

Figure 8.14 shows a continuous ECG tracing from a 20-year-old male with SVT in whom adenosine was used. Note the sudden change in rhythm. The patient experienced a sudden, "overwhelming rush of relief" with the change in rhythm.

Emergency cardioversion is employed to depolarize the atria and return the patient to a more organized rhythm. Synchronized cardioversion is the delivery of electrical current simultaneously with the QRS complex to avoid delivering a depolarizing current to the ventricles during the vulnerable period when the heart is susceptible to fibrillation. The peak of the vulnerable period, the time when it is most susceptible, is 0.20 to 0.30 second to the left of the peak of the T wave. The initial energy setting is usually 25, 50, or 100 joules (J) and varies

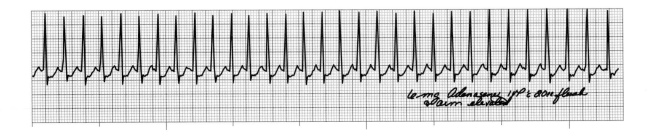

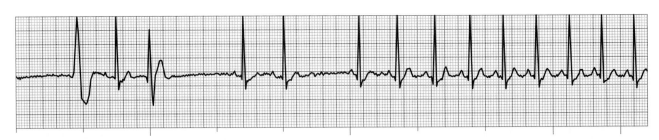

Figure 8.14 Continuous ECG tracing from a 20-year-old male who complained of increased heart rate for 4 hours while playing softball. He presented in the emergency department with chest pain and diaphoresis. The patient stated that this happens frequently, but he usually corrects the situation by holding his breath. Adenosine 6 mg was administered rapid IV push (IVP). This is an example of the variations of rhythms that occur after adenosine. The changes—which range from brief pauses to abnormal QRS complexes, some with AV conduction delay—were transient. Sinus tachycardia concludes the example. (The patient went on to sinus rhythm at about 86 bpm with a few PACs.)

with physician direction. The patient should be sedated whenever possible. **Figure 8.15** is an ECG tracing showing the conversion from SVT to sinus using synchronized cardioversion.

ATRIAL FLUTTER

Atrial flutter is a macroreentrant tachyarrhythmia and is the result of an atrial ectopic arising outside the sinus node that travels in a clockwise or counterclockwise direction, in a circular fashion usually within the right atrium. When the impulse has traveled a full circle, it reactivates the same focus again, creating a reentry loop mechanism. Thus, where one flutter wave ends, the next one arises immediately. Several flutter waves together makes out the hallmark *sawtooth* baseline. Therapeutic delay at the AV node helps prevent the many atrial impulses from conducting through to the ventricles. The ventricular response can be regular or irregular.

Atrial flutter is not considered a normal variant and is seen in patients with myocardial ischemia and may cause reentrant tachycardias. New electrocardiographic criteria are being developed for the differentiation between counterclockwise and clockwise atrial flutter through correlation with electrophysiological studies. It is not unusual for patients with frequent episodes of atrial flutter with rapid ventricular rates to undergo subsequent radiofrequency catheter ablation for ultimate relief.

In atrial flutter, atrial depolarization will be seen as sharp, positive or negative deflections at a rate of 200 to 300 bpm. The atrial P′ waves are referred to as flutter waves. In atrial flutter, the rapid atrial rate may take on a sawtooth appearance (**Figure 8.16A**), or may be visible as positive P′s (**Figure 8.16B**). In some cases of atrial flutter, lead I will not be helpful as the current of atrial activation (P′ flutter waves) is perpendicular to lead I. The ventricular rate and rhythm are a direct reflection on the AV node's ability to slow down the impulses coming to it. Remember that the physiological function of the AV node is to therapeutically delay conduction and protect ventricular response.

When atrial flutter is new to the patient, it often presents with a ventricular rate of about 150 bpm. In other words, every other atrial impulse is conducted through to the ventricles. The arrhythmia is often termed atrial flutter with 2:1 conduction. The atrial flutter waves will plot through regularly.

Atrial flutter with 2:1 conduction can be misdiagnosed as sinus tachycardia. However, in sinus tachycardia, the P and T waves are usually distinctly different from each other and do not plot through regularly. In other words, Ps plot with Ps, and Ts plot with Ts, but the

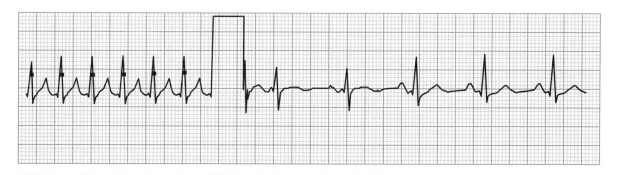

Figure 8.15 An ECG tracing showing SVT converted with synchronized cardioversion. Note the marks indicating synchrony on each of the QRS complexes. There is a 2 mV deflection indicating the delivery of electrical current. Notice that the initial deflection coincides with the expected QRS complex.

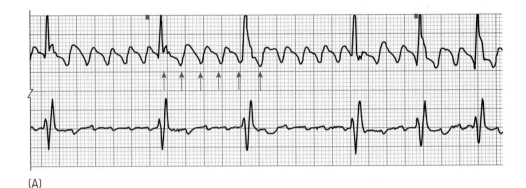

(A)

Figure 8.16A An ECG tracing shows atrial flutter with a ventricular response at 36 to 88 bpm. Note the flutter waves as they can be plotted out as negative wave forms across the tracing. The flutter waves cause occasional distortions within the QRS complex.

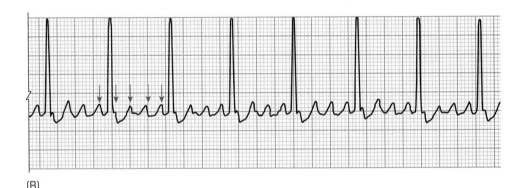

(B)

Figure 8.16B An ECG tracing showing atrial flutter with a regular ventricular response at 83 bpm. Note the flutter waves as they can be plotted out as positive wave forms across the tracing. The flutter waves cause occasional distortions within the QRS complex.

T-P-T is not rhythmic and regular. Also, looking at the negative deflections, one can plot out the flutter waves more easily.

Another clue to differentiate sinus tachycardia at 150 bpm from atrial flutter with 2:1 AV conduction is finding the P′ midway between the QRS complexes. One should suspect there are additional P′s within the QRS complex and in fact with careful assessment, be able to detect the atrial ectopic (P′). Vagal maneuvers have been shown to demonstrate the flutter as AV node conduction slows.

Finally, the patient complains of a *sudden onset* of the rapid rate and feelings of weakness and dread, which do not occur with sinus tachycardia. The ECG characteristics of atrial flutter are as follows:

- *P Wave:* There are no P waves.
- *Flutter (ff) Waves:* Atrial depolarization is regular.
- *Flutter–QRS Interval:* The flutter/QRS is usually 0.24 to 0.40 second and constant with each QRS.
- *QRS Complex:* The QRS complex duration is 0.10 second or less, most of the time. If the resulting QRS changes configuration and is greater than 0.10, which reflects the degree of refractoriness of the conduction tissue, the flutter waves will distort the QRS and T waves.

- *QRS Rate:* Ventricular rate depends on AV conduction velocity.
- *QRS Rhythm:* The ventricular response may be regular or irregular, depending on AV conduction.

Figure 8.17A and **Figure 8.17B** are examples of atrial flutter.

Causes and Consequences

Atrial flutter is relatively common in adults over 40 years of age with chronic heart disease, chronic hypertension, and myocardial ischemia. Atrial flutter is also seen in patients with valvular heart disease, acute myocardial infarction, hypoxia, quinidine excess, and pulmonary embolus, and in patients with chronic pulmonary and hepatic diseases, chronic alcohol use, and a history of smoking. The risk of mural emboli exists and patients who present with chest pain and atrial flutter should be assessed for pulmonary embolism.

AV conduction delay results in a reasonable ventricular rate in most instances. If not, and the patient is compromised, mechanical, pharmacologic, or electrical interventions may be employed. Beware of atrial flutter with a slow, regular rhythm less than 60 bpm—consider there is AV block, and the junction has taken over as the pacemaker to the ventricles. In this arrhythmia, the flutter–QRS interval will vary.

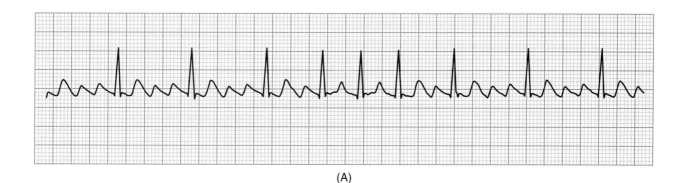

(A)

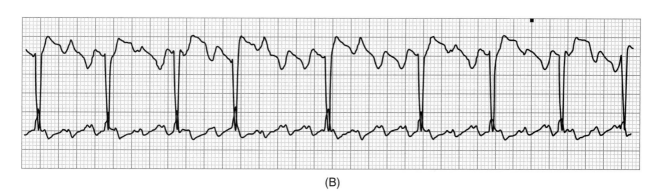

(B)

Figure 8.17 (A) ECG showing new-onset atrial flutter in a patient with negative P′. (B) is a continuous ECG tracing from a patient with recurrent atrial flutter. In the first four QRS complexes the ventricular rhythm is regular and the flutter-QRS is not consistent. Then ventricular rate increases. In this instance beware of AV dissociation and subsequent signs and symptoms associated with bradycardia. The circumstances did allow for determination of the direction of the polarity of the P′. These are examples of the difference on ECG generated by the different microreentry circuits.

Intervention

Treating patients with atrial flutter depends on their clinical condition. In some patients, the atrial flutter will convert spontaneously once the offending condition is under control. In others, administration of high-flow oxygen may be sufficient to cause the rhythm to revert back to sinus. Others may require medications and even cardioversion. However, if the rhythm persisted for longer than 48 hours, cardioversion may be associated with the theoretically increased risk of thromboembolism. In this case, anticoagulation may be recommended before attempting cardioversion.

ATRIAL FIBRILLATION

Another consequence of atrial ectopy is the occurrence of **atrial fibrillation**, a chaotic and erratic depolarization state within the atria. In contrast to atrial flutter, atrial fibrillation is one of the most commonly seen arrhythmias.

Atrial fibrillation may result from multiple reentry areas within atria. Characteristically, there is a random, irregular ventricular response. There is no organized atrial contraction, and atrial kick is lost. The greatest risk of atrial fibrillation is the formation of mural emboli.

Atrial fibrillation is classified as new onset, paroxysmal, persistent, and permanent. *New onset atrial fibrillation* is when the first episode occurs, regardless of the duration.

Paroxysmal atrial fibrillation describes an episode that begin abruptly but is self-terminating, converting within minutes, hours, or even a few days. The severity of symptoms varies depending on the patient's age and physical condition.

Persistent atrial fibrillation describes episodes that last several days or weeks. Persistent atrial fibrillation may require termination with electrical cardioversion.

Permanent atrial fibrillation describes episodes that last longer than a week and where cardioversion could not be attempted or, if cardioversion was attempted, it was not successful. Finally, if cardioversion was successful, a sinus rhythm was not maintained and the atrial fibrillation recurs and persists.

Other descriptive terms are used such as *acute, chronic, uncontrolled,* and *controlled. Acute onset* is similar to new onset and is used to describe patient signs and symptoms that require intervention. *Chronic* is a term used to describe recurrent episodes; these can be paroxysmal or persistent atrial fibrillation. *Uncontrolled* atrial fibrillation usually refers to a rapid ventricular rate that requires intervention. *Controlled* is a term that describes the optimum ventricular rate for that patient. Controlled is loosely used when first interpreting atrial fibrillation with a reasonable ventricular response, too often not being aware of patient circumstances, medical, or medication history.

While terminology and classifications are evolving, in describing the ECG of atrial fibrillation it is imperative to provide the ventricular rate range as well as patient information. The clinician is the one who decides if the rate and rhythm are controlled for that patient.

In atrial fibrillation the rate of atrial depolarization cannot be measured and results in a chaotic baseline. The atrial P′ waves are referred to as *fib* or *f waves.* Atrial kick is lost as the atria are quivering, and there is no organized atrial contraction. The onset of atrial fibrillation is usually accompanied by a rapid, irregular response, which may cause overall deterioration, myocardial ischemia, and subsequent lethal arrhythmias.

The irregular fibrillatory waves are usually easy to recognize and sometimes referred to as coarse atrial fibrillation. In other cases, the fibrillation is of such low amplitude that it is

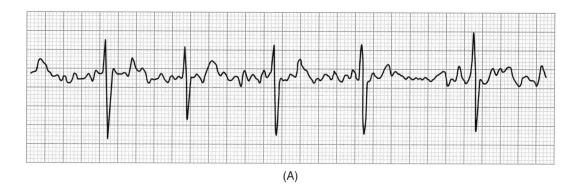

(A)

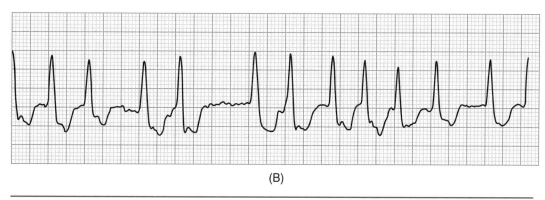

(B)

Figure 8.18 (A) ECG tracing showing narrow QRS complex with an irregular rhythm. The chaotic pattern between the QRS complexes is the atrial fibrillation. This coarse pattern is easily seen. (B) ECG tracing from a patient with narrow QRS complex with an irregular rhythm. Similar to (A), there are no identifiable P waves nor a consistent PR interval. The baseline between QRS complexes is finely distorted. This is often termed fine atrial fibrillation. There is 5 to 6 mm ST segment depression.

referred to as fine atrial fibrillation. Assessment of the tracings to determine the arrhythmia will help the practitioner with the identification. For example, in **Figure 8.18A** and **Figure 8.18B**, the QRS complexes are narrow, indicating a supraventricular origin. However, there are no identifiable P waves with consistent PR intervals, so the rhythm is not sinus in origin.

Next, the QRS rhythm in both examples is irregular, so it cannot be identified as junctional in origin. The only other option for the origin of narrow QRS is atrial. There are no flutter waves, so, by process of elimination, the rhythms are both atrial fibrillation. The ventricular rate range should be reported to provide an indication of the therapeutic blocking ability of the AV node.

The coarse or fine appearance of the fibrillatory waves has no clinical relevance.

In atrial fibrillation, the AV node is bombarded by hundreds of atrial ectopics, at varying rates and amplitudes. The AV node therapeutically and randomly conducts impulses at a varying rate of speed, so the ventricular response is irregular. When atrial fibrillation is new to the patient, the atrial rates are immeasurable, and the ventricular rhythm is irregular and often rapid. A rapid ventricular rate may compromise the patient. It is important to note the ventricular rate, as well as the patient's medication and medical history, when reporting this arrhythmia. The ECG characteristics of atrial fibrillation are as follows:

- *Fibrillatory Waves:* Atrial depolarization is erratic and irregular.
- *PR Interval:* There is no PR interval.

- *QRS Complex:* The QRS complex duration is 0.10 second or less most of the time. If the QRS changes configuration and is greater than 0.10 second this reflects an additional problem within the ventricular conduction system. The atrial fibrillation waves will often distort the QRS and T waves.
- *QRS Rate:* The rate depends on AV conduction time. Calculate and report the ventricular rate range.
- *QRS Rhythm:* The ventricular response is irregular. If the QRS rhythm is regular, there is AV block, and the source of the QRS is usually junctional in origin. This irregularity frequently occurs with digitalis toxicity.

Causes and Consequences

Atrial fibrillation does not occur in healthy subjects and should never be considered a normal variant. The patient must be assessed for chronic lung, liver, and renal diseases. Atrial fibrillation also occurs with

- Alcohol use (especially binge drinking)
- Chronic pulmonary disease
- Congestive heart failure
- Hypertensive heart disease
- Hypertrophic cardiomyopathy
- Ischemic heart disease
- Myocarditis
- Pericarditis
- Pheochromycytoma
- Rheumatic heart disease
- Thyrotoxicosis
- Valvular disease such as mitral regurgitation

Patients with coronary artery disease may develop paroxysmal atrial fibrillation in the course of acute myocardial infarction. However, atrial fibrillation may develop as a consequence of atrial dilatation (stretch) secondary to chronic congestive heart failure as well as the diseases mentioned.

For example, patients with hypertensive heart disease typically develop left ventricular and left atrial enlargement due to years of sustained high blood pressure. Other probable causes include nicotine, caffeine, and cocaine ingestion as well as long-term use of alcohol.

In some patients, atrial fibrillation occurs paroxysmally and as such lasts for only minutes, hours, or days. In other cases, the atrial fibrillation may persist for months and years. Paroxysmal atrial fibrillation is occasionally precipitated by emotional stress, excessive alcohol consumption, or excessive straining with vomiting.

As with atrial flutter, a patient with atrial fibrillation who presents with chest pain or discomfort should be thoroughly assessed as soon as possible. Without a complete diagnostic assessment it is nearly impossible to distinguish chest pain of myocardial origin from that of pulmonary embolus. Atrial fibrillation can occur within 24 hours of the onset of myocardial infarction especially in the elderly population. In inferior and right ventricular myocardial infarction increased right atrial pressure may be the cause of atrial fibrillation. The presence of ST segment elevation or depression is often difficult to discern because of the fibrillatory waves.

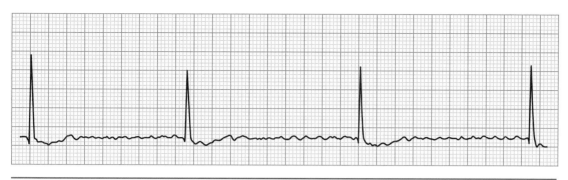

Figure 8.19 An ECG tracing from a patient in atrial fibrillation. Note the regularity of the narrow QRS rhythm. There is AV dissociation with an escape junctional rhythm. The ECG identification would be atrial fibrillation with an escape junctional rhythm at 36 bpm.

Atrial fibrillation is common after cardiac surgery involving coronary artery bypass graft and valve repair or replacement and can occur early in the postoperative period or within a month or two after discharge.

Beware of atrial fibrillation with very slow ventricular rates (**Figure 8.19**). If atrial fibrillation presents with a slow, regular rhythm less than 70 bpm, consider that there is AV block. The atria and ventricles are in dissociation, meaning atrial and ventricular functions are separate and independent. In this example, the junction has taken over as the pacemaker to the ventricles.

There are many significant consequences to atrial fibrillation. These include the predictable loss of atrial kick, diminished cardiac output, and coronary perfusion. This is complicated by rapid ventricular rates. The faster the ventricular rate, the more cardiac output will be decreased. A significant drop in cardiac output can cause congestive heart failure, hypotension, and even cardiogenic shock and myocardial ischemia and infarction.

As noted earlier, chronic atrial fibrillation, even when controlled with a reasonable ventricular rate, can result in a significant complication, the creation of a mural thrombus. The thrombi are formed by platelet aggregation in the fibrillating atria, as well as with any underlying inflammation that may exist. A mural thrombus can break off and embolize at any time, especially when the rhythm is converted to normal sinus rhythm. This sudden conversion to normal atrial contraction may cause the dislodgement of all or part of the thrombus, leading to pulmonary embolus, peripheral embolus, and stroke. For this reason, some patients with atrial fibrillation are on anticoagulants, or at least aspirin, to prevent platelet aggregation.

Stroke is another complication of atrial fibrillation as thrombi that develop inside the left atrial appendage break loose and travel forward to lodge in cerebral circulation.

Suspected Stroke Assessment and Actions

Perform a stroke assessment, establishing the time the patient was last known to be normal in presentation and behavior. Seek a higher level of care and transport to a stroke center. Consider bringing a family member or any witness to the changes in patient presentation. Assess blood glucose, CBC, electrolytes, and coagulation studies.

Intervention

Atrial fibrillation with rapid ventricular rate requires intervention. Identifying and treating the underlying cause is critical. The pharmacologic interventions with atrial fibrillation are similar to those discussed in atrial flutter. Accurate medical history, including medication history, and history of alcohol, nicotine, and stimulant use are all necessary components of the patient's history. Patients on digitalis need to be assessed to determine if indeed the digitalis has caused the symptoms and debilitation.

Conversion to sinus with medications generally takes hours or days. Some patients convert only to have atrial fibrillation recur. Other patients may never convert back to sinus rhythm. If the cause of the atrial fibrillation is the result of chronic disease, the huge, dilated atria may have become incapable of resuming normal depolarization. Long-term therapy includes antithrombotic medications and drugs to maintain a reasonable ventricular rate and rhythm.

With the relatively new onset of atrial fibrillation with cardiac compromise, and where ventricular rate is rapid and irregular and the patient hypotensive and hypoperfusing (unstable), electrical conversion may be the treatment of choice.

Electrophysiologic mapping and radiofrequency catheter ablation may be considered for patients who are medically refractory with atrial fibrillation as well as the atrial tachycardias.

Differentiation of Atrial versus Sinus and Junctional Ectopics

The approach to ECG identification of the source of the supraventricular mechanisms is uncomplicated and easy to master. **Table 8.2** describes a simple tool for differentiation of the source of the narrow QRS arrhythmia by assessing the P waves and the rate and rhythm in the atrial arrhythmias.

Table 8.2 is one approach to the process of interpreting the ECG. As with **Table 8.1**, simply use an area to the left of your ECG tracing, and write *S, J,* and *A*. Then by process of elimination, identify the source of the ectopic. Once you have defined that the ECG tracing is atrial in origin, again, use an area to the left of your ECG tracing, and write in *tach, fl, fib,* and, by process of elimination describe the arrhythmia. Tach is fast, regular, and starts suddenly; fl shows flutter waves you can count, and fib has a "junky" baseline.

Table 8.3 is an organized list of the ECG characteristics of the atrial arrhythmias, their causes, and proposed interventions.

1. Look to the left of the QRS

2. Look at the P Waves

It is *Sinus*
{ if there is
1(+) P for each QRS

It is *Junctional*
{ if there is
(−) P in front of or after each QRS or no P at all

It is *Atrial*
{ Tachy = very regular
Flutter = flutter waves you can count
Fib = junk—no identifiable Ps, QRS irregular

Table 8.2 A guideline for assessing the source of the narrow QRS complex and identifying various atrial arrhythmias.

	PAC	Flutter	Fibrillation	Tachycardia	SVT with AVN Reentry	SVT with Aberrancy
P wave	1 (+) P wave/ QRS 1 (+) P wave without a QRS	No P waves waves sawtooth >250/min	No P waves waves course or fine	Sometimes P′ wave with the QRS, sometimes independent RP > PR rate ≤250	Within the QRS distorts the QRS at its beginning or at its end	(+) P′ wave with the PAC seen at the beginning of the tach
PR interval	Different than sinus					
QRS complex	≤0.10 sec	≤0.10 sec	≤0.10 sec	≤0.10 sec	≤0.10 sec	>0.12 sec
QRS rate		60–100/min usually	60–100/min when controlled with medication	>100/min	>150/min, often >180/min	>100/min
QRS rhythm	PAC disrupts the underlying rhythm	Regular or irregular	Irregular; beware if regular and slow	Regular starts suddenly; MAT is irregular	Regular starts suddenly	Regular starts suddenly
Causes and interventions	ID and Rx the cause: normal variant atrial stretch; atrial dilation medications; stimulants: caffeine, nicotine, cocaine, illegals, and recreationals Treat the underlying pathology Discontinue the stimulants, etc.	ID cardiac and pulmonary pathologies; age, endocrine diseases; ? medications vagal maneuver may slow ventricular rate so flutter can be seen; Synch CV if unstable	ID cardiac and pulmonary pathologies; age, endocrine diseases; ? medications vagal maneuver may slow ventricular rate so the fib can be seen; Synch CV if unstable	ID cardiac and pulmonary pathologies; vagal maneuver may or may not break the tachycardia; calcium channel blockers; Synch CV if unstable	ID cardiac and pulmonary pathologies; vagal maneuver may or may not break the tachycardia; calcium channel blockers; Synch CV if unstable	ID cardiac and pulmonary pathologies; vagal maneuver may or may not break the tachycardia; Synch CV if unstable

Table 8.3 ECG characteristics of the atrial arrhythmias, their causes, and proposed interventions.

SUMMARY

Arrhythmias that are supraventricular in origin come from above the ventricles but probably occur because of atrial ectopics. Differentiation among the various sources of supraventricular tachycardia is based largely on assessment of P waves (PACs), ventricular rate, and how the arrhythmia starts off.

Atrial arrhythmias are clinically significant because they often result in a rapid ventricular response that will increase oxygen consumption, compromise cardiac output, and thus decrease coronary blood flow. Atrial contribution to cardiac output is lost, and most atrial arrhythmias indicate underlying problems such as congestive heart failure, hypoxemia, hypoxia, drug toxicity, stress, or sinus node dysfunction.

With the refinement of electrophysiologic testing, there are more and more explanations, each with its specific terminology. The basic clinical implications are the same: When the ventricular rate is too fast to maintain effective perfusion, the patient is unstable and must be treated immediately.

Reentrant tachycardias can be interrupted by the delivery of a medication designed to slow conduction and/or increase the refractoriness of the pathway. The patient may present as being stable, that is, not compromised. For example, the patient's level of consciousness (LOC) and blood pressure are not significantly altered. The patient may describe feelings of palpitation with SVT and atrial flutter and fibrillation that are new to the patient. If this is the case, the provider can continue with assessment of medical and medication history and supportive care.

Occasionally the patient will present with an altered or diminished LOC, hypotension, and hypoperfusion. This is described as being unstable. Clearly the sense of urgency for intervention is greater in the unstable patient. Usually the care is directed to slowing the ventricular response. This involves administration of medications that will slow AV conduction. If the patient is dangerously affected, then electrical intervention is in order.

Self-Assessment Exercise

Matching

Match the phrase in the left column with the lettered word or phrase in the right column, and then compare your answers with those in Appendix A.

_____ 1. Narrow QRS, regular, ventricular rate 190+ bpm

_____ 2. Narrow QRS, rate 150 bpm, positive P′ halfway between the QRS complexes

_____ 3. Negative P′ in front of each narrow QRS

_____ 4. No identifiable P waves, irregular narrow QRS

_____ 5. Sudden onset, sudden stop of narrow QRS tachycardia

A. Atrial flutter

B. Atrial fibrillation

C. Junctional rhythm

D. Junctional tachycardia

E. Paroxysmal atrial tachycardia

F. Sinus tachycardia

G. SVT

Fill in the Blanks

Complete the third column, and then compare your answers with those in Appendix A.

	Sinus Rhythm	Junctional Rhythm	PAC
P wave	1 (+)P wave/QRS	1 (−) P′ wave/QRS or no QRS	_____
PR interval	0.12–0.20 sec	≤0.12 sec	_____
QRS complex	≤0.10 sec	≤0.10 sec	_____
QRS rate	60–100/min	40–60/min	_____
QRS rhythm	Regular	Regular	_____

Complete the first and third columns, and then compare your answers with those in Appendix A.

	Atrial Tach	Sinus Tach	Junctional Tach
P wave	_____	1 (+) P wave/QRS	_____
PR interval	_____	0.12–0.20 sec	_____
QRS complex	_____	0.04–0.10 sec	_____
QRS rate	_____	100–150/min	_____
QRS rhythm	_____	Regular	_____

ECG Rhythm Identification Practice

For the following rhythms, fill in the blanks and then compare your answers with those in Appendix A.

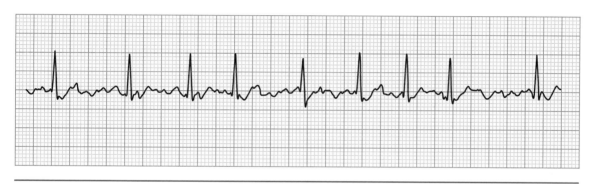

Figure 8.20

1. QRS duration _____
2. QT interval _____
3. Ventricular rate/rhythm _____
4. Atrial rate/rhythm _____
5. PR interval _____
6. Identification _____
7. Symptoms _____
8. Treatment _____

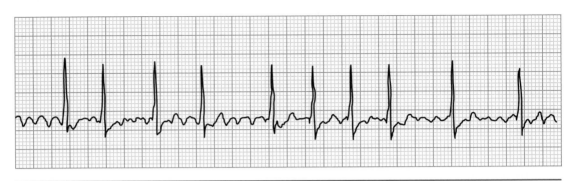

Figure 8.21

1. QRS duration _____
2. QT interval _____
3. Ventricular rate/rhythm _____
4. Atrial rate/rhythm _____
5. PR interval _____
6. Identification _____
7. Symptoms _____
8. Treatment _____

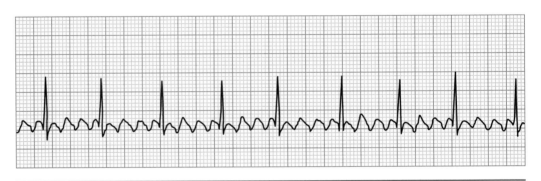

Figure 8.22

1. QRS duration _____
2. QT interval _____
3. Ventricular rate/rhythm _____
4. Atrial rate/rhythm _____
5. PR interval _____
6. Identification _____
7. Symptoms _____
8. Treatment _____

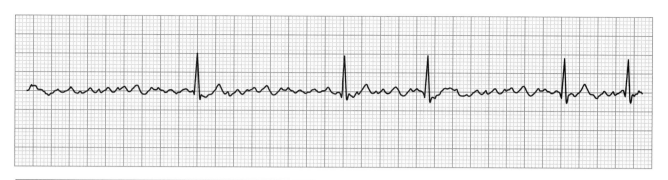

Figure 8.23

1. QRS duration _____
2. QT interval _____
3. Ventricular rate/rhythm _____
4. Atrial rate/rhythm _____
5. PR interval _____
6. Identification _____
7. Symptoms _____
8. Treatment _____

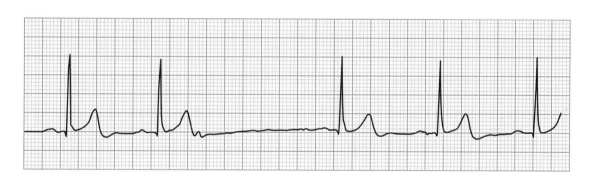

Figure 8.24

1. QRS duration _____
2. QT interval _____
3. Ventricular rate/rhythm _____
4. Atrial rate/rhythm _____
5. PR interval _____
6. Identification _____
7. Symptoms _____
8. Treatment _____

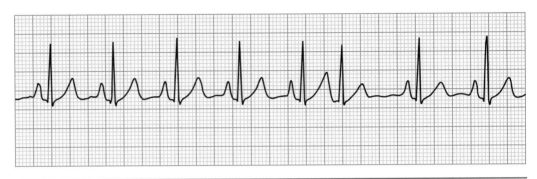

Figure 8.25

1. QRS duration _____
2. QT interval _____
3. Ventricular rate/rhythm _____
4. Atrial rate/rhythm _____
5. PR interval _____
6. Identification _____
7. Symptoms _____
8. Treatment _____

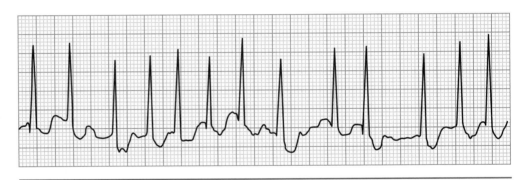

Figure 8.26

1. QRS duration _____
2. QT interval _____
3. Ventricular rate/rhythm _____
4. Atrial rate/rhythm _____
5. PR interval _____
6. Identification _____
7. Symptoms _____
8. Treatment _____

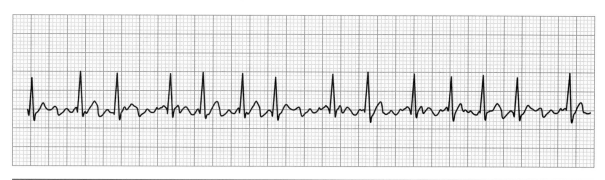

Figure 8.27

1. QRS duration _____
2. QT interval _____
3. Ventricular rate/rhythm _____
4. Atrial rate/rhythm _____
5. PR interval _____
6. Identification _____
7. Symptoms _____
8. Treatment _____

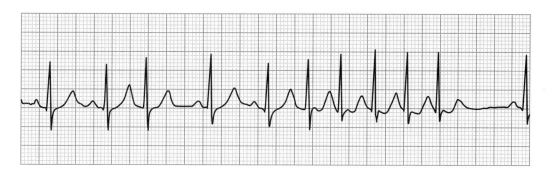

Figure 8.28

1. QRS duration _____
2. QT interval _____
3. Ventricular rate/rhythm _____
4. Atrial rate/rhythm _____
5. PR interval _____
6. Identification _____
7. Symptoms _____
8. Treatment _____

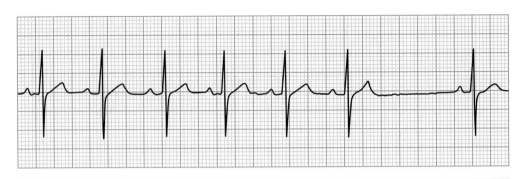

Figure 8.29

1. QRS duration _____
2. QT interval _____
3. Ventricular rate/rhythm _____
4. Atrial rate/rhythm _____
5. PR interval _____
6. Identification _____
7. Symptoms _____
8. Treatment _____

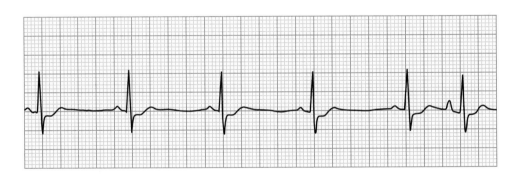

Figure 8.30

1. QRS duration _____
2. QT interval _____
3. Ventricular rate/rhythm _____
4. Atrial rate/rhythm _____
5. PR interval _____
6. Identification _____
7. Symptoms _____
8. Treatment _____

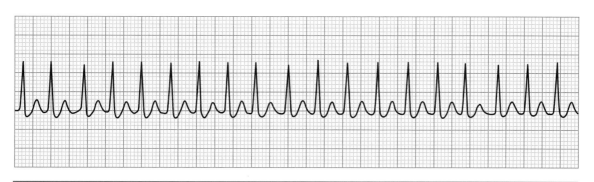

Figure 8.31

1. QRS duration _____
2. QT interval _____
3. Ventricular rate/rhythm _____
4. Atrial rate/rhythm _____
5. PR interval _____
6. Identification _____
7. Symptoms _____
8. Treatment _____

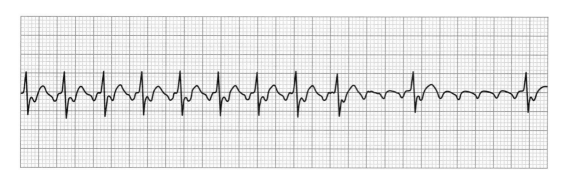

Figure 8.32

1. QRS duration _____
2. QT interval _____
3. Ventricular rate/rhythm _____
4. Atrial rate/rhythm _____
5. PR interval _____
6. Identification _____
7. Symptoms _____
8. Treatment _____

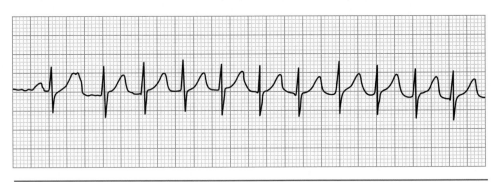

Figure 8.33

1. QRS duration _____
2. QT interval _____
3. Ventricular rate/rhythm _____
4. Atrial rate/rhythm _____
5. PR interval _____
6. Identification _____
7. Symptoms _____
8. Treatment _____

CHAPTER 9

The Ventricular Mechanisms

Premise

Any QRS different from a normally occurring QRS will be considered ventricular until proven otherwise.

Objectives

After reading the chapter and completing the Self-Assessment Exercises, the student should be able to

- Recognize the difference between QRSs that are supraventricular and ventricular in origin.
- Name the PVC in terms of its position in the cardiac cycle.
- Differentiate between ectopic and ventricular escape mechanisms.

Key Terms

accelerated
  idioventricular rhythm
  (AIVR)
asystole
end-diastolic
idioventricular rhythm
  (IVR)
interpolated
monomorphic

multiform
pairs (couplets)
polymorphic
pulseless electrical
  activity (PEA)
R-on-T
Torsades de pointes (TdP)
uniform
varying polarity

ventricular bigeminy
ventricular fibrillation
ventricular flutter
ventricular trigeminy
wide QRS complex
  tachycardia of
  uncertain origin

Introduction

Previous chapters have dealt with supraventricular arrhythmias; rhythm disturbances that arise either in the sinus node, the atria, or the AV junction, most with normal ventricular depolarization. In this chapter, we will deal with ectopics and arrhythmias that have their origin in ventricular tissue and cause abnormal ventricular depolarization.

The cells of normal ventricular musculature and conduction tissue are fast cells, due to the rapid influx of sodium. Slow cells are so named since they have extended refractory periods, and conduct and recover more slowly. Ectopic cells may be fast or slow and, in the presence of pathology, fast cells may be converted to slow cells and contribute to ectopic formation and conduction defects.

Disturbances in conduction may produce ectopic impulses by the process known as reentry. Chapter 8 defined *reentry* as the ability of an impulse to reexcite some region of the heart through which it has already passed. Reentry usually occurs when an impulse deviates around a circular conduction pathway forming a loop. There are many such potential circuits within ventricular conduction tissue where terminal Purkinje fibers attach to cardiac muscle.

When such circuits and ectopic formation occur in atrial tissue, the AV node usually protects the heart from rapid and chaotic rates. With ventricular ectopy, the vigilance of the practitioner, early recognition, and intervention are requisite forms of protection for the patient.

PREMATURE VENTRICULAR COMPLEX (PVC)

A premature ventricular complex (PVC) is a manifestation of abnormal electrical activity arising within the ventricles. PVCs are a common manifestation and frequently encountered and are regarded suspiciously since they often reflect myocardial ischemia and injury. More common problems and issues surround ventricular ectopy. The most significant factors contributing to the development of the triggered automaticity in the ventricles are:

- Adrenergic drugs
- Caffeine
- Congestive heart failure
- Electrolyte disturbances
- Hypertension
- Hypertrophy
- Hypokalemia, usually as a result of tissue hypoxia
- Hypovolemia
- Hypoxia
- Medications such as digitalis, isoproterenol, dopamine, and epinephrine
- Myocardial stretch
- Rapid rates, insufficient to provide adequate perfusion
- Slow rates, insufficient to provide adequate perfusion
- Stress
- Tissue infarction

Recognizing the PVC

By definition, the PVC occurs prior to the normally occurring QRS complex. A PVC can occur with any of the supraventricular arrhythmias. An impulse whose origin is within ventricular tissue and is outside the normal ventricular conduction system creates a QRS that is different from any supraventricular QRS. The QRS usually has an increased amplitude with its T wave of opposite polarity to its QRS. For instance, the PVC with a positive QRS will be followed by a negative T wave. Similarly, a negative QRS will be followed by a positive T wave.

The QRS morphology of the PVC is usually but not always greater in amplitude and wider than the dominant QRS. Ventricular activation that begins at a site of the ectopic ventricular focus travels across ventricular muscle mass instead of using the His-Purkinje

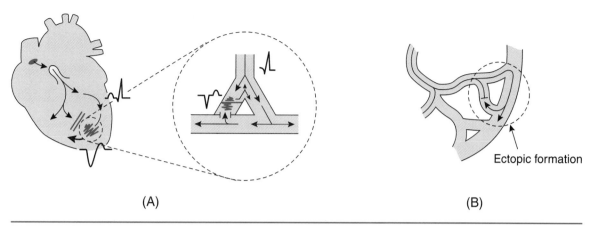

(A)   (B)

Figure 9.1 (A) The formation of a ventricular ectopic. An overall view of the conduction system with unidirectional block at a site in ventricular tissue. (B) A closer view of the focus of ventricular ectopic formation.

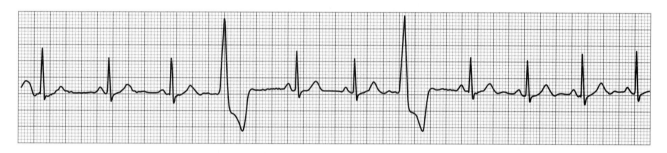

Figure 9.2 An ECG tracing of rhythm and two premature ventricular complexes (PVCs). Note the difference in morphology in the QRS complexes: The QRS of the premature complex is different from the dominant QRSs since it does not use the ventricular conduction pathways. The premature, ventricular QRS is opposite from its T wave. The sinus P waves plot through the events as sinus cadence is undisturbed. The PVCs are similar to each other and are uniform in appearance. The ECG interpretation would be sinus at 86 beat(s) per minute (bpm) with frequent, uniform PVCs.

system. Depolarization then takes longer, resulting in a broad (greater than 0.10 second) QRS complex. **Figure 9.1** illustrates the formation of ventricular ectopics. **Figure 9.2** is an ECG tracing of a sinus rhythm with a PVC.

Characteristics of a Ventricular Ectopic

Remember, the *P* in *PVC* means "premature," so, by definition, a PVC will be seen to occur prior to normally generated complexes.

- *P Wave:* That of the underlying rhythm.
- *PR Interval:* That of the underlying rhythm.
- *QRS Complex:* The QRS complex is different from the dominant rhythm and often appears bizarre in appearance in comparison with the normal QRS complexes. Often the QRS/T is greater in amplitude and duration than the dominant QRSs. However, PVCs can occur and present with diminished amplitude and narrow duration. A PVC does not have to be wide and bizarre to be ventricular in origin. The T wave of the PVC is opposite in direction from its own QRS.
- *QRS Rate:* The rate is that of the underlying rhythm.
- *QRS Rhythm:* The rhythm is that of the underlying rhythm, and its regularity will not be disturbed by the PVC.

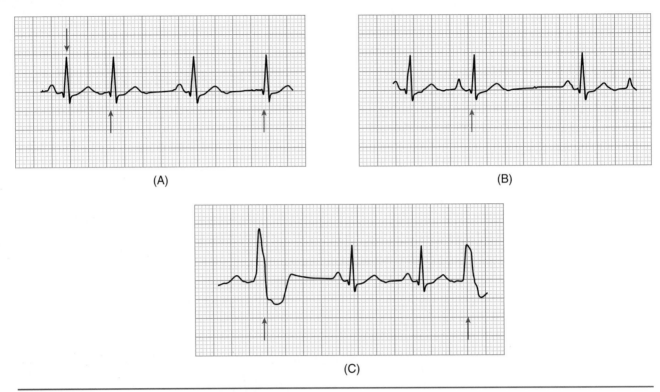

Figure 9.3 An ECG tracing showing (A) a sinus-induced QRS followed by a PJC → sinus, followed by a junctional escape complex. (B) Sinus with a PAC; and (C) sinus with PVCs. In (A) and (B), all the QRS complexes are similar as each uses the bundle branch system normally. In (C), the QRS complex of the PVC is different, and that QRS is opposite from its T wave. The PVC occurs within the ventricular musculature, outside the bundle branch system causing the abnormal configuration.

	Atrial	Junctional	Ventricular
P wave	P′ wave usually (+) or lost in the previous T	P′ wave usually (−) or none	Sinus P waves plot out regularly throughout the rhythm
PR interval	Different than sinus PR interval	≤0.12 sec if the P′ wave is visible	As with the underlying sinus mechanism
QRS complex	≤0.10 sec	≤0.10 sec	≥0.10 sec; can be ≤0.10 sec if fascicular in origin QRS is opposite in direction from its T wave

Table 9.1 Guide to ECG analysis of ectopics

Figure 9.3 is a comparison of QRS configurations that are sinus, atrial, junctional in origin, and PVCs. **Table 9.1** is a guide to ECG analysis of the ectopics.

Narrow Complex PVCs

PVCs originating within the intraventricular conduction system will be narrower than PVCs that occur outside the bundle branch system. This is because the bundle branch system will support the conduction in a different but relatively normal, rapid fashion. For a fascicular PVC, the initial wave form and the direction of the QRS will alter, depending on which fascicle is the origin.

For instance, an anterior fascicular PVC will have an inferior, rightward direction (right axis deviation) and will appear positive in lead II and negative in lead I. A posterior fascicular PVC will have a superior leftward direction (left axis deviation) and will appear negative in lead II and positive in lead I.

In either instance, the fascicular PVC will have an rSR configuration in precordial lead V_1 since the impulse originates within the left ventricular fascicles, and the right bundle branch will be the last to be activated. **Figure 9.4A** is a graphic of the ECG and ventricular conduction system showing the formation of the PVC in the left anterior fascicle (LAF) of the left bundle branch and the resulting wave forms in leads I and II. **Figure 9.4B** is a graphic of the ECG and ventricular conduction system showing the formation of the PVC in the left posterior fascicle (LPF) of the left bundle branch, and the resulting wave forms in leads I and II. **Figure 9.4C** is an ECG tracing of atrial fibrillation and a narrow-complex, fascicular PVC, confirmed on 12-lead ECG.

Variations in PVCs

PVCs are described by where they occur within the cardiac cycle.

Premature Ventricular Complex with Full Compensatory Pause. A PVC is frequently characterized by a so-called compensatory pause. The interval between the QRS complex before the PVC and the complex following the PVC is twice that of the regular cycle interval. This occurs when the PVC does not interfere with the pacemaking activity of the SA node. The sinus P waves following the PVC are not always visualized

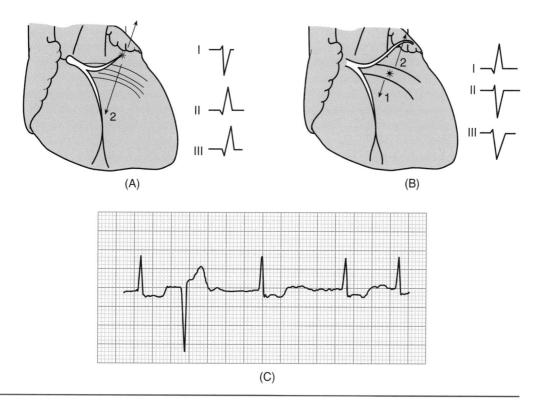

(A)   (B)

(C)

Figure 9.4 (A) The origin of a left anterior fascicular PVC and how it is visualized on ECG limb leads I, II, and II. (B) Another example of the direction of current flow of a PVC whose origin was in the area of the left posterior fascicle. (C) The ECG interpretation would be atrial fibrillation, 67 to 100 bpm, 2 mm ST segment depression and with a narrow-complex PVC. (This was confirmed on a 12-lead ECG.)

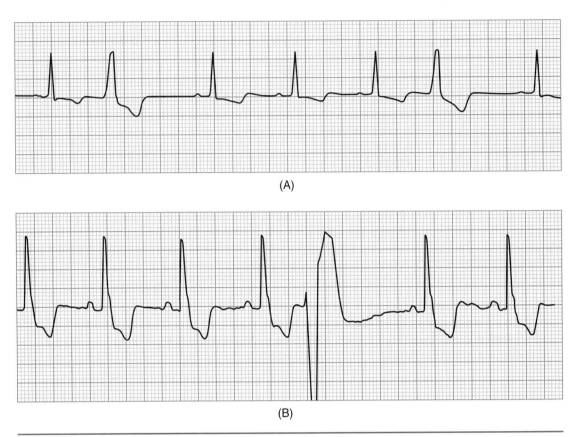

(A)

(B)

Figure 9.5 ECG tracings (A) and (B) each illustrate sinus rhythm with a PVC with compensatory pause. Note that the RR interval containing the PVC is twice the previous RR interval. Sinus P waves plot through as sinus cadence is undisturbed. The ECG interpretation for (A) would be sinus rhythm at 67 bpm with inverted T waves and a PVC. The ECG interpretation for (B) would be sinus at 71 bpm, with 5 to 6 mm ST segment depression and a PVC.

because they occur during the previous complex's refractory period. Mathematically, the distance between the sinus complex precedes the PVC, and the sinus complex that follows the PVC is equal to the sum of two consecutive sinus intervals. **Figure 9.5** consists of ECG tracings illustrating a PVC with full compensatory pause.

End-Diastolic PVC. When a PVC occurs at the end or just after a sinus P wave, it is **end-diastolic**. Remember, a sinus P wave is the last electrical event in ventricular diastole (that is, it occurs at the end of ventricular diastole, hence its name). Although the P wave preceded the PVC, that sinus P wave is not the source of the premature QRS complex.

An end-diastolic PVC is considered a relatively safe PVC in terms of electrical malfunction within the heart. It occurs far enough from the previous T wave and it can generate cardiac output of 90 to 95 percent of normal. **Figure 9.6** illustrates sinus rhythm with an end-diastolic PVC.

Interpolated PVC. When a PVC occurs between two consecutive sinus complexes, it is an **interpolated** PVC. The sinus node depolarizes at its inherent rate, and there are QRS complexes after each sinus complex. The PVC is sandwiched between two normal sinus complexes. These are often digitalis induced.

The PR interval following the interpolated PVC is typically conducted with a prolonged PR segment. This altered conduction occurs as a result of AV node delay because of

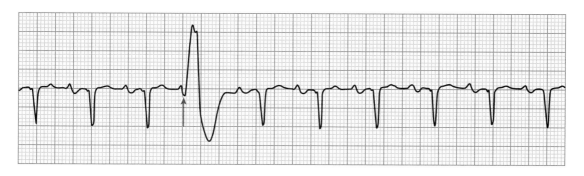

Figure 9.6 An ECG tracing showing sinus at 100 bpm with an end-diastolic PVC. Note the presence of the PVC just after the sinus P wave.

refractoriness, and the sinus is simply waiting its turn. Another less frequent cause is retrograde penetration by the PVC. This phenomenon cannot be proven on the ECG and is only inferred. It is sometimes referred to as concealed conduction. This prolongation of the PR segment may help differentiate an interpolated PVC from artifact. **Figure 9.7** is an example of a sinus mechanism with an interpolated PVC.

Uniform PVCs. When PVCs originate from one focus, they are usually **uniform** in morphology (configuration of the QRS complex and its T wave) in a given lead. Since there is only one reentrant circuit and the interval between the PVC and the preceding sinus beat is usually identical, this is known as fixed coupling and is commonly seen. PVCs from the same focus will have a similar morphology. PVCs from different foci are generated by different reentrant circuits, each with its own properties. These are called *multiformed* PVCs and the coupling cycles vary between the sinus beat and the PVC. So PVCs may have similar morphology but are not necessarily from the same focus. Verily PVCs with different morphology are not necessarily from different foci. The terms *uniform* and *multiform* are more correct when describing the morphology of a PVC. Use of multiple lead ECG can help, but electrophysiologic monitoring is a better tool for determining exact foci.

Intraventricular reentry may also cause the fixed coupling. This may occur because the normal impulse is conducted in one direction, and then, very slowly through a depressed segment of tissue, it emerges to reactivate normal tissue. If this interval is the same after each normal complex, the relationship will be established and seen as fixed coupling.

Afterdepolarization occurs when ventricular tissue is diseased or if the patient is on digitalis preparations. These afterpotentials follow the previous action potential, and if they reach their threshold, they will produce a PVC with exact coupling.

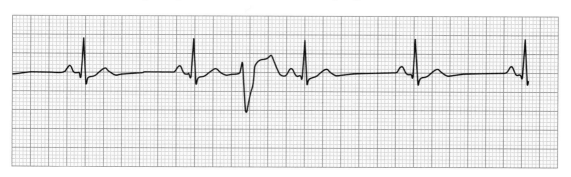

Figure 9.7 An ECG tracing showing sinus bradycardia with an interpolated PVC. Note that the sinus P waves plot through undisturbed. The ECG interpretation would be sinus bradycardia with 1 to 2 mm ST segment depression and an interpolated PVC.

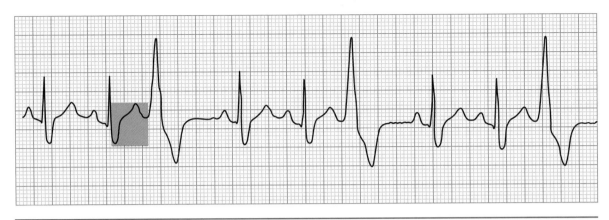

Figure 9.8 An ECG tracing showing sinus rhythm at 86 bpm with 2 mm ST segment elevation and frequent uniform PVCs. Note the similarity in the coupling intervals.

As stated earlier, uniformity in appearance and fixed coupling does not guarantee that the impulse comes from the same focus. It is possible for one focus, firing in the same direction as another focus in close proximity, to generate a PVC that is very similar. The ECG in **Figure 9.8** shows frequent uniform PVCs. Note the fixed coupling between the sinus beats and the PVCs.

Multiform PVCs. PVCs may originate in more than one focus, or a PVC may reenter (and exit) from the same focus, but depolarization occurs in a different direction. When this occurs, the PVC takes on a different appearance. The term **multiform** is recommended since a single focus can take different pathways through the ventricles and result in different QRS configurations. Just as similarity in PVC morphology does not guarantee the same focus, differences in PVC morphology do not guarantee multiple foci. **Figure 9.9** is an ECG showing the multiple PVCs of different QRS morphology. Note the difference in the coupling with the sinus beats and the PVCs.

Paired PVCs or Couplets. Pairs or **couplets** are two PVCs with similar morphology closely coupled in a row. A couplet should not be confused with coupling, which refers to the relationship of the PVC to the previous normal complex. Couplets are dangerous because the second PVC can fall on refractory tissue and cause ventricular fibrillation. **Figure 9.10** is an ECG tracing showing the occurrence of paired PVCs.

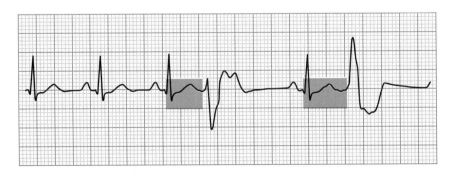

Figure 9.9 Note the difference between the PVCs. The ECG interpretation would be sinus rhythm about 78 bpm with frequent multiformed PVCs. Notice also the difference in the coupling intervals.

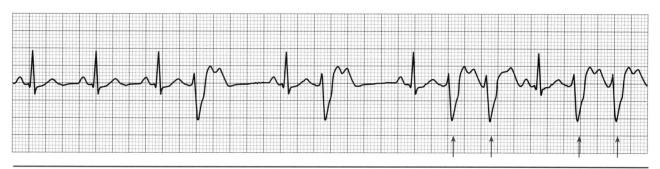

Figure 9.10 An ECG tracing showing sinus rhythm with frequent uniform PVCs and two examples of paired PVCs or couplets. Couplets indicate the beginning of reentry and should be regarded as dangerous to the patient.

Ventricular Bigeminy. Ventricular bigeminy is when every other beat is a ventricular ectopic beat—when a PVC follows every sinus beat. The pattern is sinus→PVC→sinus→PVC, and so on. When this occurs, a normal complex is followed by a PVC and the PVC is coupled with the previous QRS. The mechanism for this is thought to be reentry or afterdepolarization that may be caused by digitalis toxicity. Ventricular bigeminy can be an isolated occurrence in an otherwise healthy person.

Trigeminy occurs when every third complex is a PVC. In ventricular bigeminy or trigeminy the underlying rhythm can be sinus or junctional in origin.

Ventricular bigeminy is often seen in patients on digitalis preparations. **Figure 9.11** consists of ECG tracings from the same patient showing ventricular bigeminy (A) and trigeminy (B).

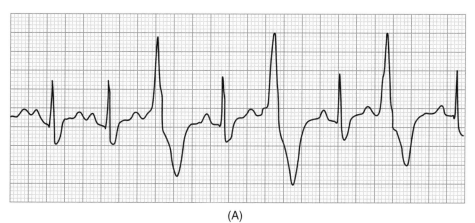

(A)

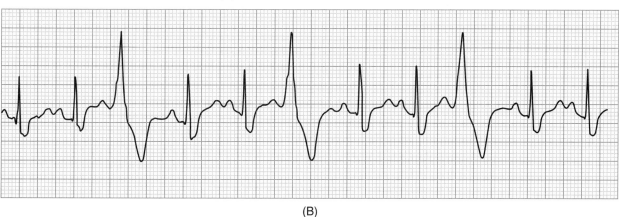

(B)

Figure 9.11 A continuous ECG tracing from a patient illustrating (A) ventricular bigeminy (every other complex is a PVC), and (B) trigeminy (every third complex is a PVC). There is 5 mm ST segment elevation.

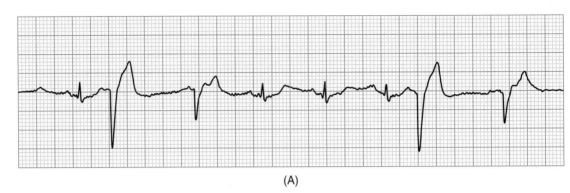

(A)

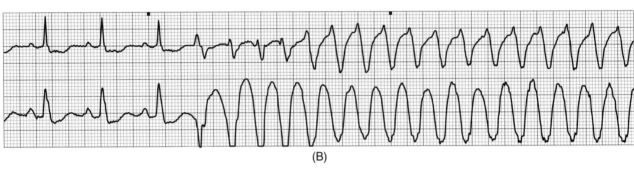

(B)

Figure 9.12 Two examples of R-on-T PVCs: (A) is an ECG tracing showing sinus rhythm with frequent R-on-T PVCs in a 61-year-old male with chest pain. Note that the PVCs are narrow, perhaps fascicular in origin. This patient later developed ventricular fibrillation. (B) is an ECG tracing from a 55-year-old patient who developed ventricular tachycardia as confirmed on 12-lead ECG. The patient responded to antiarrhythmic medication and was reportedly successfully reperfused.

R-on-T PVCs. The R-on-T phenomenon is the close coupling of the premature complex with the T wave of the preceding complex. The R wave of the PVC is superimposed onto the T wave of the preceding complex. Recall that 0.02 second to the right of the peak of the T wave is a vulnerable period, with the ability of a premature complex to initiate a dangerous and often a catastrophic arrhythmia. **Figure 9.12** is an example of ECG tracings with R-on-T PVCs.

Intervention

Assessment of the patient in whom ventricular ectopy is apparent, questioning the presence of chest pain, medical history, and medication regimen, provides a basis for interventions. Providing pain relief and reassessing the presence and frequency of the ectopics will help with the decision to use antiarrhythmia therapy. Most antiarrhythmic medications inhibit the fast sodium channels. Arrhythmias that are unresponsive to the usual therapy may be arising in slow rather than fast automatic cells. In such cases, slow channel (calcium) antagonists may be more effective.

MONOMORPHIC VENTRICULAR TACHYCARDIA

When three or more PVCs of the same polarity (**monomorphic**) occur in a row, and their rate exceeds 100 bpm, the arrhythmia is labeled ventricular tachycardia. Ventricular tachycardia may break through despite adequate sinus rate and often occurs suddenly. It is usually initiated by a PVC that is distinctly premature, but it can occur without any warning. When the ECG shows only ventricular tachycardia, it is described as sustained ventricular tachycardia or sustained v-tach. **Figure 9.13** is an ECG tracing showing ventricular tachycardia. The ECG characteristics of ventricular tachycardia are as follows:

- *P Wave:* P waves may or may not be distinguishable during ventricular tachycardia, although sinus activity, dissociated from ventricular activity, may not be affected. This means that the sinus node is depolarizing the atria in a normal manner at a rate either equal to, or slower than, the ventricular rate. Then the sinus P waves can be seen between QRS complexes. They bear no fixed relation to the QRS complexes of the ventricular tachycardia. The prudent practitioner will search for dissociated P waves.

- *PR Interval:* Sinus activity is dissociated from ventricular activity, thus a PR interval is not measurable.

- *QRS Complex:* The QRS complex duration is usually greater than 0.12 second and bizarre in appearance. The T wave may not be easily identified from the QRS complex. Sinus conduction through the AV junction may occur simultaneously with depolarization of the ventricular ectopic. When this happens ventricular tissue will be depolarized in part over the normal pathway and in part from the ventricular focus. It is as though there was a collision of forces. The resulting QRS complex will be intermediate in morphology somewhere between a normally conducted QRS and a QRS of ventricular origin. This is called a fusion beat. The prudent practitioner will search for fusion beats.

- *QRS Rate:* The ventricular rate is between 100 and 170 bpm. Three or more consecutive PVCs greater than 100 bpm constitute ventricular tachycardia.

- *QRS Rhythm:* The rhythm is regular or very slightly irregular.

An ectopic pacemaker in the ventricle often produces a wide QRS complex tachycardia. Ventricular tachycardia may terminate spontaneously. The more rapid the ventricular tachycardia, the greater the incidence of instability in the heart and certainly in the patient. Ventricular tachycardia of greater than 120 bpm is often an unstable situation.

Intervention

When ventricular tachycardia persists, and the patient is hemodynamically stable, antiarrhythmic medications may be employed. If the rhythm does not convert, or if the patient is considered unstable, then electrical cardioversion or defibrillation may be required to terminate the arrhythmia.

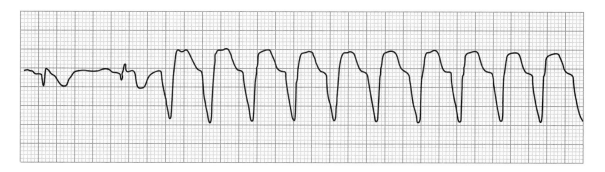

Figure 9.13 An ECG tracing showing ventricular tachycardia. There are two sinus beats followed by the onset of a sustained ventricular tachycardia.

Any wide QRS complex tachycardia should be treated as ventricular tachycardia until proven otherwise. The initial intervention for wide complex tachycardia is as though the rhythm is ventricular tachycardia until multiple lead ECG and clinical analyses are completed.

INTERMITTENT VENTRICULAR TACHYCARDIA

During sinus, atrial, or junctional rhythms, there may be a run or salvo of three PVCs in a row. For instance, the clinician may see three PVCs in a row—that is, a burst of ventricular tachycardia—then two more sinus complexes, followed by more PVCs. **Figure 9.14** illustrates two rhythms each with episodes or runs of ventricular tachycardia.

Wide QRS Complex Tachycardia of Uncertain Origin

Differentiation between ventricular tachycardia and SVT with aberrant conduction or use of a bypass tract is difficult. Vagal maneuvers and drug interventions that slow AV conduction may help, and with persistent occurrences, electrophysiologic testing should be done.

Wide QRS complex tachycardia of uncertain origin should be considered to be ventricular tachycardia until proven otherwise. One of the first clues may be that it is described

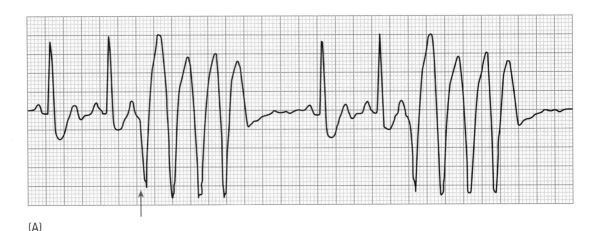

(A)

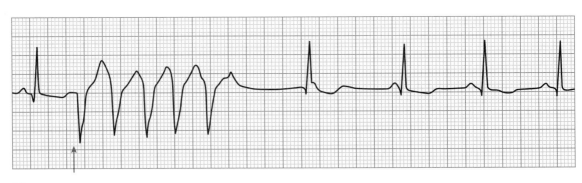

(B)

Figure 9.14 Two ECG tracings, each showing sinus mechanisms with runs of ventricular tachycardia, each beginning with R-on-T PVCs.

as "it looks too good to be v-tach." The patient should be treated as though it were ventricular tachycardia, regardless of age or circumstance—that is, if stable, consider ventricular antiarrhythmic medications; if unstable with a pulse, consider sedation and synchronized cardioversion.

Utilization of multiple-lead ECG is helpful in many instances:

- QRS complex if negative in leads I, II, and III and positive in aVR (northwest axis deviation).
- Precordial negative concordance. That is, all the QRS complexes in V_1 through V_6 are negative.
- Random presence of sinus P waves.
- Random presence of fusion beats.

Figure 9.15 displays a 12-lead ECG showing positive polarity (northwest axis deviation), and **Figure 9.16** illustrates a 12-lead ECG showing precordial negative concordance.

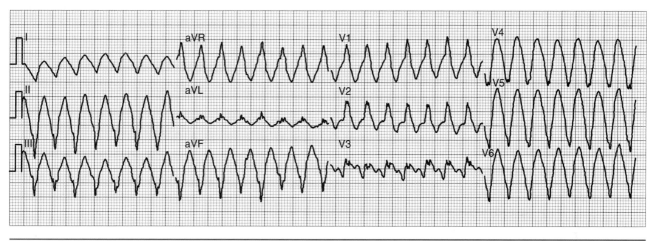

Figure 9.15 Twelve-lead ECG showing RBBB pattern (QRS >140 milliseconds [ms]) and northwest axis (negative polarity in leads I, II, and III and positive polarity in aVR)—hallmarks in identifying ventricular tachycardia. (Courtesy Roger D. White, MD, Mayo Clinic, Rochester, MN.)

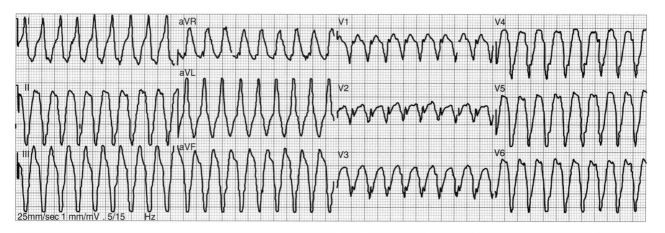

Figure 9.16 Precordial concordance typical of ventricular tachycardia. All QRS complexes in the precordial leads are negative in polarity. Also, there is northwest axis, that is, negative polarity in leads II, III, and aVF, and positive polarity in aVR. (Courtesy Roger D. White, MD, Mayo Clinic, Rochester, MN.)

POLYMORPHIC VENTRICULAR TACHYCARDIA

Polymorphic ventricular tachycardia occurs when the ventricular activation sequence varies. It can be seen in patients with normal hearts, but more frequently with chronic coronary artery disease and acute myocardial ischemia. The ECG displays ventricular tachycardia of **varying polarity, that is, some are positive in configuration and some are negative.** It can be intermittent or sustained and of rapid rate. **Figure 9.17A** shows polymorphic ventricular tachycardia, and **Figure 9.17B** shows polymorphic ventricular tachycardia, specifically Torsades de pointes (TdP).

Torsades de Pointes (TdP)

Torsades de pointes (TdP) is a form of **polymorphic** ventricular tachycardia that is frequently associated with a long QT interval. TdP creates a spindlelike pattern on the ECG that appears to undulate in relation to the baseline. For example, there will be QRS complexes of one polarity followed by complexes of the opposite polarity separated by complexes of an intermediate form. The alteration in polarity usually occurs gradually and is repeated several times in succession. TdP is frequently initiated by a PVC occurring on a prolonged T or TU wave. The rate range of the TdP is greater than 170 bpm, and usually 250 to 350 bpm.

Torsades de pointes is a French term meaning "twisting of the points." Beginning in 1966 the term was used to describe this ECG rhythm as different from other ventricular tachycardias. *Pointes* refers to the QRS complexes. In some clinical settings *Torsade* is used to describe a single episode, whereas *Torsades* is the plural form describing more than

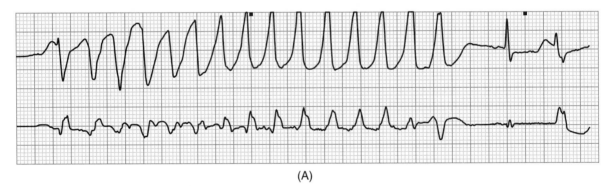

(A)

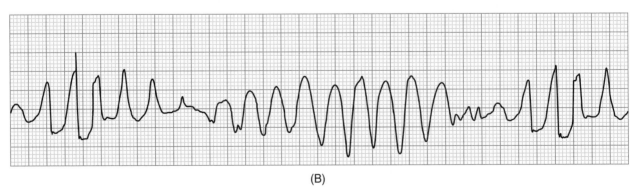

(B)

Figure 9.17 Two ECG tracings showing polymorphic ventricular tachycardia. (A) The rhythm spontaneously converted after reportedly being managed with intravenous (IV) magnesium. (B) Torsade de pointes. The patient was unstable with a pulse and responded to defibrillation.

one episode of this specific tachycardia. *Torsades de pointes* indicates that more than one sequence is seen. Most clinicians opt for the short form: TdP.

The Mechanism of TdP

Early afterdepolarization are cyclic changes in cellular membrane potential and delay or interrupt repolarization. Individuals with congenital prolonged QT intervals are candidates for TdP. Medications and over-the-counter (OTC) drugs that alter potassium or sodium currents during repolarization can cause perilous forms of ventricular tachycardia, specifically TdP.

Runs of TdP often terminate and recur. Patients are often unstable but many retain carotid pulses. Repeated episodes are progressively longer and the patient becomes progressively unstable. Left untreated, this arrhythmia may deteriorate into ventricular fibrillation.

TdP can be misinterpreted as ventricular fibrillation. Ventricular fibrillation is chaotic without any characteristic spindle effect, and the QRS rate is immeasurable. Clinically, some patients with TdP have pulses, and patients in ventricular fibrillation are pulseless.

Presence of renal disease, intrinsic cardiac disease, central nervous system (CNS) abnormalities such as subarachnoid hemorrhage, and intracranial trauma can generate TdP. Additional conditions that may prolong the QT interval include but are not limited to bradycardia, cirrhosis, congestive heart failure, diabetes mellitus, hypocalcemia, hypokalemia, and hypomagnesemia. Abnormalities such as hypothyroidism, hyperparathyroidism, hyperaldosteronism, pheocromocytoma, and hyperaldosteronism have been implicated in prolongation of the QT and onset of TdP.

Female gender has been identified as a risk for TdP. The longer QR interval in women makes them more susceptible to effects of drugs that prolong ventricular repolarization. The use of potassium channel blockers has been implicated in TdP in women.

ECG rhythm disturbances that may deteriorate into TdP include severe bradyarrhythmias such as complete AV block with idioventricular rhythm.

The list of drugs causing prolonged QT interval and thus putting the patient at risk for TdP grows every day. Drugs such as quinidine, procainamide, disopyramide, amniodarone, and aprindine cause a prolonged QT interval. Psychotropic drugs, such as phenothiazines and tricyclic antidepressants, can also cause prolonged QT intervals. Organophosphate poisoning is another cause of prolonged QT intervals resulting in TdP. Recent studies have highlighted erythromycin-related antibiotics as well as as levofloxacin, ketoconazole, antihistamine agents, astemizole, and terfenadine. The phenothiazines are reported as contributing to a high incidence of arrhythmias and reported deaths through similar effects on conduction.

Other causes of TdP include nonsedating antihistamines and some OTC supplements. The use of liquid protein and other quick-weight-loss products has been implicated in electrolyte depletion–induced TdP. Prolonged QT alone does not absolutely preclude TdP. However, the instances of occurrence are frequent enough to warrant vigilant observation.

Intervention

Treatment begins with assessment of serum electrolytes and correction of potassium and magnesium abnormalities. Magnesium is currently the drug of choice. The use of magnesium IV with an infusion may be indicated because of its effectiveness in stabilizing membrane potential. Where TdP is caused by other than cardiac drugs, treatment includes administration of the antidote specific to the offending drug.

The ECG characteristics of TdP are as follows:

- *P Wave:* P waves can be identified if the underlying rhythm is sinus.
- *PR Interval:* There is a measurable PR interval if the underlying rhythm is sinus.
- *QRS Complex:* There are discrete QRS complexes with an underlying rhythm. However, with TdP there are no describable QRS complexes.
- *QRS Rate:* The rate is undeterminable.
- *QRS Rhythm:* Unless there is an underlying rhythm TdP presents as chaotic, with multiple twists.

Initial treatment for the unstable patient in sustained TdP is defibrillation and often requires multiple defibrillation attempts. Magnesium sulfate is frequently administered. TdP frequently recurs or persists with increasing duration even after conversion. When this happens, definitive treatment is to initiate transcutaneous pacing at a more rapid rate than the TdP, thus preventing its recurrence. This is called *overdrive pacing.* Overdrive pacing should be initiated only between episodes of TdP. Overdrive pacing *does not* stop the TdP but may assist in preventing recurrence.

VENTRICULAR FLUTTER

This rhythm is rarely seen because it deteriorates rapidly into ventricular fibrillation. The ECG characteristics of ventricular flutter are:

- *P Wave:* P waves may not be distinguishable during ventricular flutter, although atrial activity, dissociated from ventricular activity, may not be affected. The ventricular rate is too fast to discern the P waves.
- *PR Interval:* Since atrial activity is dissociated from ventricular activity, a PR interval is not visible.
- *QRS Complex:* The QRS complex duration is usually greater than 0.12 second and bizarre in appearance. The T wave may not be separated from the QRS complex.
- *QRS Rate:* The ventricular rate is 250 to 350 bpm; thus sinus activity cannot be determined.
- *QRS Rhythm:* The rhythm is regular or slightly irregular. In ventricular **flutter**, undulating waves are seen rising and falling.

When the ventricular rate is this fast, the patient is unstable. The rhythm requires immediate unsynchronized cardioversion. Any atrial activity may be unaffected. Left untreated this arrhythmia is usually short-lived, deteriorating into ventricular fibrillation within a very short time. **Figure 9.18** is an example of ventricular flutter with a ventricular rate at 272 bpm.

VENTRICULAR FIBRILLATION

Multiple, disorganized complexes characterize ventricular fibrillation and cause cardiac arrest. Ventricular fibrillation may be of sudden onset or may follow PVCs, ventricular tachycardia, and ventricular flutter, or it can occur without any warning ectopic.

Ventricular **fibrillation** is a terminal rhythm. This means that there is no natural conversion to a normal rhythm and there are no intermittent episodes of ventricular fibrillation.

Clinically, there is no pulse and no cardiac output with ventricular fibrillation. Occasionally, there are erratic movements in the patient's extremities, or agonal breath sounds may accompany this rhythm. The practitioner should not presume that because these movements

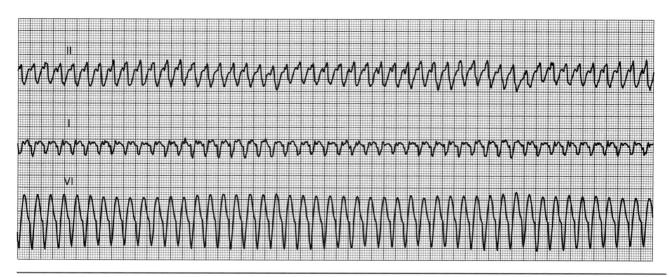

Figure 9.18 A 12-lead ECG of ventricular flutter, ventricular rate calculated at 272 bpm.

occur, the rhythm must not be ventricular fibrillation. These are terminal events accompanying the fibrillation and ensuing death.

Ventricular fibrillation may be confused with artifact; for example, when the patient is unresponsive, in a seizure state, or shivering. Assess and confirm pulses and responsiveness. The ECG characteristics of ventricular fibrillation are as follows:

- *P Wave:* P waves are unidentifiable.
- *PR Interval:* There is no measurable PR interval.
- *QRS Complex:* There are no discrete QRS complexes.
- *QRS Rate:* The rate cannot be determined.
- *QRS Rhythm:* The rhythm is chaotic, with multiple, disorganized contractions of the ventricles.

Figure 9.19 shows three ECG examples of ventricular fibrillation.

Coarse versus Fine Ventricular Fibrillation

Despite the chaos, ventricular fibrillation has a direction to the flow of current. It is easily recognized in a lead parallel to that flow of current and often referred to as coarse. If the flow is off in another direction, the amplitude may be diminished. There is no clinical difference between *fine* versus *coarse* ventricular defibrillation. *Coarse ventricular fibrillation* does not imply a more easily converted rhythm; nor does *fine ventricular fibrillation* imply a more lethal situation. **Figure 9.20A** and **Figure 9.20B** illustrate ventricular fibrillation of varying amplitudes.

If the fibrillation is of low amplitude, frequently called fine v-fib, it may be confused with asystole. It is vital to confirm on several leads to differentiate between ventricular fibrillation and asystole.

Once ventricular fibrillation is confirmed, whether fine or coarse, immediate defibrillation is the treatment of choice.

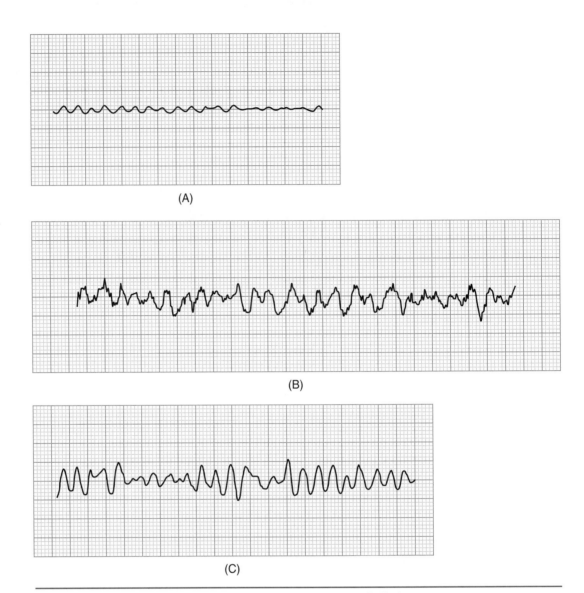

(A)

(B)

(C)

Figure 9.19 ECG tracings from three patients, each with ventricular fibrillation.

VENTRICULAR ESCAPE: IDIOVENTRICULAR RHYTHM

With abnormal ventricular depolarization, the ventricular pacemaker is not as efficient as the supraventricular pacemakers. It is the lowest of the series of pacemakers and may become dominant when the higher pacemakers have failed. It may be an "escape" or "safety" rhythm and should never be suppressed.

Idioventricular rhythm (IVR) appears in the presence of depressed conduction and the ventricles assume the control of the rhythm. The ventricles have the ability to initiate impulses at 20 to 40 bpm. The rhythm is usually regular.

Idioventricular rhythm is clinically significant because it is slow and usually does not produce effective perfusion. IVR may accelerate or progress to ventricular tachycardia or fibrillation.

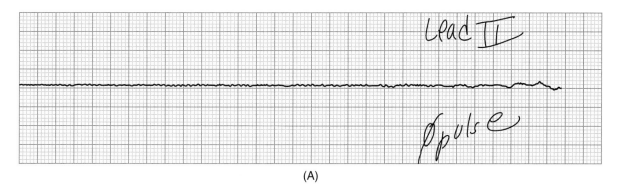

(A)

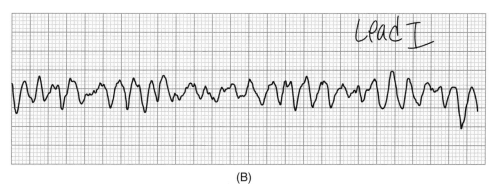

(B)

Figure 9.20 ECG tracings from the same patient. (A) An apparent asystole or fine ventricular fibrillation. (B) Ventricular fibrillation confirmed on lead I.

Initial therapies should be directed to accelerating the more normal rhythms and subsequently the ventricular rate. For instance, blocking the vagus with atropine may provoke the sinus or junction to generate potential and take control. The ECG characteristics of idioventricular rhythm are as follows:

- *P Wave:* P waves may not be present. If they are, they are independent of the IVR.
- *PR Interval:* There is no measurable PR interval.
- *QRS Complex:* The QRS complex duration is usually greater than 0.10 second, often greater than 0.12 second. However, a ventricular ectopic that occurs within the ventricular fascicles can elicit a narrower than expected QRS.
- *QRS Rate:* The inherent rate of the ventricular pacemaker is 20 to 40 bpm.
- *QRS Rhythm:* The rhythm is usually regular.

Figure 9.21 shows examples of idioventricular rhythm.

ACCELERATED IDIOVENTRICULAR RHYTHM (AIVR)

Accelerated idioventricular rhythm (AIVR) is three or more successive complexes in a row, with a rate between 40 and 100 bpm. AIVR often begins with a long coupling interval and terminates when the sinus rate emerges at a time when it can conduct through to the ventricles. The ECG characteristics of AIVR are as follows:

- *P Wave:* P waves may not be present. If they are, they are independent of the AIVR.
- *PR Interval:* There is no measurable PR interval.
- *QRS Complex:* The QRS complex duration is usually greater than 0.10 second, often greater than 0.12 second. When the origin of a ventricular ectopic is within the ventricular fascicle, the QRS may not exceed 0.12 second.
- *QRS Rate:* The accelerated rate of the ventricular pacemaker is 40 to 100 bpm.
- *QRS Rhythm:* The rhythm is usually regular.

Figure 9.22 is an example of atrial fibrillation progressing to accelerated idioventricular rhythm.

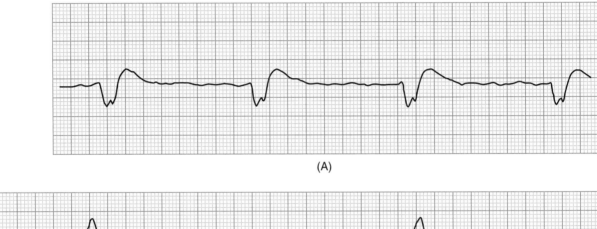

(A)

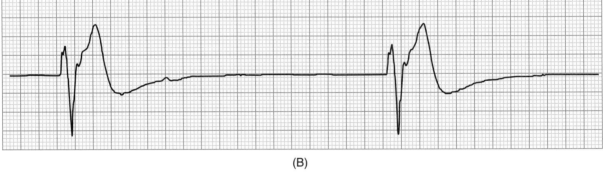

(B)

Figure 9.21 (A) ECG tracing showing idioventricular rhythm at 37 bpm. (B) An idioventricular rhythm at 16 bpm. Both patients were pulseless and did not respond to epinephrine, atropine, or transcutaneous pacing.

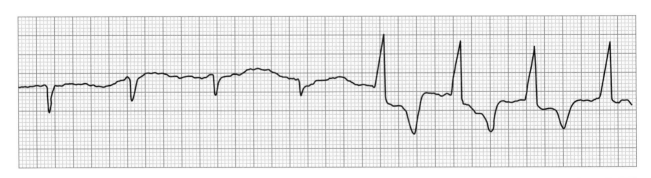

Figure 9.22 An ECG tracing showing atrial fibrillation with an accelerated junctional rhythm at 67 bpm progressing to an accelerated idioventricular rhythm at 75 bpm.

Causes

Accelerated idioventricular rhythm occurs when an area of enhanced automaticity exists within the ventricular conduction system. When the rate is similar to the underlying sinus rate, it will begin and end with ventricular fusion beats. Fusion beats are created when ventricular and supraventricular forces collide or fuse and create a different QRS. Fusion beats at the onset show the progressive dominance of the ventricular focus; fusion beats at the end of AIVR show the return to dominance by the supraventricular pacemaker.

With abnormal ventricular depolarization, the ventricular pacemaker is not as efficient as the supraventricular pacemakers. An idioventricular escape mechanism is the lowest of the series of pacemakers and may become dominant when the higher pacemakers have failed. It may be an escape or safety rhythm and should not be suppressed. It can be seen post myocardial infarction or post reperfusion procedures.

Intervention

In most cases, intervention for idioventricular rhythm or AIVR with slower rates calls for acceleration of some higher order of rhythm. The use of atropine may block the action of the vagus so that sinus or junctional escape rhythms may surface and take over. The application of the transcutaneous pacemaker is also appropriate.

ASYSTOLE

Asystole occurs when there are no ventricular complexes, indicating the ventricles are inactive. There is cardiac electrical activity, hence no contractions of the myocardium, and therefore no cardiac output or blood flow. In some instances, the atria continue to beat in their own time. Any hope for an escape pacemaker of some kind to take over is minimal. **Figure 9.23** shows a continuous ECG tracing from a patient with ventricular fibrillation who deteriorated into asystole.

Asystole versus Fine Ventricular Fibrillation

Ventricular fibrillation is the result of chaotic activity within the ventricular system. Many fibers are depolarizing, and there is no effective perfusion. When the flow of current is largely parallel to the monitoring lead, the fibrillation is easily recognized. However, when the flow of current is at right angles to the monitoring lead, the ECG may look like asystole. Switch to leads I and III to differentiate asystole from ventricular fibrillation.

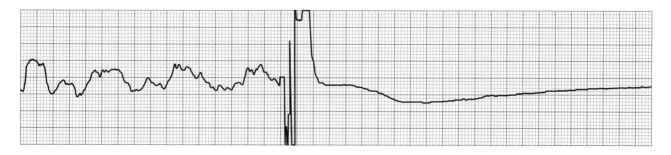

Figure 9.23 A continuous ECG tracing in a patient who was defibrillated. The resulting asystole was confirmed with two leads.

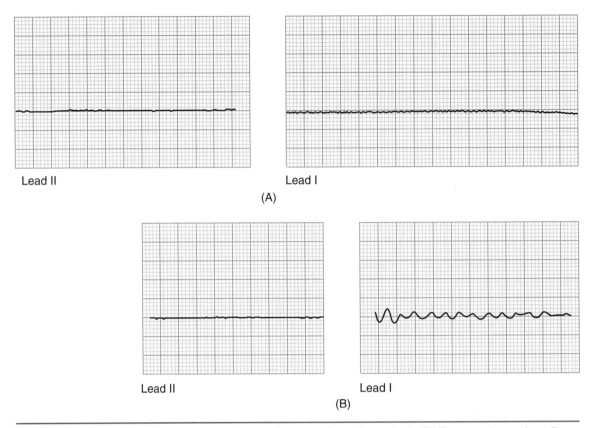

Figure 9.24 (A) An ECG in a patient where the asystole was confirmed in two leads. (B) The asystole was, in reality, ventricular fibrillation as confirmed in a second lead.

Figure 9.24A shows asystole in lead II and confirmed in lead I. **Figure 9.24B** shows asystole in lead II confirmed as v-fib in lead I.

Intervention

Do not defibrillate patients in asystole. Intervention for patients with confirmed asystole includes cardiopulmonary resuscitation (CPR), airway management, and multiple approaches using drugs and devices to initiate and enhance myocardial activity. This includes the use of epinephrine, possibly atropine, and transcutaneous or transvenous pacing. Although the use of atropine and pacing is rarely thought to be beneficial, application and documented lack of response can be comforting to the patient's family, assuring them that everything possible was attempted.

PULSELESS ELECTRICAL ACTIVITY

There are tragic circumstances where the ECG of a patient in cardiac arrest continues to display an identifiable rhythm but the patient is unresponsive and does not have a palpable pulse, thus the term **pulseless electrical activity (PEA)**. The actual ECG rhythm in such cases may present as sinus rhythm, any of the atrial arrhythmias, AV junctional rhythm, or any of the AV blocks. There may be ectopy of any origin or frequency.

Despite the presence of electrical function (as seen by the ECG), with PEA there is no mechanical response and no cardiac output, pulse, or blood pressure.

Causes

Electrical mechanical dissociation (EMD), as one explanation, is a catastrophic, physiologic event for which there is little recourse. EMD occurs with extremes in electrolyte imbalance and drug overdose. There are other conditions, termed mechanical impediments to cardiac filling and subsequent systole, that result in a similar circumstance. These include hypovolemia, tension pneumothorax, pulmonary embolus, severe hypovolemia, extremes of body temperature, and/or hypoxemia, all of which, in excess, can deprive the myocardium of adequate mechanical abilities. **Figure 9.25** is a documented example of a clearly distinct atrial fibrillation in a patient with PEA due to massive pulmonary embolus and cardiac tamponade confirmed on postmortem examination.

Another mechanical impediment causing PEA is cardiac tamponade. *Tamponade* is the compression of the heart resulting from fluid collecting in the pericardial space and limiting the heart's normal range of motion. For example, pericardial effusion may act to mechanically "choke off" the heart by preventing it from adequately filling, therefore inadequately pumping. Tamponade may be reversible, for example, when diagnosed quickly and pericardiocentesis is successful.

PEA has been known to occur in cases where the myocardium has sustained injury that may or may not be reversible. This can occur with blunt force trauma to the chest. In most instances of this type, acute changes are seen in the 12-lead ECG that include ST elevation, inverted T waves, and often deep Q waves in the anterior precordial leads.

Intervention

Treatment for PEA includes CPR, airway management, and multiple approaches using drugs and devices to initiate and enhance myocardial activity. The treatment also should be directed to identification of the cause of the mechanical impairment to circulation. Vasopressin is a potent vasopressor that may be useful. As with asystole the use of epinephrine is encouraged and, if the ECG rhythm is a bradycardia, atropine and pacing may be considered. As in asystole, the documented evidence of the lack of response may be a comfort to the patient's family.

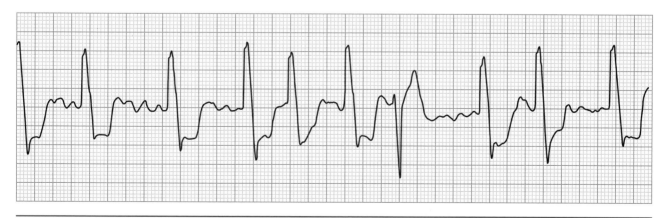

Figure 9.25 An ECG showing atrial fibrillation ventricular rate range of 60 to 100 bpm and a PVC. However, this is a documented example of a patient who was pulseless. Pulmonary embolus and cardiac tamponade were confirmed on autopsy.

	PVC*	IVR	AIVR	V-Tach	V-Fib	Asystole
P wave		Independent or none	Independent or none	Independent or none	Unable to see	Independent or none
PR interval						
QRS complex	≥0.10 sec	≥0.10 sec	≥0.10 sec	≥0.10 sec	≥0.10 sec	≥0.10 sec
QRS configuration	QRS/T wave	QRS/T wave	QRS/T wave	QRS/T wave		
QRS rate		20–40/min	41–100/min	>100/min		
QRS rhythm		Regular	Regular	Regular		

Table 9.2 Guide to ECG analysis of the ventricular mechanisms.

*P waves, PR interval, and QRS rate and rhythm are as with the underlying rhythm.

SUMMARY

Ventricular ectopics can be idiopathic; however, in a patient who has chest pain or other signs of acute coronary syndrome, they are often signs of myocardial ischemia and hypoxia. PVCs frequently deteriorate into arrhythmias that are life-threatening. **Table 9.2** summarizes the characteristics of ECG changes with ventricular mechanisms.

PVCs and the ventricular arrhythmias were the foundation for prehospital medicine and the initiation of coronary care units. The need for vigilance, rapid recognition and intervention of the ventricular ectopics, their sequelae, and their implications to patient welfare were great concern and remain so to this day.

Differentiation of the origins of wide QRS complex tachycardias is critical. We have seen examples of 12-lead ECGs that demonstrate the criteria for differential interpretations of these arrhythmias. The use of multiple-lead ECGs has become a necessary, frequent, and dependable technique for determining the source of the tachycardia and selecting appropriate interventions.

Self-Assessment Exercises
Fill in the Blanks

Complete the third and fourth columns, and then compare your answers with those in Appendix A.

	Sinus Rhythm	PJC	PAC	PVC
P wave	1 (+) P wave/QRS	1 (−) P wave/QRS or no P wave/QRS	_____	_____
PR interval	0.12–0.20 sec	≤0.12 sec	_____	_____
QRS complex	≤0.10 sec	≤0.10 sec		
QRS rate	60–100/min	N/A	_____	_____
QRS rhythm	Regular	Disturbs sinus	_____	_____

Complete the first and third columns, and then compare your answers with those in Appendix A.

	Atrial Tach	Sinus Tach	Ventricular Tach
P wave	_____	1 (+) P wave/QRS	_____
PR interval	_____	0.12–0.20 sec	_____
QRS complex	_____	≤0.10 sec	_____
QRS rate	_____	100–150/min	_____
QRS rhythm	_____	Regular	_____

ECG Rhythm Identification Practice

For the following rhythms, fill in the blanks and then compare your answers with those in Appendix A.

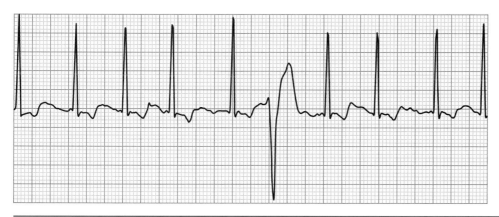

Figure 9.26

1. QRS duration _____
2. QT interval _____
3. Ventricular rate/rhythm _____
4. Atrial rate/rhythm _____
5. PR interval _____
6. Identification _____
7. Symptoms _____
8. Treatment _____

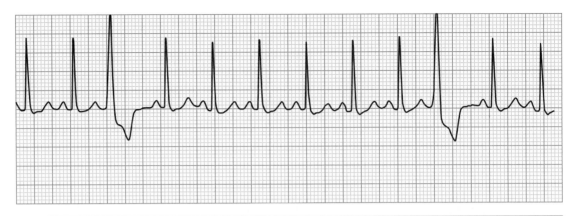

Figure 9.27

1. QRS duration _____
2. QT interval _____
3. Ventricular rate/rhythm _____
4. Atrial rate/rhythm _____
5. PR interval _____
6. Identification _____
7. Symptoms _____
8. Treatment _____

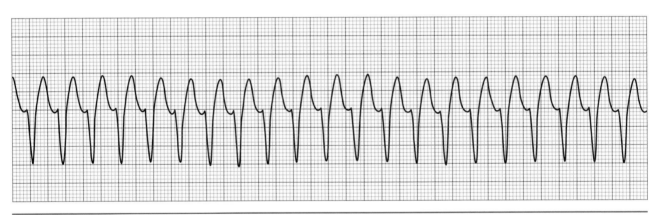

Figure 9.28

1. QRS duration _____
2. QT interval _____
3. Ventricular rate/rhythm _____
4. Atrial rate/rhythm _____
5. PR interval _____
6. Identification _____
7. Symptoms _____
8. Treatment _____

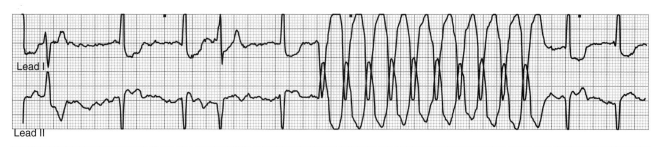

Figure 9.29

1. QRS duration _____
2. QT interval _____
3. Ventricular rate/rhythm _____
4. Atrial rate/rhythm _____
5. PR interval _____
6. Identification _____
7. Symptoms _____
8. Treatment _____

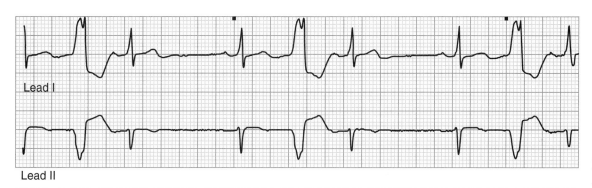

Figure 9.30

1. QRS duration _____
2. QT interval _____
3. Ventricular rate/rhythm _____
4. Atrial rate/rhythm _____
5. PR interval _____
6. Identification _____
7. Symptoms _____
8. Treatment _____

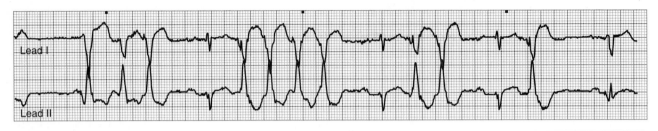

Figure 9.31

1. QRS duration _____
2. QT interval _____
3. Ventricular rate/rhythm _____
4. Atrial rate/rhythm _____
5. PR interval _____
6. Identification _____
7. Symptoms _____
8. Treatment _____

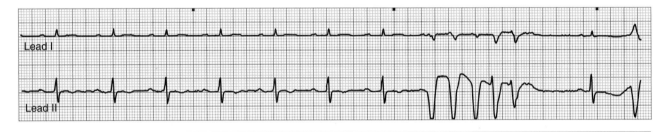

Figure 9.32

1. QRS duration _____
2. QT interval _____
3. Ventricular rate/rhythm _____
4. Atrial rate/rhythm _____
5. PR interval _____
6. Identification _____
7. Symptoms _____
8. Treatment _____

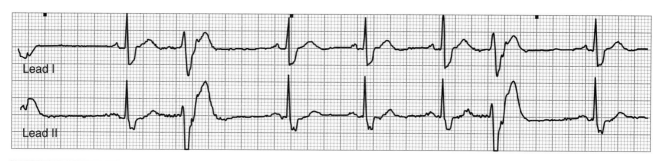

Figure 9.33

1. QRS duration _____
2. QT interval _____
3. Ventricular rate/rhythm _____
4. Atrial rate/rhythm _____
5. PR interval _____
6. Identification _____
7. Symptoms _____
8. Treatment _____

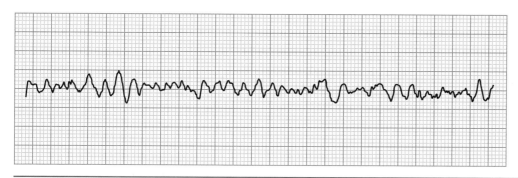

Figure 9.34

1. QRS duration _____
2. QT interval _____
3. Ventricular rate/rhythm _____
4. Atrial rate/rhythm _____
5. PR interval _____
6. Identification _____
7. Symptoms _____
8. Treatment _____

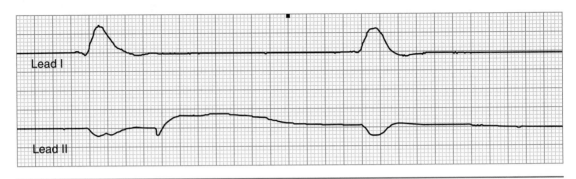

Figure 9.35

1. QRS duration _____
2. QT interval _____
3. Ventricular rate/rhythm _____
4. Atrial rate/rhythm _____
5. PR interval _____
6. Identification _____
7. Symptoms _____
8. Treatment _____

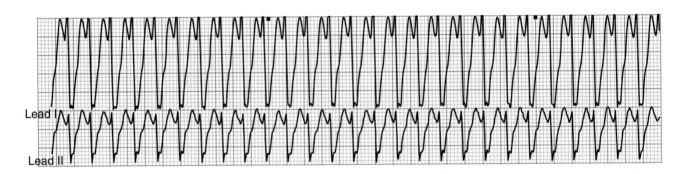

Figure 9.36

1. QRS duration _____
2. QT interval _____
3. Ventricular rate/rhythm _____
4. Atrial rate/rhythm _____
5. PR interval _____
6. Identification _____
7. Symptoms _____
8. Treatment _____

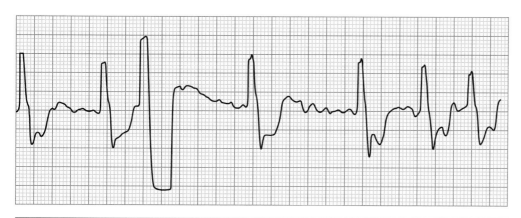

Figure 9.37

1. QRS duration _____
2. QT interval _____
3. Ventricular rate/rhythm _____
4. Atrial rate/rhythm _____
5. PR interval _____
6. Identification _____
7. Symptoms _____
8. Treatment _____

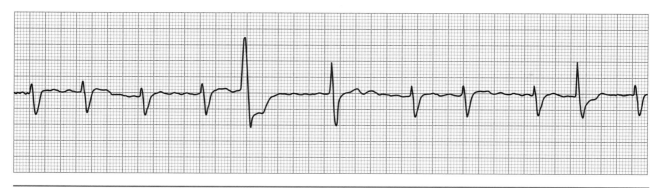

Figure 9.38

1. QRS duration _____
2. QT interval _____
3. Ventricular rate/rhythm _____
4. Atrial rate/rhythm _____
5. PR interval _____
6. Identification _____
7. Symptoms _____
8. Treatment _____

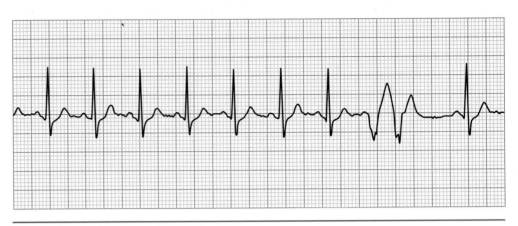

Figure 9.39

1. QRS duration _____

2. QT interval _____

3. Ventricular rate/rhythm _____

4. Atrial rate/rhythm _____

5. PR interval _____

6. Identification _____

7. Symptoms _____

8. Treatment _____

AV Conduction Defects

Premise

- In the AV conduction defects, pathology exists or a medication has been taken that causes an unnatural conduction delay.
- The naming of most other arrhythmias gives an easy-to-recognize indication as to the source, pacer, or ectopic and the resulting fast or slow heart rate. The titles of the AV conduction defects are less clear and can be mastered if you keep in mind the components of the heart's electrical conduction system and the pathology reflected by their ECG measurements.

Objectives

After reading the chapter and completing the Self-Assessment Exercises, the student should be able to

- Identify the ECG patterns of the AV conduction defects.
- Realize the implications of the defects.

Key Terms

advanced AV block	nodal	Type II AV block
first-degree AV block	Mobitz	Wenckebach
complete AV block	second-degree AV block	
infranodal	Type I AV block	

Introduction

Recall that electrical activation normally begins with the SA node, and the wave of depolarization spreads out and downward throughout the atria to the AV junction. In the AV junction, there is a natural delay in the AV node and then the impulse travels down the His bundle and its branches and fascicles throughout the ventricles. This natural delay is especially helpful in atrial flutter and fibrillation when the AV node functions in a therapeutic manner, protecting the ventricles from a rapid and chaotic atrial rate.

In the AV conduction defects, the conduction of the normal wave front can be delayed or blocked at any point after atrial depolarization. This can occur within the AV node (**nodal**) or below the His bundle (infranodal) and may involve one, two, or all of the fascicles and the bundle branches. In the previous chapters, each of the arrhythmias was identified by (1) the pacemaker (sinus) or ectopic (junctional or atrial) and (2) the resulting ventricular heart rate and rhythm.

For example, in sinus tachycardia, the pacemaker is in the sinus node, and the heart rate is greater than 100 beats per minute. In atrial tachycardia, the ectopic that is controlling the heart is within atrial tissue, and the heart rate is greater than 100 beats per minute.

When identifying the AV conduction defects, the name of the arrhythmia does not always define the specific pathology. The prudent practitioner must be vastly certain of which defects are involved. This involves knowing the patient history and physical assessment and results of other diagnostic tools.

Type, Wenckebach, or *Mobitz* describes the ECG patterns and characteristics. The terms *nodal, infranodal,* and *fascicular* describe the defect's probable anatomical location. In other words, the ECG is the clue, not the diagnosis.

Precise identification of the source of the conduction disturbance is done with the His-bundle electrocardiogram. For example, prolonged atrium-His interval or the absence of His-bundle signal indicate AV nodal block, while a prolonged His-V interval or the absence of a signal from the ventricles following a His signal indicates bilateral bundle defect. This study would be appropriate when the patient has recurrence of the "blocks" or a more precise identification of the site of the disease is in the best interest of the patient.

When learning the AV conduction defects the student must learn by rote, the specific term associated with the ECG evidence of the conduction defect. The analysis of the ECG should include all the information as an aid to focusing on the problem until clinical verification can be attained. So the interpretation shall include

- The pacemaker, sinus or atrial
- The sinus or atrial rate
- The ventricular (QRS) rate and rhythm
- The QRS duration and configuration
- The description of the patterns of the PR interval(s).

The ECG identification of the defects should not simply be a process of algebraic ratios, but include a clear description of all the components of the arrhythmia. Too often, blatant shortcuts lead to errors in interpretation.

There are three categories for consideration:

1. *First-degree AV block,* where there is delay in conduction
2. *Second-degree AV block,* where there is intermittent conduction delay
   a. *Type I:* Typically group beating with progressively prolonged PR intervals.
   b. *Type II:* Sudden missing or dropped QRS complexes.
   c. *2:1:* Every other QRS complex is missing, thus 2:1 cannot be categorized as either Type I or Type II.
   d. *Advanced:* More than one QRS complex is missing, without warning.
3. *Complete AV block,* where there is
   a. *No conduction* (therefore **no** PR interval).
   b. A junctional or ventricular escape rhythm controlling the ventricles.

FIRST-DEGREE AV BLOCK

The word *block* in describing this arrhythmia is a misnomer—*block* usually implies no conduction. Through the process of time and simplicity in categorization, the term prevails and will continue here. **First-degree AV block** implies conduction delay within the AV node or the His bundle.

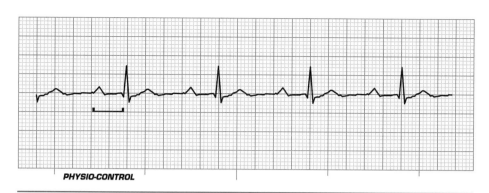

Figure 10.1 An ECG tracing illustrating a sinus rhythm at 60 per minute with a consistently prolonged (0.32 second) PR interval. The ECG interpretation would be sinus at 60 per minute with first-degree AV block.

Recall that the time taken by the spread of depolarization from SA node activation, through the atria and the AV node up to ventricular activation is seen on the ECG as the PR interval and the two events occur within 0.20 second. A P wave of prolonged duration as with atrial hypertrophy may cause a distortion in the P wave and result in a PR interval greater than 0.20 second.

Interference with AV conduction results in a lengthening of the PR segment and thus the PR interval. When this lengthening of the PR interval is consistently greater than 0.20 second, this is first-degree AV block.

ECG Characteristics

ECG characteristics of first-degree AV block are

- *P Wave:* The P waves are positive, of normal duration, and are uniform if the SA node is the pacemaker. Every P wave is followed by a QRS complex.
- *PR Interval:* The PR interval is greater than 0.20 second and *constant* from beat to beat. The PR can extend to greater than 0.60 second.
- *QRS Complex:* The duration is 0.10 second or less.
- *QRS Rate:* The rate is dependent on the basic rhythm. If the basic rhythm is sinus, the rate is constant between 60 and 100 beats per minute; greater than 100 per minute is tachycardia and less than 60 is bradycardia.
- *QRS Rhythm:* The rhythm is usually regular.

Figure 10.1 is an ECG tracing of first-degree AV block.

Table 10.1 shows the comparison in ECG configurations between sinus rhythm and first-degree AV block. Note the only difference is the PR interval.

	Sinus	First-Degree AV Block
P wave	1 (+) P wave/QRS	1 (+) P wave/QRS
PR interval	**0.12–0.20 sec**	**>0.20 sec and consistent**
QRS complex	0.10 sec	0.10 sec
QRS rate	60–100/min	60–100/min
QRS rhythm	Regular	Regular

Table 10.1 Comparison in ECG characteristics of sinus rhythm and sinus with first-degree AV block.

Causes

First-degree AV block is, of itself, not critical. Clinically, though, it must always be assessed in terms of the patient's presentation, chief complaint, and past medical history.

First-degree AV block is seen with

- Advancing age
- Conditioned athletes
- Electrolyte disturbances
- Endocarditis
- Inferior wall myocardial infarction
- Medications such as beta-blockers, calcium channel blockers, or digitalis
- Myocarditis
- Pericarditis
- Right coronary artery disease

Intervention

Typically, the overall heart rate is within normal limits, the patient's signs and symptoms are not related to the rate, and no intervention is required. There may be a temptation to intervene if a bradycardia is present; however, the risk of accelerating the sinus rate may provoke a higher degree of block if the AV node cannot accommodate with an increased rate of conduction. Atropine is a consideration, but increasing sinus rate may not result in increased AV conduction.

SECOND-DEGREE AV BLOCK

In **second-degree AV block**, one or more sinus impulses fail to reach the ventricles, thus the descriptive term *intermittent*. Sometimes the impulse is conducted and sometimes it is not. When sinus beats are conducted the PR may be normal or prolonged but *always the same when the cycle resumes;* that is, the first sinus conducted beat after the drop. First, plot out the cadence of the P waves to differentiate between a nonconducted PAC and an AV block. In the AV conduction defects, sinus P waves will plot through.

Second-degree AV block is categorized as one of two types: Type I and Type II. However, the clinician must bear in mind that the designation of Type I and Type II second-degree AV block is based on *patterns seen on the ECG*, not on the physiologic site of the block. The clinician should determine the site of the pathology before attempting treatment of the patient.

SECOND-DEGREE AV BLOCK TYPE I (MOBITZ I)

Type I, also termed **Wenckebach** or **Mobitz,** is characterized on the ECG by the progressive prolongation of the PR interval (specifically the PR segment) until a P wave does not conduct, causing a pause in the rhythm. The cycle then recurs so that there are groups that make up this phenomenon. The greatest increase usually occurs with the second PR in the group. RR intervals decrease progressively despite the increasing PR intervals.

Type I AV block frequently involves the AV node; however, there are instances when the disease is infranodal, within the His bundle or within the proximal portions of the bundle branches.

The QRS complex is within normal limits when the defect is nodal or within the His bundle. When the disease is below the His bundle, the QRS complex is wider or of a specific configuration reflecting bundle branch or fascicular block and a 12-lead ECG is necessary to confirm the problem (see Chapter 11).

ECG Characteristics

- *P Wave:* The P waves are positive, uniform, and plot out. The sinus rate is usually within normal limits.
- *PR Interval:* There is a progressive increase in PR interval until one P wave is blocked. The PR interval after the blocked beat may be normal or prolonged, but it will be consistent (Wenckebach periodicity).
- *QRS Complex:* The QRS complex duration is 0.10 second or less.
- *QRS Rate:* The ventricular rate will be less than the sinus rate because of the non-conducted sinus P waves.
- *QRS Rhythm:* The ventricular rhythm is irregular because of the progressive shortening of the RR interval and the block. The RR interval that includes the blocked P wave is usually less than twice the normal cycle length.
- *Wenckebach Periodicity:* The cycle may repeat itself with variations in the numbers of conducted beats. This results in groups that begin and end with a P wave, called *Wenckebach periodicity* or the *Wenckebach phenomenon.*

In summary, second-degree Type I AV block with Wenckebach periodicity is characterized by the following:

- There is group beating.
- The group begins and ends with a P wave.
- There is one more P wave than QRSs within the group.
- The PR after the missed QRS is the same regardless of the numbers of PQRST complexes in the group.
- The greatest increase in the PR interval occurs within the second PR interval of the group.
- There are irregular or decreasing RR intervals.

Figure 10.2 and **Figure 10.3** are ECG tracings showing sinus rhythm with second-degree AV block Type I Wenckebach.

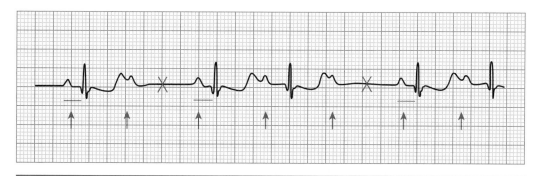

Figure 10.2 In this ECG tracing, first plot out the P waves and determine these are not blocked PACs. Note that after the missed QRS complex, the PR interval is the same. The QRS in each example is within normal limits. The PR interval is progressively longer until the sinus P does not conduct into the ventricles. The *X* indicates the dropped QRS complexes. There is group beating and the group begins and ends with a P wave. The ECG interpretation would be sinus at 86 per minute; ventricular rate range of 43–86 per minute; second-degree AV block, Type I Wenckebach; QRS at 0.08 second.

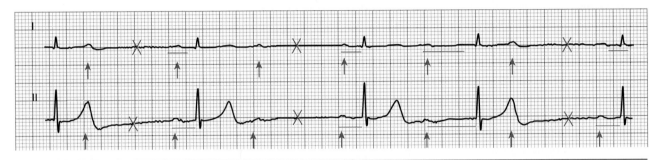

Figure 10.3 An ECG tracing in two leads showing second-degree AV block. The P waves plot through. The PR lengthens progressively, but the PR is constant after the missed beat. The *X* indicates the dropped QRS complexes. The QRS is within normal limits at 0.08 second. There is group beating. The ECG interpretation would be sinus at 67 per minute with second-degree AV block, Type I Wenckebach; QRS at 0.04–0.06 second, ventricular rate 30–57 per minute. Note that one PR interval measures 0.60 second. This is not junctional escape—it is an example of the extent of the conduction delay in this patient.

Causes

The causes of second-degree AV block Type I are

- Increased vagal tone, such as in athletes or during sleep.
- Cardiomyopathy.
- Autoimmune or inflammatory conditions, such as neonatal lupus erythematosus, myocarditis, endocarditis, Lyme disease, and rheumatic fever.
- Drug toxicity from medications or other substances also frequently causes second-degree AV block. These include excessive doses of digoxin, beta-blockers, calcium channel blockers, and Vaughan-Williams Class III agents (e.g., sotalol, amiodarone).
- Thyrotoxicosis is a cause possibly exacerbated by beta-blocker therapy.
- Hypothyroidism, either primary or drug induced.
- Inferior wall myocardial infarction.

Intervention

Early reperfusion usually resolves and sinus rhythm should return. However, until reperfusion can be accomplished, and if the block is accompanied by hypotension and hypoperfusion, transcutaneous or transvenous pacing may be indicated. The use of atropine may provoke a higher degree of AV block. Pressors may be a consideration if electronic pacing does not improve perfusion.

SECOND-DEGREE AV BLOCK TYPE II (MOBITZ II)

Type II AV block is characterized *on the ECG* by a constant PR interval following a blocked P wave. Conducted P waves may display a normal QRS complex if the site of block is within the bundle of His, or more commonly, a bundle branch block pattern if it is more distal. When the pathology in Type II is usually below the AV node and the term **infranodal** is often used again, to describe the *anatomic location* of the block. Remember, *Type II* and *Mobitz II* refer to an *ECG pattern*. It is best to describe the pattern, including sinus and ventricular rates, the PR interval. the duration, and morphology of the QRS complex.

A hallmark of this type of second-degree AV block is that the PR interval does not lengthen before a dropped beat. More than one nonconducted sinus beat may occur in succession.

ECG Characteristics

- *P Wave:* The P waves are positive, uniform, and plot out. The sinus rate is usually within normal limits.
- *PR Interval:* This interval may be normal or prolonged, but it will remain consistent.
- *QRS Complex:* Duration is greater than 0.10 second when the block is infranodal and below the bundle of His. The QRS complex may present as rS, rsR', or a broad, notched QRS when involving the bundle branch system. When the QRS suggests fascicular or bundle branch block a 12-lead ECG should be taken to clarify the site of the defect.
- *QRS Rate:* The ventricular rate will be less than the sinus rate because of the non-conducted P waves.
- *QRS Rhythm:* The ventricular rhythm is most often irregular, with pauses corresponding to the nonconducted beats.

Figure 10.4A and **Figure 10.4B** are examples of second-degree AV Type II. Note that the sinus rate is faster than the ventricular response and the PR intervals are consistent.

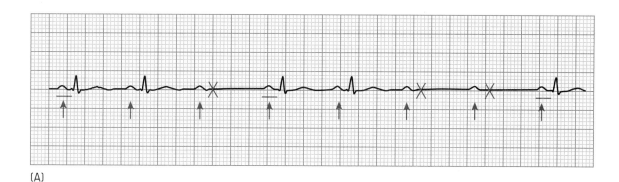

(A)

Figure 10.4A An example of second-degree Type II. The sinus rate is 75 per minute and the ventricular response is 27–75 per minute. The *X* marks the missing QRS complexes. The PR intervals are consistent at 0.18 second. There is no Wenckebach periodicity. The QRS complex is 0.08 second. The interpretation would be sinus at 75 per minute, ventricular rate 27–75, second-degree AV block probably Type II, and QRS at 0.08 second.

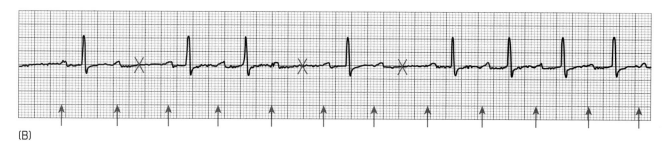

(B)

Figure 10.4B An example of second-degree AV block. Note that the PR intervals (0.36 second) are consistent. There is no Wenckebach periodicity. Sinus rate is 75 per minute.. The ventricular rate range is 40–75 per minute, with the QRS at 0.08 second. This is an example of Type II. There were four conflicting interpretations to this tracing.

Causes

Anterior wall myocardial infarction (AWMI) is the primary cause of Type II AV conduction defects. Second-degree AV block Type II is clinically significant because it is

- Often associated with pathology and accompanied with a fall in cardiac output
- Often associated with Stokes-Adams syncope
- A precursor of and often deteriorates into complete AV block dependent on a ventricular escape pacemaker, which will be too slow and unreliable to maintain systemic perfusion

Intervention

Often the patient presents with syncope and/or near-syncopal episodes. Temporary transcutaneous or transvenous pacing is in order. If indeed the patient is subsequently diagnosed with fibrotic disease, permanent pacing may be the treatment of choice.

2:1 BLOCK

A 2:1 block cannot be classified as either Type I or Type II because only one PR interval is available for analysis before the block. However, careful analysis of the PR interval can provide information that may help define the source of the problem.

ECG Characteristics

- *P Wave:* The P waves are positive, uniform, and plot out. The sinus rate is usually within normal limits.
- *PR Interval:* This interval may be normal or prolonged, but it will remain consistent.
    - If the PR of the conducted beat is 0.18 second or less, the block may be below the AV node.
    - If the PR interval of the conducted beat is greater than 0.28 second, the block may be within the AV node.
- *QRS Complex:* Duration may be greater than 0.10 second when the block is infranodal or below the bundle of His. The QRS complex morphology may be an rS, an rsR′, or a broad, notched QRS when involving the bundle branch system. When the QRS suggests fascicular or bundle branch block a 12-lead ECG should be taken to clarify the concern.
- *QRS Rate:* The ventricular rate will be one-half the sinus rate because of the nonconducted P waves.
- *QRS Rhythm:* The ventricular rhythm is regular.

Figure 10.5A and **Figure 10-5B** are ECG examples of 2:1 block.

ADVANCED OR HIGH-GRADE AV BLOCK

Second-degree **advanced** (or high-grade) **AV block** can be interpreted when the sinus rate is reasonable, but two or more consecutive sinus impulses are not conducted and the conducted P waves have consistent PR intervals. Again, it is best to describe the pattern and include the sinus and ventricular rates as well as the duration and morphology of the QRS complex.

Figure 10.6 is an ECG tracing showing a sinus mechanism with two consecutive non-conducted P waves. In this example, the P waves plot through regularly. Where there is a missed QRS complex, the PR after the missed beat is constant.

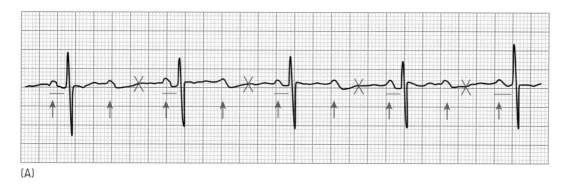

(A)

Figure 10.5A An ECG with a sinus rate at 100 per minute with a ventricular response at 50 per minute and the PR intervals consistent at 0.16 second. The ECG interpretation should be sinus at 100 per minute, ventricular rate at 50 per minute (2:1 block), with consistent PR interval at 0.16 second and QRS at 0.08 second.

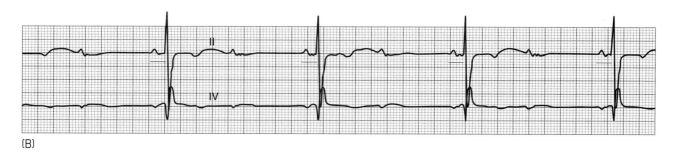

(B)

Figure 10.5B In this ECG you can see the sinus rate is twice the ventricular. The P waves plot out and the PR is consistent. This is an example of second-degree AV block (2:1). A 12-lead ECG is necessary to confirm the site of the conduction defect. The interpretation would be second-degree AV block 2:1, sinus rate 57, ventricular rate 28, a fixed PR of 0.16 second, QRS at 0.16 second, with a broad terminal S wave in lead II and an inverted T wave.

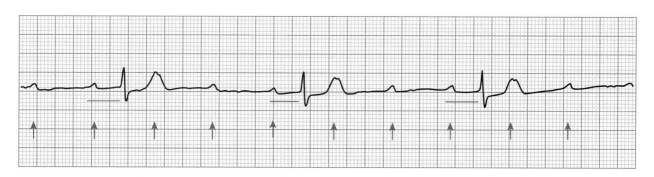

Figure 10.6 An ECG tracing illustrating advanced or high-grade AV block. The sinus rate is 86 per minute; the ventricular rate is 30 per minute. There are two P waves that do not conduct. The conducted beats have consistent PR intervals. The ECG interpretation would be sinus at 86 per minute with second-degree AV block, ventricular rate at 30 per minute; QRS is 0.08 second.

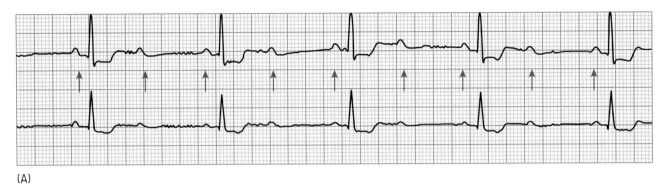

(A)

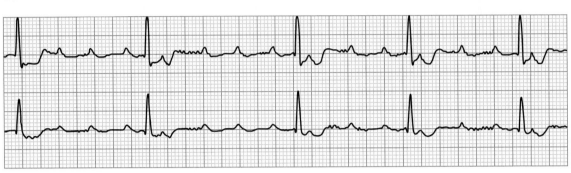

(B)

Figure 10.7 (A) The ECG shows the sinus rate that is twice that of the ventricular response. The PR interval is consistent at 0.20 second. The interpretation would be second degree AV block, atrial rate 86/minute, ventricular rate 43/minute with 2:1 conduction, QRS = 0.08 second. (B) The patient received atropine and while the atrial rate increased (150/minute), the ventricular rate range changed to 37–48/minute and the PR interval was prolonged.

Intervention

Interpretation should not be focused solely on a single ECG monitoring lead. Assessment using a multiple lead ECG (and an in-hospital His-bundle ECG) correlated with patient presentation and past medical and medication history is crucial to safe patient interventions.

Prematurely treating with agents that will increase the sinus rate may not increase AV conduction. In fact, the use of such agents can result in rapid sinus rates with complete AV block or provoke the use of accessory pathways, and cause abnormal ventricular conduction and possibly ventricular tachycardia.

Patients with any form of second-degree AV block complicated with a bradycardia who are hypotensive and hypoperfusing should be considered for transcutaneous or transvenous pacing while further investigation continues for a transient or reversible cause. Patients with a structural heart disorder will probably benefit from an implanted pacemaker.

Figure 10.7A and **Figure 10.7B** are ECG tracings reportedly from a patient who received atropine because of the bradycardia. Note the change in sinus rate and the PR interval.

Too often ECG phrases and patterns without a thorough analysis of the ECG can lead to errors in judgment. For example, **Figure 10.8** is an example of the hazards of hasty interpretation. At first glance the rhythm was identified as an "obvious Wenckebach Type I moving into 2:1 which we know is Type II so you can see that the site of the defect has changed." This is an example of a very common mistake of assuming that all 2:1 is Type II. The tracings are continuous and in (A), plotting out the P waves reveals that as the sinus rate increases there is progressive decrease in AV conduction (Wenckebach periodicity). In (B) the sinus

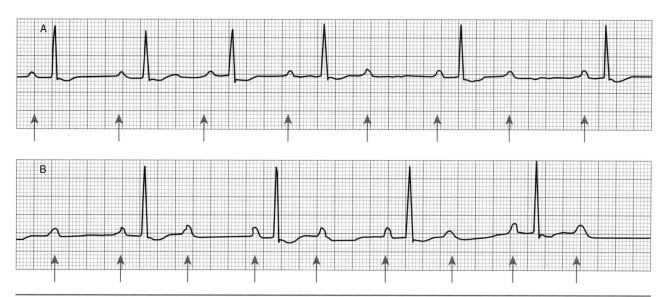

Figure 10.8 An example of incorrect interpretation. The strips are continuous. The rhythm was first identified as an "obvious Wenckebach Type I moving into 2:1 Type II...... the site of the defect has changed." Carefully examine the ECG: in tracing (A). Plotting out the P waves and the PR intervals reveals a sinus rate of 60 bpm; however, when the sinus rate increased to 73/minute, there was a decrease in conduction. The ventricular rate range changed from 60 to 37 bpm. The bottom tracing (B) show sinus continuing at 73/minute, second-degree AV block, 2:1 conduction, a ventricular rate at 39 bpm.

rate continues but AV conduction does not improve, giving rise to 2:1 conduction. Given the top tracing, the evidence supports this as Type I. The patient did not change the site of his conduction defect.

Table 10.2 summarizes ECG configuration in Type I and Type II second-degree AV blocks.

Type I Wenckebach or Mobitz	Type II
Pathology is AV nodal if PR of the conducted beat is >0.28 sec.	Pathology is infranodal if the PR of the conducted beat is ≤0.18 sec.
Associated with IWMI, digitalis, and chronic AV lesions.	Lesion is infranodal.
Nature is ischemic, reversible, sometimes transient.	Associated with AWMI or chronic lesions within the bundle branch system.
P waves plot though; PR interval may prolong prior to the missing QRS; PR after the dropped QRS is constant.	P waves plot through; dropped QRS is preceded by a fixed PR interval.
Ventricular rhythm can be regular or irregular (Wenckebach periodicity).	Ventricular rhythm can be regular or irregular.
In the presence of sinus bradycardia, usually responds to pharmacologic intervention.	Usually does not respond well to pharmacologic intervention and may provoke transition to complete AV block.
Rarely requires electronic pacing; however, pacing is preferred to pressors.	Usually requires electronic pacing.

Table 10.2 Summary of differences in pathology and ECG characteristics and interventions in Types I and II second-degree AV block.

COMPLETE AV BLOCK

Pathology involved in AV block can progress in severity until all the sinus impulses are completely blocked or may be the first occurrence and an indication the patient has a conduction defect. Regardless of the site of the lesion, there is no conduction through to the ventricles; there is *no* PR interval. The patient presentation will reflect the bradycardia and diminished cardiac output. When the disease is infranodal or a result of anterior wall myocardial infarction, the patient is subject to hemodynamic compromise, and syncopal and near-syncopal episodes are common occurrences. Hypoperfusion with this arrhythmia is the rule rather than the exception. Hence, rapid intervention with electronic pacing is usually necessary to manage these patients. Any patient with a history of unexpected episodes of falling or syncopal and near-syncopal episodes should be assessed for complete AV block, particularly in the aging population.

In **complete AV block,** the sinus rate is different, faster, and *independent* of the ventricular rate. There is no relationship between P and QRS; thus there is *no* PR interval. The atria, remaining under the control of the SA node, or in atrial flutter or fibrillation, are beating at their own intrinsic rate and are completely dissociated from the ventricles.

ECG Characteristics

The ECG characteristics of complete AV block are as follows:

- *P Wave:* The P waves are positive and uniform in lead II and are not associated with the QRS complexes. The sinus rate is independent and faster than the escape ventricular rate.
- *PR Interval:* Since there is no relationship between the P waves and the QRS complexes, there is *no* PR interval to measure.
- *QRS Complex:* Depending on the site of impulse formation, the QRS complex duration may be normal, with the pacemaker in the AV junction, or greater than 0.12 second with the QRS opposite in direction from the T wave, when the pacemaker is from the ventricle.
- *QRS Rate:* When complete AV block occurs at the level of the AV node (nodal), an escape junctional rhythm will usually take over and control the ventricular rate at 40 to 60 beats per minute. When complete AV block occurs below the His bundle (infranodal), the ventricular rhythm will be controlled by a ventricular escape mechanism ranging between 20 and 40 beats per minute.
- *QRS Rhythm:* The ventricular rhythm is regular since the escape pacemaker is from the AV junction or an escape ventricular focus.

The patient presentation is a good clue to the site of the disease. Patients with a junctional escape rhythm usually have adequate rate and perfusion, whereas patients with idioventricular rhythm are clearly compromised.

Figure 10.9A, **Figure 10.9B**, and **Figure 10.9C** are examples of complete AV block.

Causes

Complete AV block is caused by progressive fibrotic disease within the AV node, or with inferior or anterior wall myocardial infarction. In atrial fibrillation with complete AV block, the cause is usually medication induced (see Chapter 8).

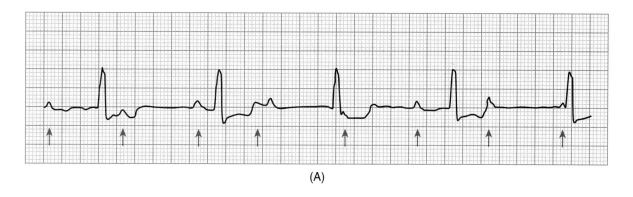

(A)

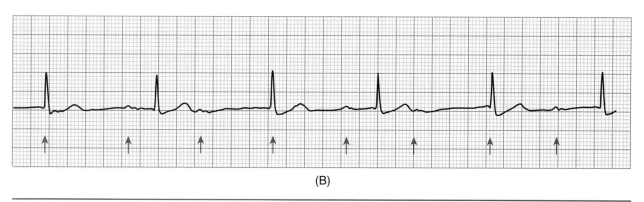

(B)

Figure 10.9A and Figure 10.9B These ECG tracings are examples of complete AV block. In (A), sinus rate is 75 per minute and the independent ventricular rate is 50 per minute. In (B), the sinus rate is 75 per minute and ventricular rate is 50 per minute. Both are examples of complete AV block—that is, the sinus and ventricular rates are independent of each other (AV dissociation).

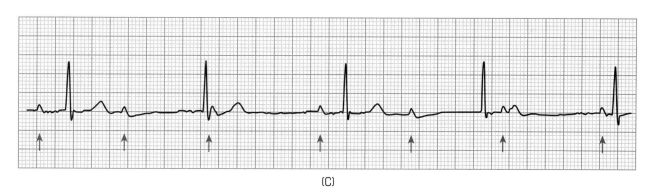

(C)

Figure 10.9C An ECG illustrating complete AV block, probably at the level of the AV node since the QRS is 0.06 second. The sinus rate, although irregular, is faster than the QRS rate, and the P waves and QRS complexes are independent of each other. There are no consistent PR intervals, and the ventricular rhythm is regular. This is an example of AV dissociation. The ECG interpretation would be sinus at 50 per minute with complete AV block, a junctional rhythm with a ventricular rate at 40 per minute.

Table 10.3 summarizes the ECG configurations in AV block.

	First-Degree AV Block	Second-Degree AV Block Type I* (Wenckebach or Mobitz Type I)	Second-Degree AV Block 2:1*	Second-Degree AV Block Type II* (Mobitz Type II)	Complete AV Block
	Every P has a QRS	**Missing a QRS**	**Missing a QRS**	**Missing a QRS**	**AV dissociation***
P wave		(+) P wave/QRS	(+) P wave/QRS	(+) P wave/QRS	Independent and regular
PR interval	>0.20 sec	Progressively prolonged PRI after the missed QRS is the same (constant)	Can be < or > than 0.20 sec PRI after the missed QRS is the same (constant)	Can be < or > than 0.20 sec PRI after the missed QRS is the same (constant)	No PR interval
QRS complex	≤0.10 sec usually**	<0.10 sec usually**	≤0.10 sec usually**	>0.10 sec usually	≤0.10 sec with junctional escape >0.10 sec with ventricular escape
QRS rate	Same as sinus rate	Ventricular rate slower than sinus	Ventricular rate slower than sinus	Ventricular rate slower than sinus	Ventricular rate slower than sinus
QRS rhythm	Regular	Irregular Group beating	Regular	Regular or irregular	Regular

Table 10.3 Summary of the ECG characteristics in AV block.
*Misses a QRS. The PR after the missed QRS is constant.
** In the absence of preexisting BBB.
***P waves are independent of QRS complex in rate and rhythm.

SUMMARY

The AV conduction defects are categorized as first-, second-, and complete AV block. First-degree AV block presents as a fixed PR interval greater than 0.20 second, with the segment being prolonged. There may be disease within the AV junction, usually within the AV node.

Second-degree AV block is divided into Type I (Wenckebach or Mobitz I), Type II (Mobitz II), 2:1 conduction, and advanced. In Type I there is group beating, with lengthening PR intervals. The PR intervals are constant after the missing QRS. The sinus rhythm is regular while the ventricular rate is slower and irregular. The group begins and ends with the sinus P wave.

Type II usually presents with a QRS greater than 0.20 second and a configuration that represents intraventricular conduction delay. The PR after the missed QRS is constant and may be normal or prolonged. Type 2:1 occurs without warning, no group beating, and no two conducted P waves in a sequence, and the lesion could be in the AV node, with the His bundle or the penetrating portions of the bundle branch system. A wide QRS complex suggests Type II. Twelve-lead ECG is necessary for correct interpretation and identification of the defect. Advanced AV block by definition is when two or more consecutive P waves are not conducted. Again, assessment of the QRS morphology and 12-lead ECG is necessary. In all instances, patient assessment with detailed attention to patient history and presentation is critical.

Complete AV block is characterized by complete inability of sinus impulses to conduct through to the ventricles. There is independent function so that P waves plot through, there is *no* PR interval, and the ventricles are under control of either a junctional or ventricular escape rhythm.

Interpretation of the ECGs for the AV blocks must include sinus and ventricular rates, as well as QRS duration and configuration and 12-lead ECG for confirmation.

Self-Assessment Exercises
Fill in the Blanks

Complete the second and third columns, and then compare your answers with those in Appendix A.

Block Type I	Sinus Rhythm	First-Degree AV Block	Second-Degree AV
P wave	1 (+) P wave/QRS	1 (+) P wave/QRS	_____
PR interval	0.12–0.20 sec	>0.20 sec	_____
QRS complex	≤0.10 sec	≤0.10 sec	_____
QRS rate	60–100/min	_____	_____
QRS rhythm	Regular	_____	_____

Complete the second and third columns, and then compare your answers with those in Appendix A.

Block Type II	Sinus Rhythm	Complete AV Block	Second-Degree AV
P wave	1 (+) P wave/QRS	Sinus Ps plot through	_____
PR interval	0.12–0.20 sec	No PRI	_____
QRS complex	≤0.10 sec	≤0.10 sec	_____
QRS rate	60–100/min	_____	_____
QRS rhythm	Regular	_____	_____

ECG Rhythm Identification Practice

For the following rhythms, fill in the blanks and then compare your answers with those in Appendix A.

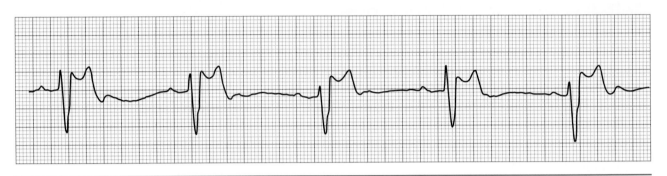

Figure 10.10

1. QRS duration _____
2. QT interval _____
3. Ventricular rate/rhythm _____
4. Atrial rate/rhythm _____
5. PR interval _____
6. Identification _____
7. Symptoms _____
8. Treatment _____

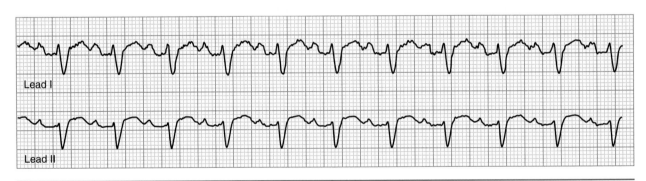

Lead I

Lead II

Figure 10.11

1. QRS duration _____
2. QT interval _____
3. Ventricular rate/rhythm _____
4. Atrial rate/rhythm _____
5. PR interval _____
6. Identification _____
7. Symptoms _____
8. Treatment _____

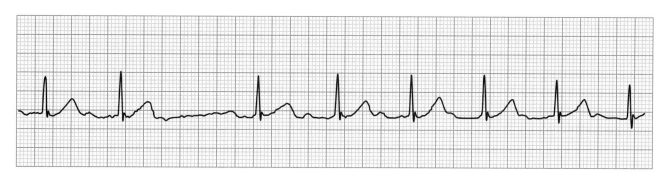

Figure 10.12

1. QRS duration _____
2. QT interval _____
3. Ventricular rate/rhythm _____
4. Atrial rate/rhythm _____
5. PR interval _____
6. Identification _____
7. Symptoms _____
8. Treatment _____

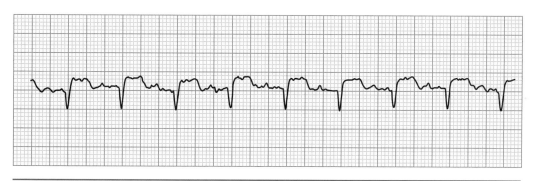

Figure 10.13

1. QRS duration _____
2. QT interval _____
3. Ventricular rate/rhythm _____
4. Atrial rate/rhythm _____
5. PR interval _____
6. Identification _____
7. Symptoms _____
8. Treatment _____

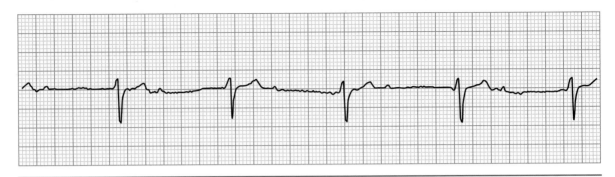

Figure 10.14

1. QRS duration _____
2. QT interval _____
3. Ventricular rate/rhythm _____
4. Atrial rate/rhythm _____
5. PR interval _____
6. Identification _____
7. Symptoms _____
8. Treatment _____

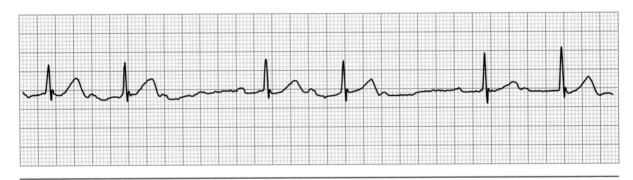

Figure 10.15

1. QRS duration _____
2. QT interval _____
3. Ventricular rate/rhythm _____
4. Atrial rate/rhythm _____
5. PR interval _____
6. Identification _____
7. Symptoms _____
8. Treatment _____

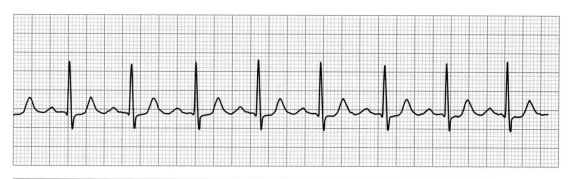

Figure 10.16

1. QRS duration _____
2. QT interval _____
3. Ventricular rate/rhythm _____
4. Atrial rate/rhythm _____
5. PR interval _____
6. Identification _____
7. Symptoms _____
8. Treatment _____

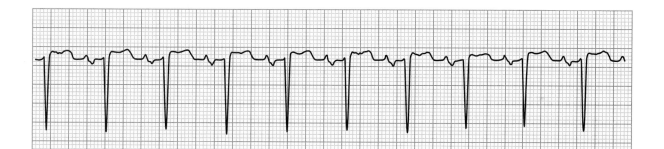

Figure 10.17

1. QRS duration _____
2. QT interval _____
3. Ventricular rate/rhythm _____
4. Atrial rate/rhythm _____
5. PR interval _____
6. Identification _____
7. Symptoms _____
8. Treatment _____

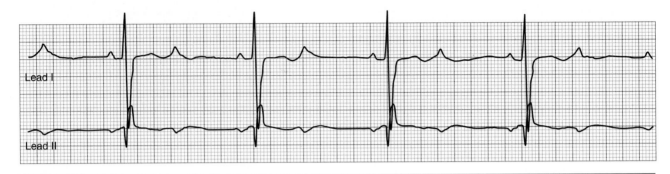

Figure 10.18

1. QRS duration _____
2. QT interval _____
3. Ventricular rate/rhythm _____
4. Atrial rate/rhythm _____
5. PR interval _____
6. Identification _____
7. Symptoms _____
8. Treatment _____

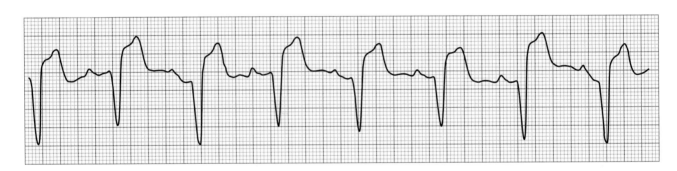

Figure 10.19

1. QRS duration _____
2. QT interval _____
3. Ventricular rate/rhythm _____
4. Atrial rate/rhythm _____
5. PR interval _____
6. Identification _____
7. Symptoms _____
8. Treatment _____

Intraventricular Conduction Defects

Premise

The levels of the ventricular conduction system can be easily tracked using the 12-lead ECG.

Objectives

After reading the chapter and completing the Self-Assessment Exercise, the student should be able to

- Identify the arterial perfusion of the bundle branches.
- Identify the ECG changes in right bundle branch block.
- Identify the ECG changes in left anterior and left posterior fascicular block.
- Identify the ECG changes in bifascicular block.
- List the clinical implications for each of the ventricular conduction defects.

Key Terms

bifascicular block	fascicular block	trifascicular block
bundle branch block	hemiblock	ventricular activation
fascicle	intrinsicoid deflection	time (VAT)

Introduction

An intraventricular conduction defect is the result of impaired conduction of electrical impulses through one or more of the divisions of the intraventricular conduction system. The primary conduction pathways that make up the intraventricular conduction system are the right bundle branch and the left main branch. The left main bundle, also known as the common left bundle, divides into bundles of fibers called a fascicle. The primary fascicles are the left anterior (LAF) and left posterior fascicle (LPF). The septal fibers that extend from the left main branch vary in length and breadth, and are not recognized as comprising a true fascicle. **Figure 11.1** illustrates the intraventricular conduction system.

When conduction through one or more of the bundle branches is impaired, there is a delay in the conduction pattern. One or parts of the ventricle can depolarize out of normal sequence, the ramifications of which include abnormal ventricular wall motion.

To understand the implications of **bundle branch block**, it is critical to know the anatomy of the intraventricular conduction system and the arterial supply to the right and left bundle branches. Bundle branch block of any kind can occur without infarction. However, if

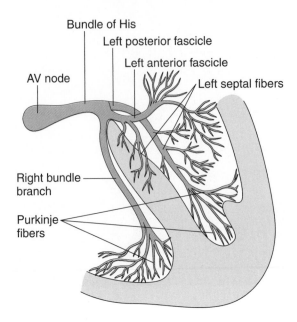

Bundle of His

Left posterior fascicle

Left anterior fascicle

Left septal fibers

AV node

Right bundle branch

Purkinje fibers

Figure 11.1 Illustration of the conduction system from the AV node through to the His-Purkinje fibers.

a patient presents with a myocardial infarction and the dominant blood vessel to the electrical conduction system is affected, the clinician should be able to anticipate the intraventricular conduction defects, predict the implications, and prepare accordingly.

THE BUNDLE BRANCHES AND ARTERIAL PERFUSION

Recall that the right bundle branch is a long fiber that begins at the level of the bundle of His and threads through the intraventricular septum to the base of the anterior papillary muscle of the right ventricle. The left anterior descending coronary artery perfuses the anterior myocardium and the anterior two-thirds of the septum. Its septal branch perfuses the proximal right bundle branch and the anterior division of the left bundle branch.

The left bundle branch divides into two primary fascicles: anterior and posterior. The more distal anterior fascicle has its origin in the bundle of His and threads through to the anterior superior endocardial surface and to the papillary muscle of the mitral valve. The anterior fascicle receives blood from the left anterior descending coronary artery and the right coronary artery (RCA). The posterior fascicle also has its origin in the bundle of His and runs from the bundle to the posterior papillary muscle of the left ventricle. Perfusion to the posterior fascicle is by the RCA. The perforating arteries of the left anterior descending coronary artery also perfuse the posterior fascicle.

The RCA is responsible for perfusion to the posterior one-third of the septum. The AV nodal branch of the RCA perfuses the AV node and the bundle of His. As a result, occlusion in anterior wall myocardial infarction is a common cause of right bundle branch block (RBBB) while the left bundle branch block (LBBB) is seen with anterior wall myocardial infarction.

Arterial occlusion is one cause of a conduction disorder occurring in the bundle branch system. If the occlusion is not complete, the resulting ECG may show signs and symptoms of intermittent conduction defects. However, one of the more common causes of LBBB is longstanding left ventricular hypertrophy with resulting thickening of heart muscle. Common causes of left ventricular hypertrophy include hypertensive heart disease, valvular heart disease, and as a sequela to open-heart surgery.

The presence of axis deviation on the ECG is recognized by many investigators as associated with delayed activation of tissue surrounding or near the infarcted area. The clinical significance of this phenomenon is the risk of sustained ventricular tachycardia.

NORMAL SEQUENCE OF VENTRICULAR DEPOLARIZATION AND THE QRS VECTOR

Impulse propagation, usually from the sinus node, results in depolarization of the ventricular muscle and is responsible for the various components of the QRS vector—the wave form of depolarization. The first portion of the ventricular muscle to be activated is the junction of the middle and lower segments of the interventricular septum on the endocardial surface of the left ventricle. This depolarization wave causes vectorial forces that are oriented anteriorly, to the right, and superiorly or inferiorly. There is a counterclockwise rotation in the horizontal and left sagittal planes and a variable rotation in the frontal plane. From this point, the activation front proceeds rapidly toward the apex of the heart, speaking to both the right and left ventricular surfaces.

Because the left ventricle has greater muscle mass than the right, the depolarization forces responsible for activation of the left ventricle dominate the electrical field of the heart. As a result, the activation process is oriented primarily posteriorly, inferiorly, and to the left, corresponding to the anatomical position of the left ventricle. Simultaneous depolarization of the right and left free walls occurs well into the inscription of the QRS complex.

It is important to reemphasize that activation of the left ventricle is the result of impulse transmission through the two main branches of the left bundle, which has a short main trunk and bifurcates early into the anterior and posterior divisions or fascicles. The anterior branch provides conduction fibers to the anterior-superior aspects of the left ventricle and the posterior branch provides conduction fibers to the posterior-inferior aspects of the left ventricle. As the activation wave spreads inferiorly and posteriorly through the branches of the left bundle, it causes a simultaneous depolarization of the inferior and lateral aspects of the left ventricle.

Anatomically, the right bundle is a single trunk that bifurcates late into the Purkinje fibers. Occasionally, the time for completion of the left and right ventricular activation is not identical; in the majority of cases this is due to late activation of the outflow tract of the right ventricle or of the upper third of the interventricular septum. This disparity in the activation process may cause some vectorial forces that are oriented anteriorly and to the right. This is reflected on the ECG by the presence of an R′ in lead V_1 and a small S wave in leads V_5 or V_6. However, this pattern should not be interpreted as representative of a conduction abnormality of the right bundle or incomplete RBBB as it is a normal event.

The entire ventricular activation process takes about 100 milliseconds or 0.10 second. **Figure 11.2** illustrates the sequence of ventricular activation with QRS vectors superimposed from 10 to 100 milliseconds.

ECG CHANGES IN BUNDLE BRANCH BLOCK

In bundle branch block, the ST segment and T wave are usually in the opposite direction from the terminal portion of the QRS complex, primarily because repolarization of the ventricles is severely disturbed by this conduction defect. When bundle branch block is

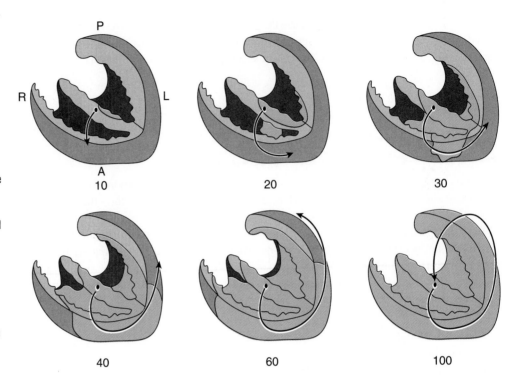

Figure 11.2 Sequence of ventricular activation as seen in the horizontal plane with QRS vectors superimposed at 10, 20, 30, 40, 60, and 100 milliseconds. From the point of view of lead II, the Q wave occurs over 10 to 20 milliseconds; the R wave over the next 30 to 40 milliseconds; and the S wave over the remaining 60 to 100 milliseconds. From the point of view of lead V_1, the small initial R wave occurs over 10 to 20 milliseconds and a negative S wave over the next 30 to 100 milliseconds. The progressive clearing in each model corresponds to the segments of myocardium that are being depolarized. (A = anterior; P = posterior; R = right; and L = left.)

confirmed, these changes are called secondary T waves. On the other hand, segments and T waves that are the same polarity as the terminal portion of the QRS are called primary ST-T-wave changes, and indicate myocardial ischemia.

Rate-Related Bundle Branch Block. Occasionally, when heart rate increases as with stress testing, for example, bundle branch block will occur at a particular rate. In this case, the bundle branch may still be in a refractory period and unable to conduct the increased rate of incoming impulses normally. Rate-related bundle branch block is usually transient and once the heart rate returns to a normal, slower pace, the QRS will appear normal at 0.10 second. This a called rate-dependent (or rate-related) bundle branch block. Rate-dependent bundle branch block may be RBBB or LBBB. When it develops at a faster heart rate, it is referred to as tachycardia-dependent, and at a slower heart rate it is called as bradycardia-dependent. Rate-dependent bundle branch block is important because this entity has to be differentiated from patients who present with new-onset BBB in the course of myocardial ischemia, injury, and infarction.

Right Bundle Branch Block

Significant alterations in the sequence of right ventricular depolarization occur when impulse propagation through the right main bundle is interrupted. The initial spread of activation, however, is normal during the first 40 milliseconds. The initial 10 to 20 milliseconds of ventricular depolarization represent septal depolarization, which is normally oriented to the right and anteriorly, because this area is supplied by the conduction fibers from the left bundle. Therefore, in RBBB, the beginning of the QRS complex is usually unchanged. What this means is there is a small R wave present in V_1 as the wavefront crosses the septum. There is a small Q wave in V_6; normal activation of the left ventricle follows, producing an S wave in V_1 and an R wave in V_6. When the wave of electrical activity reaches the right bundle, the normal rapid conduction is halted. To depolarize the right ventricle, the impulse must travel through myocardial tissue rather than specialized conduction pathways. This takes time. Consequently, the QRS represents terminal conduction delay in the form of a late, broad R wave (R′) in V_6 and a broad S wave in leads I, III, V_5, and V_6. The triphasic rsR′ is seen in leads V_1 and V_6. **Figure 11.3** is a graphic illustration of and its associated ECG changes.

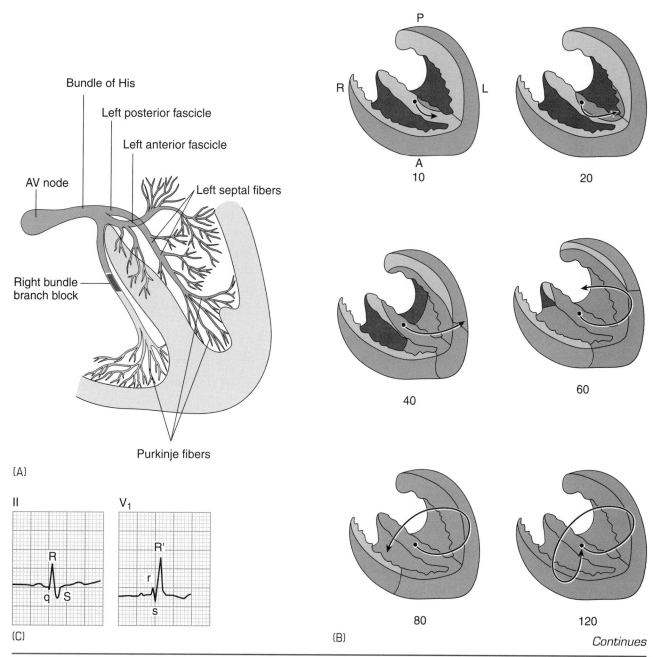

(A)

(C)

(B)

Continues

Figure 11.3 (A) Right bundle branch block; (B) shows the QRS complexes reflective of right bundle branch block; (C) shows the sequence of ventricular activation from 10 to 120 milliseconds. The QRS vector is superimposed on the heart with the corresponding cleared areas of the ventricles as they are being depolarized. Note the counterclockwise rotation of the QRS with delayed terminal appendage oriented anterior and to the right, occurring between 80 and 120 milliseconds. Also notice that completion of depolarization takes 120 milliseconds or 0.12 second; (D) is a 12-lead ECG of right bundle branch block, showing the changes in the QRS complex in leads V_1 and V_2. The QRS complex is prolonged, greater than 0.10 second. There is a broad terminal S wave (shaded) in leads I, II, aVL, V_5, and V_6. The inverted T waves (arrow) seen in right precordial leads V_1 to V_3 are secondary T-wave inversions.

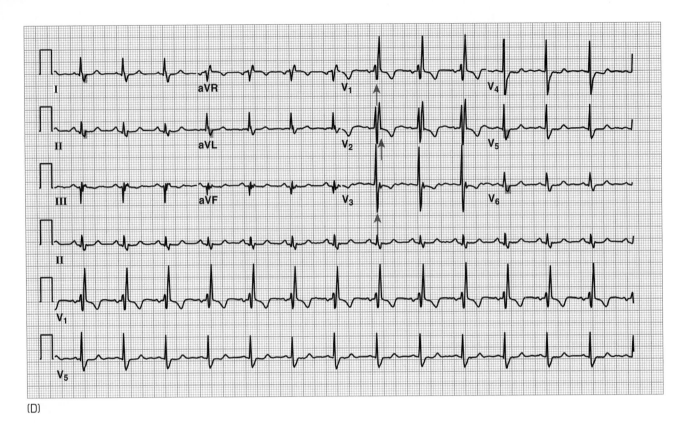

(D)

Figure 11.3 Continued

Causes of RBBB are:

- Acute heart failure
- Anterior myocardial infarction
- Cardiomyopathy
- Congenital lesions
- Ischemic RCA disease
- Legnegre's disease
- Lev's disease
- Normal variant
- Rheumatic heart disease
- Surgical correction of tetrology of Fallot
- Surgical correction of a ventricular septal defect
- Syphilis
- Trauma
- Tumors

Incomplete Right Bundle Branch Block. The term *complete bundle branch block* does not imply an irreversible condition. As previously discussed, RBBB can occur when related to an increase in activity and heart rate. When this happens, the morphology of RBBB remains but the QRS may be less than 0.12 second.

The clinical significance of incomplete right bundle branch block (IRBBB) remains controversial. ECG changes representative of IRBBB include:

- QRS complex less than 0.12 second
- rsR′ complex in V_1

IRBBB in conditioned athletes may be related to an increase in muscle mass at the tip of the right ventricle. Once the activity is discontinued, the ECG signs of IRBBB disappear. Of the reported 14 percent of athletes affected with this phenomenon, 10 percent are between 20 and 35 years old.

Right Bundle Branch Block and Acute Myocardial Infarction. RBBB ECG patterns do not conflict with the patterns of infarction. The initial forces of left-to-right septal activation are intact, so when an infarction occurs, the resulting Q waves and ST segment elevation are visible.

RBBB that occurs within days of anterior wall myocardial infarction has a high risk of progressing to involve left anterior fascicular block (LAFB) and complete AV block. If MCL_1 or V_1 are the monitoring leads, the progressive involvement of the left bundle will be missed, since fascicular block is only diagnosed in the limb leads. In the case of anterior wall infarction, it is difficult to determine if the RBBB is new or preexisting without obtaining previous records and 12-lead ECGs.

To summarize, ECG changes representative of RBBB include:

- QRS complex greater than 0.10 second, 0.12 second, or more
- Triphasic complex, Rsr' in V_1 and Qrs in V_6
- Small q and broad S waves (qS) in leads I, aVL, and V_6
- ST-T-wave changes

These changes in the terminal part of the QRS are all due to the late depolarization over right ventricular tissue.

Left Bundle Branch Block

Complete left bundle branch block (CLBBB) results when there is total interruption of transmission of the electrical impulse through the left main bundle or of the two main branches of the left bundle. LBBB is usually caused by occlusion in the left main branch or a simultaneous block in both anterior and posterior fascicles. It is usually the result of left anterior descending coronary artery disease. In LBBB, the normal wave of depolarization is altered.

The sequence of left ventricular activation is markedly altered. Transmission of the impulse to the left ventricle occurs through excitation of the right septal mass, which is supplied by branches of the right bundle. Thus, the activation wave crosses the intraventricular septum in a right-to-left direction. It follows, then, that the right ventricle depolarizes before the left. It is generally accepted that most of the conduction abnormalities of this type happen due to a delay in transmission across the intraventricular septum, as with anteroseptal myocardial infarction.

The normal septal Q wave is not recorded in leads I, V_5, and V_6 with the abnormal septal depolarization. If Q waves are recorded in the presence of LBBB, the possibility of concurrent problems such as infarction should be considered.

Recall the left bundle is thick and broad and has a blood supply from both right and left coronary arteries. Consequently, LBBB in a patient with diagnosed myocardial infarction usually reflects underlying heart disease because a very large lesion is required to block the left bundle branch. LBBB without underlying heart disease is very rare. **Figure 11.4** illustrates LBBB and its associated ECG changes.

Causes of LBBB include:

- Acute heart failure
- Acute myocardial infarction
- Cardiomyopathy

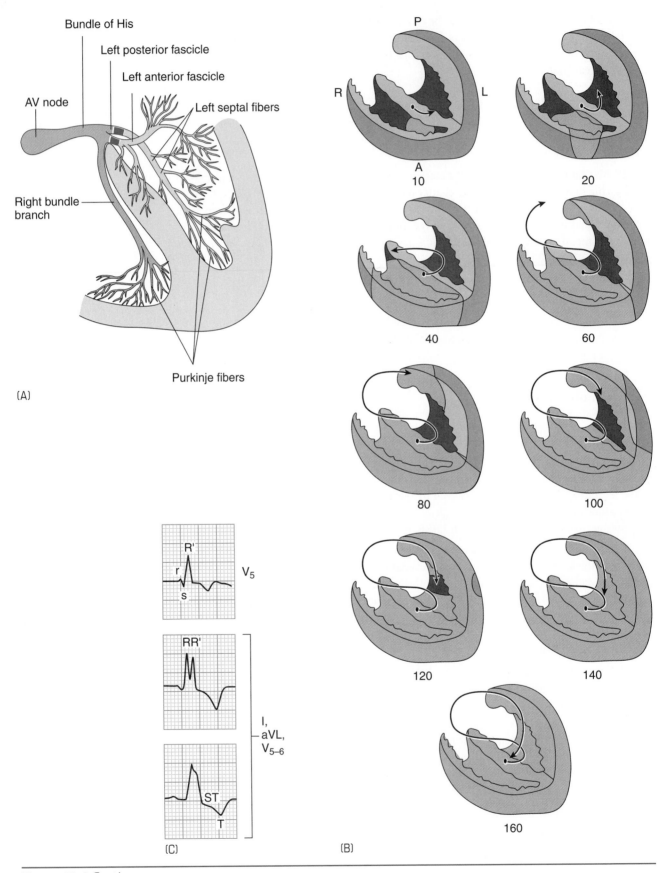

(A)

(B)

(C)

Figure 11.4 *Continues*

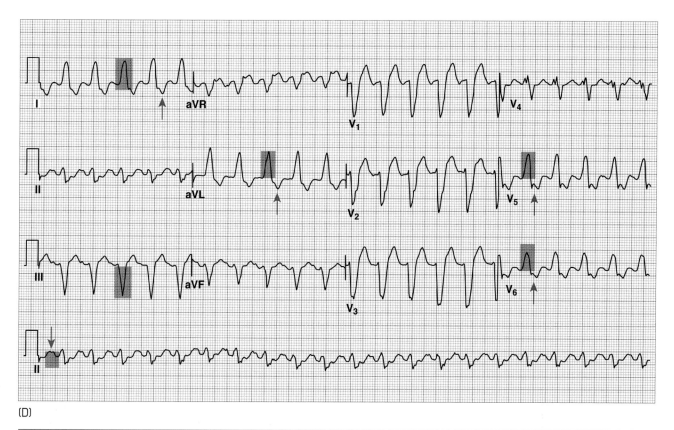

(D)

Figure 11.4 (A) Left bundle branch block. (B) The QRS complex that reflects the ECG changes associated with left bundle branch block is slurred and prolonged, greater than 0.12 second. (C) The sequence of ventricular activation from 10 to 160 milliseconds. The QRS vector is superimposed on the heart with the corresponding cleared areas of the ventricles as they are being depolarized. Note the near figure eight pattern reflecting the abnormal depolarization. Also note that completion of depolarization is 160 milliseconds or 0.16 second. (D) The broad, positive QRS complex in leads I, II, and aVL and the broad negative deflection in lead III reflect the direction of septal depolarization from right to left.

- Congenital lesions
- Ischemic LCA disease
- Legnegre's disease
- Lev's disease
- Rheumatic heart disease
- Syphilis
- Trauma
- Tumors

ECG criteria for diagnosing LBBB are:

- QRS greater than 0.12 second
- QS or rS complexes in V_1
- Monophasic R wave in V_5 and V_6
- Notched or slurred QRS
- No Q or S waves in leads I, aVL, or V_6
- Ventricular activation time that exceeds 0.02 second in V_1 and 0.04 second in V_6
- Secondary ST-T-wave changes in the left precordial leads V_5 and V_6

Incomplete Left Bundle Branch Block.

An ECG showing the pattern of left bundle branch block with a QRS of less than 0.12 second may indicate an incomplete left bundle branch block (ILBBB). However, cause for this type of conduction defect remains controversial. It has been suggested that LBBB occurs when transmission of the electrical impulse through the left main bundle is partially interrupted. This produces an abnormal sequence of ventricular activation, with the right ventricle activating slightly earlier than the left through the intact right bundle branch. This blockage causes various degrees of delay through the left bundle, resulting in degrees of abnormalities in the QRS vector. These are particularly evident during the initial 30 milliseconds, meaning that ventricular activation time is delayed.

The time from the beginning of the initial inscription of the QRS to the point where the impulse arrives under a particular electrode of a lead measure is called the **ventricular activation time (VAT)**. The corresponding deflection produced is called the **intrinsicoid deflection**. V_1 measures VAT for the right ventricle, which is normally 0.02 second because the right ventricle is thin-walled. It is measured from the beginning of the small R wave to the peak of that small R wave.

V_6 measures VAT for the left ventricle, which is usually 0.04 second. It is calculated from the beginning of the QRS to the peak of the R wave. Recall that the left ventricle is thicker than the right and it takes longer for the impulse to arrive under the V_6 electrode. In LBBB, the VAT exceeds 0.02 second in V_1 and 0.04 second in V_6. **Figure 11.5** shows the measurement of the ventricular activation time in V_1 and V_6.

Left Bundle Branch Block Resulting from Myocardial Infarction.

LBBB can result from arterial occlusion and concomitant with a myocardial infarction. Though left bundle branch block can be a preexisting disease, it most commonly occurs after anterior wall myocardial infarction.

In LBBB, septal activation has to be reversed. Recall that the left bundle branches are incapable of conduction; therefore, depolarization of the right ventricle appears first, followed by the left. Consequently, any Q waves that originate because of left ventricular problems are obscured. Without clear Q waves, it's really difficult to confirm the diagnosis of myocardial infarction.

Many clinicians believe that the ECG is not helpful in diagnosing an MI in the presence of LBBB. When LBBB is present, an upright T wave in V_5 and V_6 may indicate ischemia

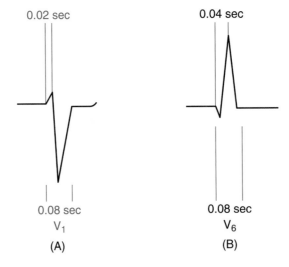

Figure 11.5 (A) VAT time for the right ventricle measured from the beginning of the QRS to the peak of the small R wave in V_1; (B) VAT time for the left ventricle measured from the beginning of the QRS to the peak of the R wave in V_6.

in that area. This is because the ST segment and T wave in LBBB are usually opposite in polarity from the terminal portion of the QRS (a secondary T wave). When the ST segment and T wave are of the same polarity of the terminal portion of the QRS, (a primary T wave), this is an acute sign of a possible ischemia. Therefore, with ECG changes of LBBB and positive T waves are present in a lead with a negative terminal QRS, the clinician must suspect an acute MI is in progress. Other ECG findings with LBBB and myocardial infarction are:

- Decrease in R wave amplitude over left ventricular leads
- Q waves in I, aVL, or V_6 greater than 0.04 second, which may indicate anteroseptal or lateral wall myocardial infarction
- ST segment and T-wave displacement, affecting the normal ST segment convex appearance

While these changes may be useful indicators, there is no way to diagnose an acute myocardial infarction in the presence of LBBB using the ECG. Nevertheless, the presence of LBBB should alert the clinician to the possibility of an MI. The patient who presents with acute chest pain, shortness of breath, diaphoresis, pallor, and all the clinical findings of an acute MI should be treated appropriately. In these circumstances, the ECG is a valuable tool that must be supported with clinical correlation.

FASCICULAR BLOCKS

The main left bundle divides early into the anterior-superior and the posterior-inferior branches. Conduction abnormalities through the left anterior branch result in a marked degree of frontal plane left axis deviation (LAD) called left anterior **fascicular block** (LAFB) or left anterior **hemiblock** (LAH). Similarly, a conduction abnormality through the left posterior branch results in a marked degree of frontal plane right axis deviation (RAD) and is called left posterior fascicular block (LPHB) or left posterior hemiblock (LPH). The anatomic distribution of this branch makes isolated LPFB rare.

Left Anterior Fascicular Block

Blood to the left anterior fascicle is supplied from the septal branch of the left anterior descending coronary artery. In some instances, there is an additional blood supply from the AV nodal branch of the right coronary artery. LAH can be congenital or can occur with hypertensive heart disease, aortic valve disease, and cardiomyopathy. LAH can also be intermittent, rate-related, or transient. Clinically, the most common cause is arterial occlusion involving the ventricular septum, with acute anterior myocardial infraction, but it can also occur with inferior wall myocardial infarction.

The sequence of ventricular activation in LAFB causes delayed activation of the superior aspect of the left ventricular wall. The abnormal ventricular activation process causes large, late ventricular forces oriented superiorly and to the left. The activation process begins in the inferior-posterior aspects of the left ventricle, which depolarizes first through the intact left posterior-inferior branch.

Patients with fascicular block must be closely monitored for **bifascicular block** (RBBB and LAH). The QRS is usually 0.10 second and presents with an rS in leads II, III, and aVF. The negative amplitude of the QRS is most prominent in lead III and the axis is shifted to the far left. There may be small Q waves in leads I and aVL. **Figure 11.6** illustrates ECG changes with LAFB.

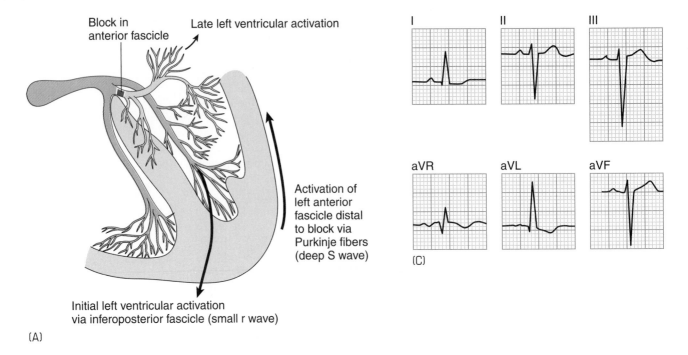

Block in anterior fascicle

Late left ventricular activation

Activation of left anterior fascicle distal to block via Purkinje fibers (deep S wave)

Initial left ventricular activation via inferoposterior fascicle (small r wave)

(A)

(C)

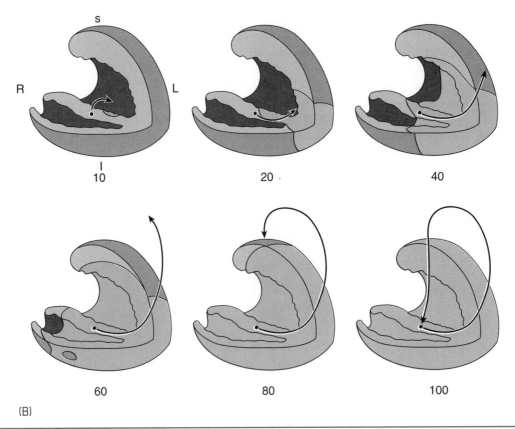

(B)

Figure 11.6 *Continues*

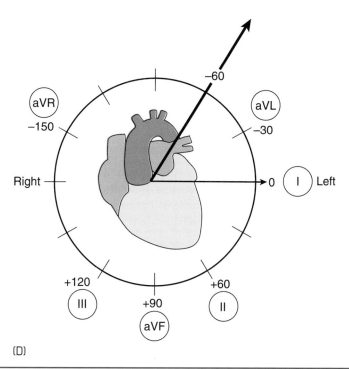

(D)

Figure 11.6 (A) Left anterior fascicular block (LAFB). (B) The sequence of activation from 10 to 100 milliseconds. QRS vectors in the frontal plane with the corresponding areas of the ventricles being depolarized in patients with left anterior fascicular block (LAFB, also known as left anterior hemiblock, or LAH). The QRS vector is superimposed on the heart with the corresponding darkened areas of the ventricles as they are being depolarized. Note the normal inferior orientation of the QRS during the first 10 to 20 milliseconds. The QRS vectors continue with counterclockwise rotation causing a marked superior displacement of the maximum forces of the QRS; left axis deviation. (C) Associated ECG changes. Note that the QRS complex is an rS configuration in leads II, III, and aVF; the Rs configuration in leads I and aVL. (D) The circle plotting the mean flow of current as affected by LAFB. The QRS in lead III is most negative of the limb leads and leads I and aVL are positive, with lead I the most positive. The darker of the two arrows is directed superior and the arrow to the left indicates a superior, leftward shift.

The ECG characteristics of LAFB include:

- QRS complex usually at 0.10 second
- LAD of –40 degrees or more
- rS in leads II, III, and aVF, with no terminal R wave
- Small Q waves in leads I and aVL due to the shift of initial forces inferiorly and to the right
- A terminal r or R in aVR

Left Anterior Fascicular Block and RBBB

Left anterior fascicular block (LAFB, or LAH) can occur with RBBB because the structures involved are similar and share much of the same blood supply. On the ECG RBBB is recognized in V_1; if the S wave is greater than the R wave, then LAD is present. When RBBB is concomitant with an LAFB, it is called bifascicular block. Often the LAH obscures the RBBB.

ECG characteristics of bifascicular block are:

- QRS complex usually at 0.10 second
- RBBB pattern with left axis deviation (RBBB + LAH)
- RBBB pattern with right axis deviation (RBBB + LPH)

Left Anterior Fascicular Block and Myocardial Infarction

If some portion of the anterior wall is involved with inferior wall myocardial infarction, or if the AV nodal artery is affected as with proximal RCA disease, LAH may obscure the ECG signs of MI. The Q wave one would anticipate will be missing from leads II, III, and aVF. In addition, inferior wall MI and LAH can each cause left axis deviation. With inferior wall MI an axis shift is usually leftward to about 30 degrees. This is due to the loss of inferior forces. If the axis is 60 degrees, concomitant LAFB (LAH) is probably the cause.

An analytical assessment can still be made. Recall that LAH with or without inferior wall myocardial infarction will produce deep S waves in lead II but no terminal r wave. In aVR a terminal r or R will occur with LAFB (LAH).

Left Posterior Fascicular Block

Left posterior fascicular block (LPFB), also called left posterior hemiblock (LPH), is caused by an obstruction of the posterior-inferior division of the LBBB. Isolated LPFB is rare since it is shorter and thicker than the anterior fascicle and has a dual blood supply. LPFB has more serious clinical implications since it implies compromise to both the right and left coronary arteries as well as damage to large areas of myocardial muscle and to the electrical conduction system in the left ventricle. In patients with posterior or lateral wall myocardial infarction LAFB (LPH) is often associated with RBBB.

When left posterior fascicular block is present, the sequence of activation is characterized by initial depolarization of the anterior-superior aspect of the left ventricle. This causes the QRS forces to be oriented superiorly and to the right or left. Late activation of the posterior-inferior walls of the left ventricle results in large forces oriented inferiorly and to the right. The left ventricle is depolarized by a left anterior fascicle and right axis deviation is obvious. There are tall R waves in lead III, and an rS wave in leads I and aVL. Right axis deviation can be caused by other conditions; for instance, right ventricular hypertrophy, chronic obstructive lung disease, and lateral wall myocardial infarction. Each of these has to be ruled out clinically before making the diagnosis of LPFB. **Figure 11.7** is an illustration of ECG changes with LPFB.

COMPLETE LEFT BUNDLE BRANCH BLOCK

With complete left bundle branch block (CLBBB), the QRS axis is usually within normal limits or a mild degree of left axis deviation (LAD). CLBBB with marked degree of LAD could represent the result of complete block of the anterior division of the left bundle, with partial block of the posterior division. CLBBB and a marked degree of right axis deviation (RAD) probably represents a complete block of the posterior division with a partial block of the anterior division. In isolated complete LAH, there is a marked degree of left axis deviation, usually secondary to complete block of the anterior division of the left bundle. Isolated left posterior hemiblock usually shows a marked degree of RAD that is due to complete block of the posterior division of the left bundle.

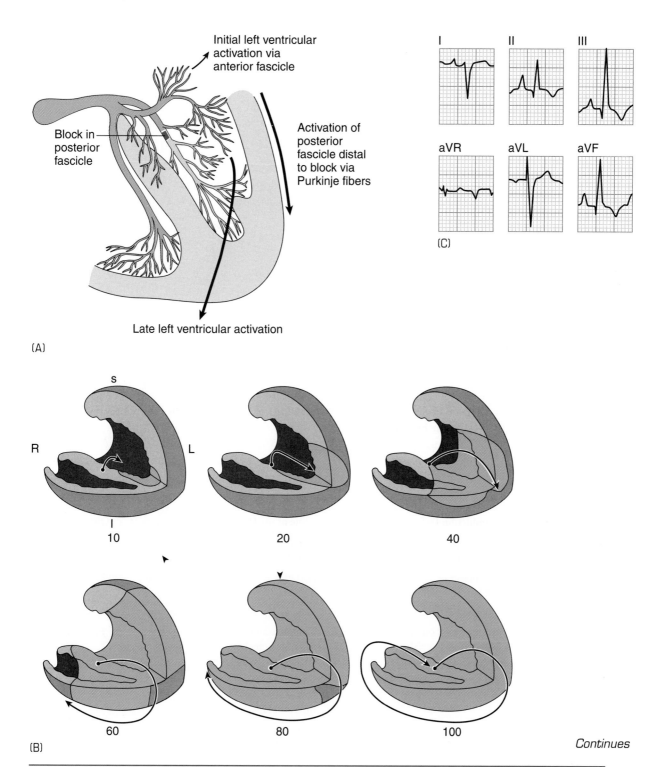

Figure 11.7 (A) Left posterior fascicular block; (B) the sequence of activation from 10 to 100 milliseconds. QRS vectors are shown with the corresponding area of the ventricles being depolarized in patients with left posterior hemiblock. The QRS vector is superimposed on the heart with corresponding darkened areas of the ventricles as they are being depolarized. Note the superior orientation of the QRS during the first 10 to 20 milliseconds. The QRS vectors continue and the result is the anterior and rightward orientation of the maximum QRS forces. (C) The associated ECG changes. The QRS complex is prolonged, greater than 0.10 second; note the rS configuration in leads I and aVL and the Rs configuration in leads II, III, and aVF. (D) The QRS in lead III is most positive of the limb leads; leads I and aVL are negative, with lead I the most negative. The circle plotting the mean flow of current as affected by LPFB. The longer, darker arrow is directed inferior and to the right indicating a rightward shift.

Continues

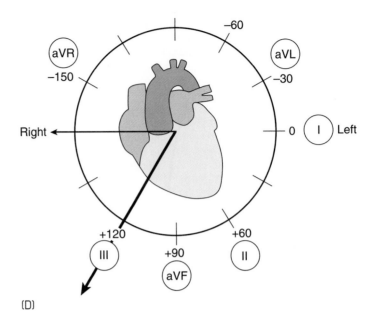

Figure 11.7 Continued (D)

Figure 11.8 summarizes the implications of various levels of conduction defects within the left bundle branch.

Table 11.1 provides an overview of conduction abnormalities of the left bundle, indicating the site of the conduction defect, the direction of the QRS axis, and the duration of the QRS complex.

Conduction Defect	Site of the Defect	QRS Axis	QRS Duration
Left anterior fascicular block (aka left anterior hemiblock)	Anterior-superior branch	−45° or more	0.12 sec or less
Left posterior fascicular block (aka left posterior hemiblock)	Posterior-inferior branch	+100° or more	0.12 sec or less
Complete left bundle branch block	Left main branch	−30° or less	0.14 sec or more
Complete left bundle branch block with left axis deviation	Complete anterior-superior branch	−45° or more	0.14 sec or more
Complete left bundle branch block with right axis deviation	Complete posterior-inferior branch Partial superior-inferior branch	+110° or more	0.14 sec or more

Table 11.1 Summary of conduction abnormalities of the left bundle, with site of defect, direction of axis, and duration.

TRIFASCICULAR BLOCK

A block located in each of the three main fascicles on the bundle branch system is called a **trifascicular block**. If the block is complete, the patient will be left with an escape ventricular pacemaker below the lesions. Assessment of the ECG involves reviewing leads II, III, and

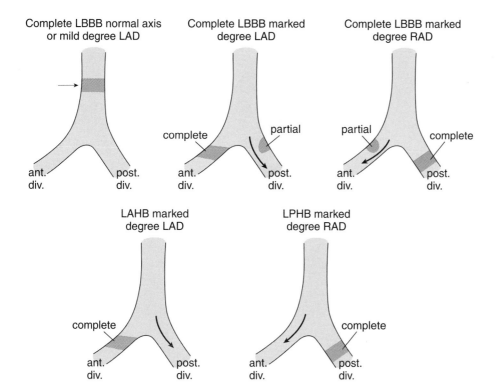

Figure 11.8 Types of left bundle branch conduction defects and associated axis deviations.

aVF for axis shift with LAH as well as assessment of the PR interval for signs of complete AV block. Lead V₁ should be assessed for RBBB. In addition, the clinician should look for the following:

- rS in leads II, III, and aVF, with no terminal R wave
- Small Q waves in leads I and aVL due to the shift of initial forces inferiorly and to the right
- Occurrence of a terminal r or R in aVR

SUMMARY

Structure and function are related throughout the human body. The heart is especially revealing when there is the slightest alteration in its electrical system. Without the flow of electric impulses, the muscular pump fails to be effective. The 12-lead ECG reveals in its entirety the framework of the heart's critical action potential. Nutrition via arterial blood flow is as important to the bundle branch system as it is to the myocardium. It is important to differentiate whenever possible a bundle branch block that is a result of variance of rate or myocardial ischemia, injury, or infarction.

Self-Assessment Exercise
ECG Rhythm Identification Practice

Identify the ECG criteria listed below each ECG. Use the Lewis circle to help with calculation of axis. Then compare your answers with those in Appendix A.

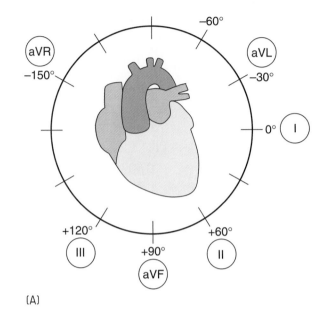

(A)

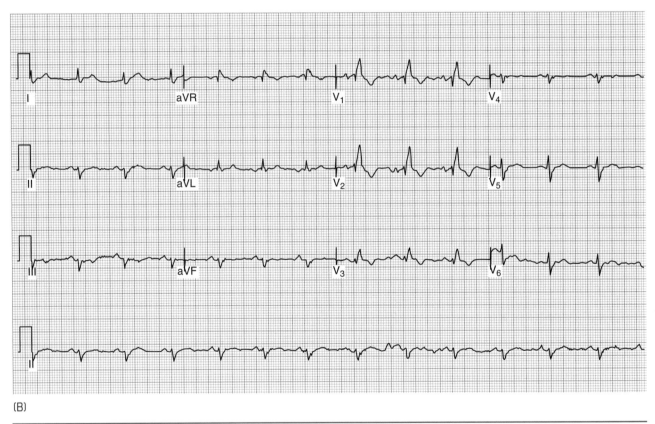

(B)

Figure 11.9

1. What is the underlying rhythm?

2. What are the acute changes? _____

3. What is your interpretation? _____

4. What can happen next? _____

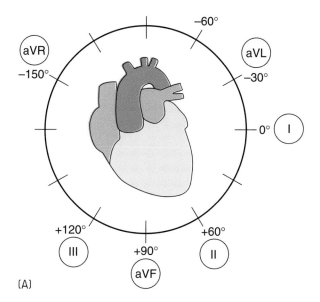

(A)

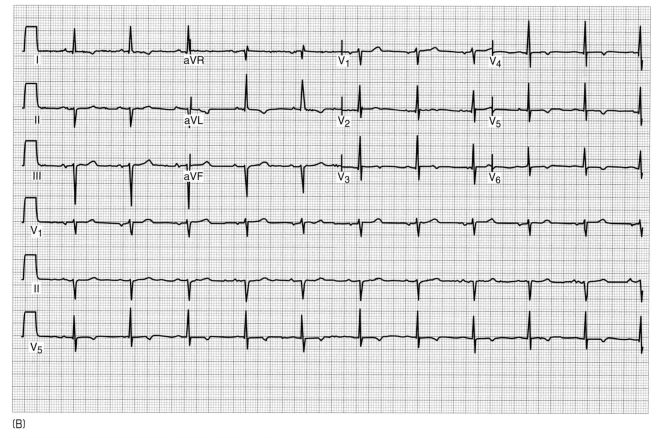

(B)

Figure 11.10

1. What is the underlying rhythm? _____

2. What are the acute changes? _____

3. What is your interpretation? _____

4. What can happen next? _____

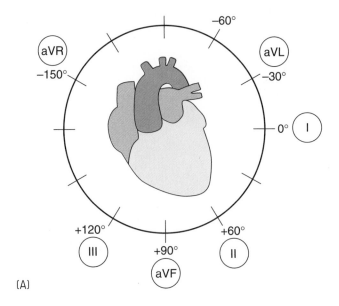

(A)

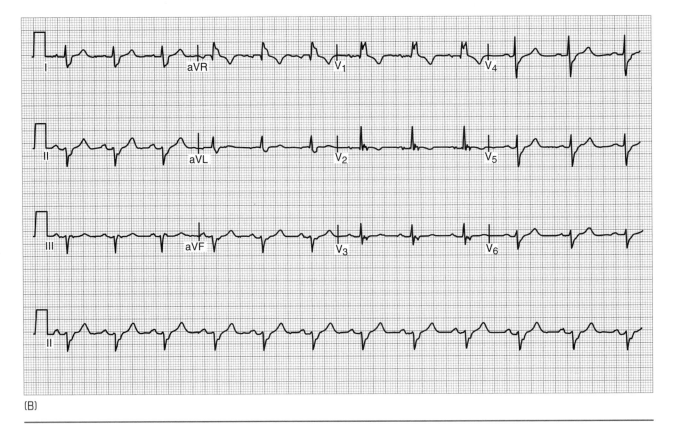

(B)

Figure 11.11

1. What is the underlying rhythm? _____

2. What are the acute changes? _____

3. What is your interpretation? _____

4. What can happen next? _____

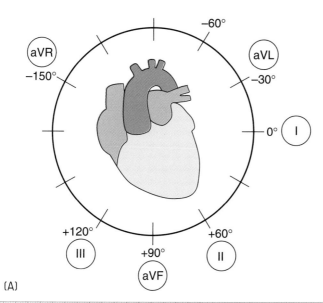

(A)

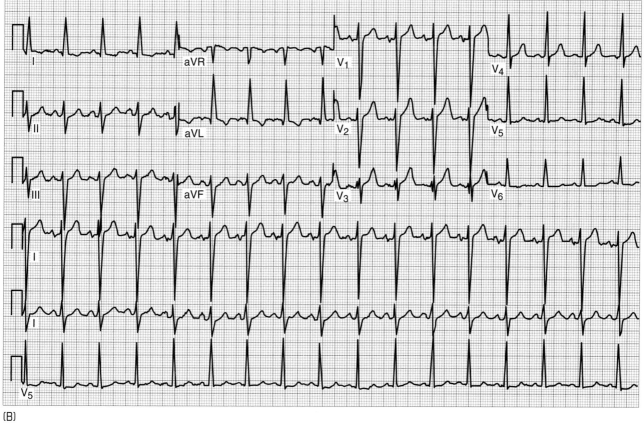

(B)

Figure 11.12

1. What is the underlying rhythm? _____

2. What are the acute changes? _____

3. What is your interpretation? _____

4. What can happen next? _____

Chamber Enlargement and Hypertrophy

Premise
Increased amplitude of ECG wave forms does guarantee the diagnosis of hypertrophy or chamber enlargement.

Objectives
After reading the chapter and completing the Self-Assessment Exercise, the student should be able to
- Identify the ECG characteristics of left and right atrial enlargement.
- Identify the ECG patterns seen in ventricular hypertrophy.
- Identify the ECG signs of ventricular strain pattern.

Key Terms
hypertrophy	P pulmonale	specificity
P mitrale	sensitivity	

Introduction
Patients who have atrial or ventricular hypertrophy or atrial or ventricular enlargement can have otherwise normal ECGs. ECG changes can be masked in patients who are obese and those patients who have chronic obstructive lung disease. Air and fatty tissue are very poor electrical conductors, so these changes may be masked or lost to the clinician using the ECG as a diagnostic tool. Patients with normal hearts may show ECG changes indicative of enlargement of atria and the ventricles or even hypertrophy, because they have a very thin chest wall or simply as a normal variant.

RIGHT ATRIAL ENLARGEMENT
Recall that P waves represent atrial depolarization. In right atrial enlargement, the P wave in lead II is 3 mm or greater in amplitude and may have a normal duration. Such P waves are referred to as **P pulmonale**. Right atrial enlargement (RAE) is frequently accompanied by right ventricular hypertrophy (RVH). **Figure 12.1** is an illustration of the increased amplitude of a P wave.

P pulmonale

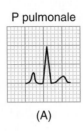

(A)

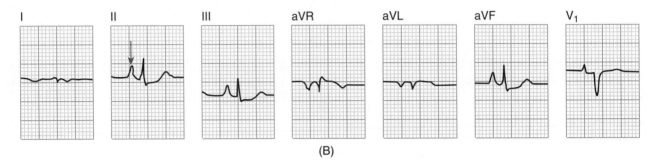

I   II   III   aVR   aVL   aVF   V₁

(B)

Figure 12.1: (A) PQRST complex with a P wave of 3 mm and 0.08 second; (B) frontal plane ECG tracing showing increased P-wave amplitude significant for P pulmonale.

The most frequent causes for RAE are:

- Pulmonary hypertension
- Pulmonary emboli
- Chronic pulmonary disease
- Pulmonary valve disease
- Tricuspid valve disease

LEFT ATRIAL ENLARGEMENT

The presence of left atrial enlargement (LAE) is revealed on the terminal configuration of the P wave. First of all, the P wave is increased to about 0.12 second or more and may have a notched or diphasic appearance in lead II and V₁. This is called **P mitrale** and suggests LAE. **Figure 12.2** contains ECG tracings showing the increased duration and change in morphology of a P mitrale.

The most frequent causes for LAE are:

- Systemic hypertension
- Aortic valve disease
- Mitral valve disease
- Left ventricular failure

Figure 12.2 ECG tracings showing changes in P-wave morphology associated with P mitrale. (A) A notched P wave is visible in lead I; (B) a diphasic P wave is seen in lead V₁.

P Mitrale

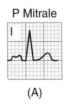

(A)

Diphasic P wave in lead V₁

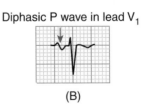

(B)

VENTRICULAR HYPERTROPHY

In ventricular hypertrophy the increase in muscle mass, secondary to hemodynamic effects of pressure or volume load, exaggerates the vectorial forces generated by the left ventricle. For instance, mitral valve disease causing insufficiency can promote retrograde blood flow and chamber enlargement. As a result, the increased workload will cause an increase in left ventricular mass called **hypertrophy**. While many patients may have hypertrophy and it goes unnoticed, the following are criteria that, if present, are diagnostic of hypertrophy.

- QRS amplitude (voltage criteria; i.e., tall R waves in LV leads, deep S waves in RV leads)
- Widened QRS/T angle (i.e., *left ventricular strain pattern*, or ST-T oriented opposite to QRS direction)
- Leftward shift in frontal plane QRS axis
- Evidence for left atrial enlargement (LAE)
- Delayed intrinsicoid deflection in V_6 (i.e., time from QRS onset to peak R is 0.05 second or more)

Figure 12.3 illustrates the relative size of the ventricle with hypertrophy.

Right Ventricular Hypertrophy

Because left ventricular activity overshadows the right, when RVH is visible on the ECG the condition is extremely severe. The most useful clue to RVH is right axis deviation and abnormalities in V_1 (recall that V_1 faces the right ventricle). The most frequent causes for right ventricular hypertrophy are:

- Congenital heart disease such as pulmonary stenosis, tetralogy of Fallot, and Eisenmenger's syndrome
- Congenital defects with ventricular overload
- Mitral insufficiency with pulmonary hypertension, mitral stenosis
- Primary pulmonary disease
- Pulmonary vascular hypertension
- Pulmonary emboli
- Pulmonary stenosis

ECG changes that are criteria for RVH include:

- Right axis deviation
- R-wave height to S-wave depth ratio greater than 1 in V_1

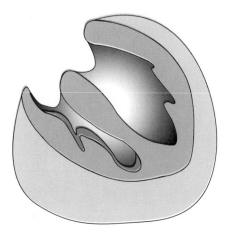

Figure 12.3 An illustration of the change in the relative size of the right ventricular wall with hypertrophy. Note the thickness in the myocardial layer, as well as the affected septum and the papillary muscles. Also note the change in volume capacity of the affected ventricle.

- R wave is greater than or equal to 7 mm in V$_1$
- S wave is greater than or equal to 7 mm in V$_5$ and V$_6$
- R wave in V$_1$ plus the S wave in V$_5$ or V$_6$ is greater than 10 mm
- Slight increase in QRS duration
- rSR' (RBBB pattern) or qR with R wave greater than 10 mm or qRS pattern in V$_1$
- Right ventricular strain pattern
- Associated right atrial enlargement
- R in aVR 5 mm or more
- R in aVR is greater than the Q in aVR

Figure 12.4 illustrates the sequence of activation in RVH.

Left Ventricular Hypertrophy

Left ventricular muscle mass in the normal human heart is roughly 2 to 3 times thicker than right ventricular muscle mass. This is due to the force with which blood is pumped into systemic circulation, which can be 10 times greater than blood flow to the pulmonic circulation. The QRS complex depicted on a normal ECG represents depolarization of the ventricles and reflects left ventricular muscle mass. It follows, then, that left ventricular enlargement will be represented on the ECG by changes in the duration of the QRS complex in some of the leads.

Common causes of left ventricular hypertrophy (LVH) include:

- Systemic arterial hypertension
- Aortic stenosis or insufficiency
- Coarctation of the aorta
- Hypertrophic cardiomyopathy
- Primary pulmonary disease
- Mitral insufficiency

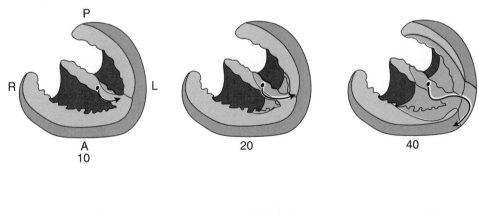

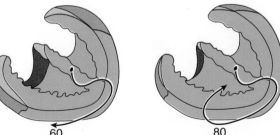

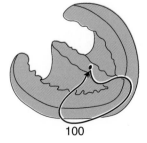

Figure 12.4 Sequence of ventricular activation from 10 to 100 milliseconds as displayed in the horizontal plane in RVH. The QRS vector is superimposed on the heart with the corresponding cleared areas of the ventricles as they are being depolarized.

There are major criteria for assessment of the ECG and determinants of left ventricular hypertrophy. One example is the *Estes criteria*, which assigns points. Greater than 5 points is considered *diagnostic* and at least 4 points in considered *probable*.

- **2 points** Direction of the QRS vector (left axis deviation)
- **1 point** QRS duration ≤0.10 second
- **1 point** QRS morphology (delayed intrinsicoid deflection in V_5 or V_6) >0.05 second
- ST abnormalities
  - **3 points** without digitalis
  - **1 point** with digitalis
- **3 points** Voltage criteria (any of the following)
  - R or S waves in limb leads ≥20 mm
  - S wave in V_1 or V_2 ≥30 mm
  - R wave in V_5 or V_6 ≥30 mm

Changes in the QRS

In LVH, the QRS vector is directed somewhat more leftward and more posterior, greater than 30 degrees. **Figure 12.5** illustrates the change in the relative size of the left ventricular wall. The ECG leads show changes reflecting the hypertrophy. **Figure 12.6** illustrates the sequence of activation in LVH. Measurement and shape of the QRS (0.10 second or less) are rarely changed as a result of the sequence of depolarization remaining the same. Remember that the duration of the QRS complex reflects the ventricular conduction system, not the size of the ventricles.

Voltage Criteria. There are several ways to determine the presence of LVH using the 12-lead ECG, and many point systems for more elaborate identification. It is best to work with a method that uses two levels of certainty: voltage criteria and secondary ST-T changes.

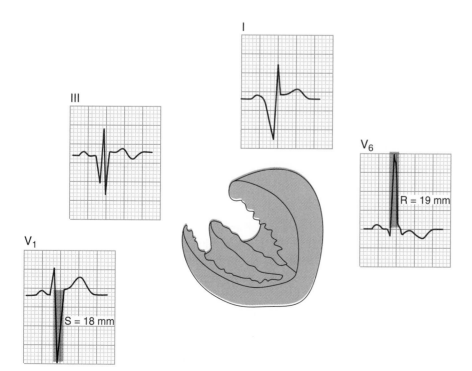

Figure 12.5 Illustration of the heart showing excessive thickness of the left ventricle and the septum. The ECG leads demonstrate evidence of LVH by voltage criteria: $SV_1 + RV_6 = >35$ mm.

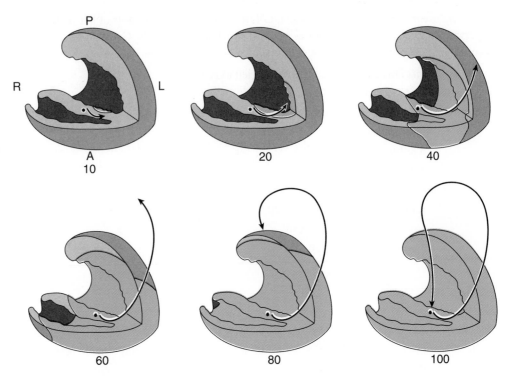

Figure 12.6 Sequence of ventricular activation from 10 to 100 milliseconds as displayed in the horizontal plane in left ventricular hypertrophy. The QRS vector is superimposed on the heart with the corresponding cleared areas of the ventricles as they are being depolarized. The extension of the QRS loop reflects the amplitude of the QRS as affected by hypertrophy.

The clinician should not favor any one criterion, but adapt to the patient circumstance by taking into consideration individual variables. In fact, using voltage criteria alone can result in a false negative identification.

The most common changes in the ECG are:

- The increased voltage of the mean QRS vector is reflected in the tall R waves in leads I and/or aVL, V_3 or V_6.
- Deep S waves in V_1 may also be seen.
- The amplitude of the R wave is greater than 27 mm in V_5 or greater than 25 mm in V_6. (This application has merit for patients older than 35 years.)

There are many methods that can be used to determine voltage. The methods outlined here include the following:

- Index of Lewis
- R-wave height
- Sokolow-Lyon criteria
- R/S voltage criteria
- Cornell voltage criteria

There are natural instances of increased amplitude in the QRS complexes of young persons with slight builds who tend to have a higher voltage. The Lewis criteria can differentiate in such cases, with fewer false positives. Also, if left anterior fascicular block is present, the increased voltage criteria will correct for this factor. The *index of Lewis* criteria are outlined as follows:

Net positive deflection in lead I in mm

+ Net negative deflection in lead III in mm

= >21 mm = left ventricular hypertrophy

The *height of the R wave* in aVL should measure greater than 13 mm as a criterion for hypertrophy. Although this system is straightforward, there are frequent false positives. Most authorities recommend use of the index of Lewis or Sokolow-Lyon to confirm the interpretation using R-wave height as a sole measure.

The *Sokolow-Lyon criteria* are very popular, but not recommended for patients under the age of 35 years:

- Look at leads V_1, V_5, and V_6.
- When the S wave in V_1 plus the wave in V_5 or V_6 is 35 mm or greater, it is positive for LVH:
  - (SV_1 + RV_5 or RV_6 = >35 mm is indicative of LVH)

Figure 12.7 shows a 12-lead ECG illustrating the relative size of QRS complexes consistent with LVH.

The *R/S Voltage Criteria* include any of the following:

- The R wave in aVL is greater than 11 mm.
- The S wave in V_1 (SV_1) plus the R wave in V_5 (RV_5) or the R wave in V_6 (RV_6) is greater than 35 mm.
- The R wave in V_5 or V_6 is greater than 25 mm.

The specificity is greater than 95 percent using these criteria, but the sensitivity is low, less than 30 percent.

To assess the ECG using the *Cornell voltage criteria*:

- Add the height of the R wave in aVL and the depth of the S wave in V_3.
- If the result is greater than 28 mm in males or greater than 20 mm in females, LVH is present.

This test has a sensitivity, or true positive rate, of about 42 percent and specificity, or true negative rate, of about 96 percent.

Axis. In LVH there is

- Leftward, posterior shift.
- Poor R-wave progression across the precordium.
- Occasionally, there is loss of terminal rightward forces manifested by the presence of secondary ST and T-wave abnormalities.

Figure 12.8 is a 12-lead ECG from an adult patient showing left atrial enlargement (lead II) and LVH SV_1 + RV_5 = 47 mm.

LVH with Left Bundle Branch Block.
Most patients with left bundle branch block (LBBB) may also have anatomic LVH, making the increased duration of the QRS difficult to determine. Some authors found that the sum of the S-wave amplitude in V_2 and the R-wave amplitude in V_6 of 4.5 mV or more had an 86 percent and a 100 percent specificity to detect LVH in patients with LBBB.

LVH with Right Bundle Branch Block.
The sensitivity of ECG criteria for LVH decreases in the presence of right bundle branch block (RBBB). A useful sign when these two exist is the presence of left atrial enlargement. The presence of a P-wave terminal force in V_1 increases the sensitivity for LVH to over 70 percent with an approximate specificity of 80 percent. A Sokolow index of greater than or equal to 3.5 mV is 100 percent specific for LVH in patients who are not obese.

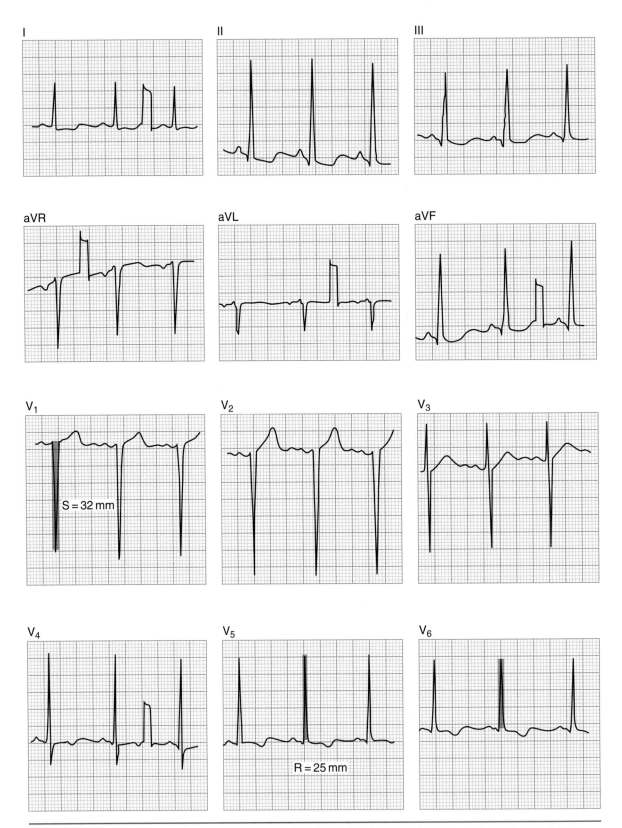

Figure 12.7 A 12-lead ECG illustrating QRS complexes (shaded) with left ventricular hypertrophy. Look at leads V_1, V_5, or V_6. Add the values of the S wave in V_1 plus the value of the R wave in V_5 or V_6. Note the value is greater than 35 mm and, therefore, is indicative of LVH.

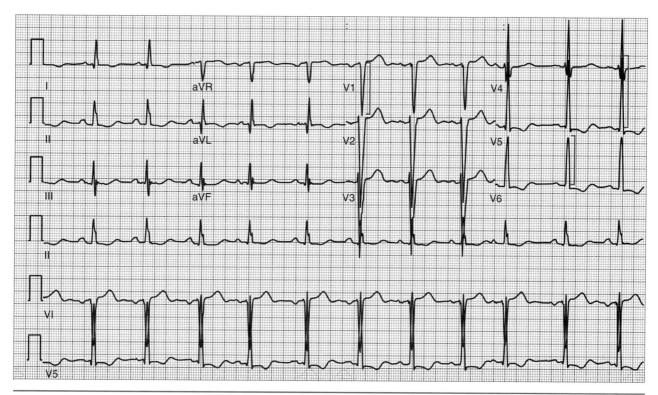

Figure 12.8 Twelve-lead ECG showing left atrial enlargement (lead II) and left ventricular hypertrophy: $SV_1 + RV_5 = 47$ mm.

Ventricular hypertrophy involving *both ventricles* is difficult to interpret on the ECG. However, if the patient history and presentation signal the problem and there is ECG evidence of left atrial enlargement, the following may help with the interpretation:

- R/S ratio in V_5 or V_6 less than 1.0 mm.
- S in V_5 or V_6 greater than 6.0 mm.
- Right axis deviation 90 degrees or more.
- Criteria for both LVH and RVH are met.
- Criteria for LVH are met and either right axis deviation *or* right atrial enlargement is present.

Ventricular Strain Pattern

Ventricular strain is denoted by ST segment and T-wave changes that are frequently seen with ventricular hypertrophy. The reason for these changes is not altogether clear. It is thought that perhaps conduction delays in repolarization through the thickened walls play an important role, as does ischemia due to the increase in muscle fiber diameter.

Left Ventricular Strain. Left ventricular strain manifests on the ECG with:

- ST segment depression and asymmetrical T-wave inversion in leads that face the affected ventricle, I, aVL, V_5 and V_6.
- The affected ST segments have a downsloped appearance, frequently referred to as hockey stick in shape.
- Reciprocal ST elevation in upright T waves is seen in V_1 and V_2, which face the right ventricle; therefore, LVH with a strain pattern will cause 1.0 to 2.0 mm of ST elevation in V_1 and V_2 and may be mistaken for an acute injury pattern.

Left ventricular strain pattern

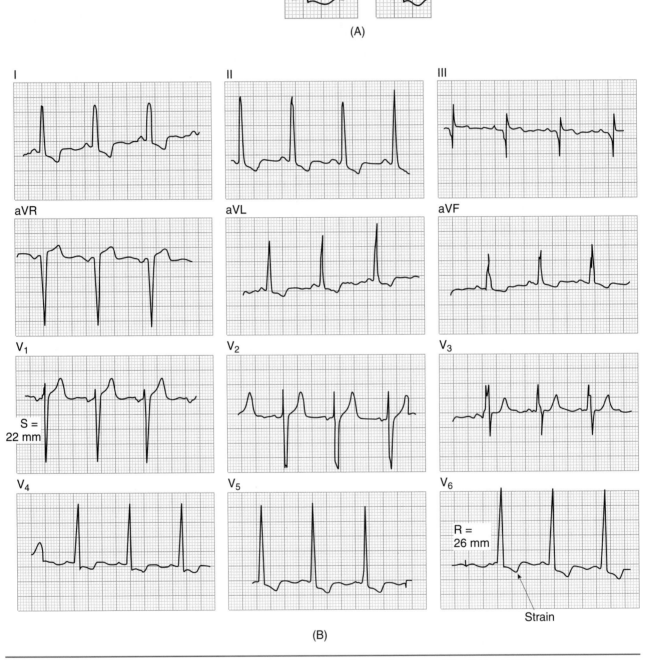

(A)

(B)

Figure 12.9 (A) ECG complexes illustrating the ST-T-wave changes seen in a strain pattern; (B) a 12-lead ECG in left ventricular hypertrophy. Note the deep S waves in V$_1$, increased R-wave amplitude in V$_5$ and V$_6$, with ST-T-wave changes reflecting strain in V$_6$. (C) A 12-lead ECG in RVH. Note the increased amplitude (shaded) of R waves in lead III and deep S waves in I and aVL. Lead V$_5$ has been minimized to "make it fit" for mounting purposes. Note that the QRS in V$_5$ is half the true illustration of that lead, while V$_1$ shows the characteristic ST-T-wave strain pattern.

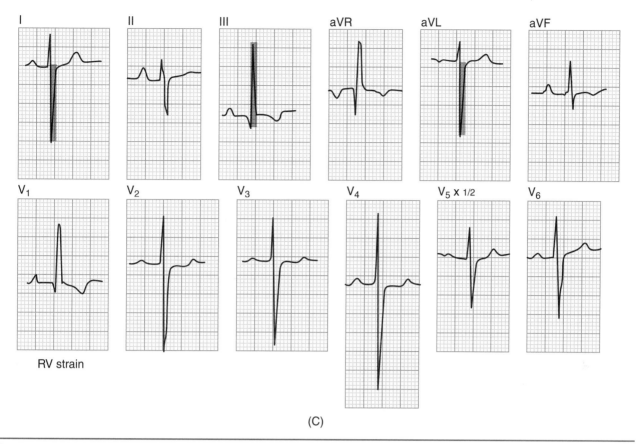

RV strain

(C)

Figure 12.9 Continued

Right Ventricular Strain. Right ventricular strain shows the same kind of ST segment changes in left ventricular strain, but in different leads. In right ventricular strain, leads V_1, V_2, II, III, and aVF show ST segment depression with asymmetrical T-wave inversion. **Figure 12.9** shows two 12-lead ECGs illustrating ventricular hypertrophy and strain.

There are several ECG changes with ventricular strain. Secondary ST-T-wave changes, sometimes referred to as left ventricular strain pattern, are the most suggestive criteria. The spatial changes can be approximated by identifying:

- Sagging ST segments and inverted T waves in every lead with a tall R wave
- A rising ST and upright T in every lead with a deep S wave

SUMMARY

The ECG diagnosis of hypertrophy and strain is not realistic without a 12-lead ECG. However, clinical presentation and medical history are vital in validating changes with the 12-lead ECG in the clinical setting. The 12-lead ECG is very revealing in regard to all four of the heart's chambers and affords the clinician the ability to interpret nonacute conditions. The assessment of increased amplitude can support the diagnosis of chamber enlargement due to chronic disease. Confirmation by use of 12-lead ECG is a valuable tool in diagnosing the existence of chamber hypertrophy. Awareness of the existence of chamber abnormality may alter choice of intervention and affect long-term outcome.

In this chapter we have discussed tools for assessing atrial and ventricular enlargement. Atrial enlargement is infrequently seen, and occurrence of right atrial enlargement is more common than left. Ventricular hypertrophy must be substantiated with clinical assessment and history. Ventricular changes are more commonly encountered and many measurement criteria exist. As with any other diagnosis, the use of the ECG as a tool requires a consistent approach, remembering that vigilance and verification with clinical assessment are critical.

Self-Assessment Exercise
ECG Rhythm Identification Practice

Identify the ECG criteria listed below each ECG, and then compare your answers with those in Appendix A.

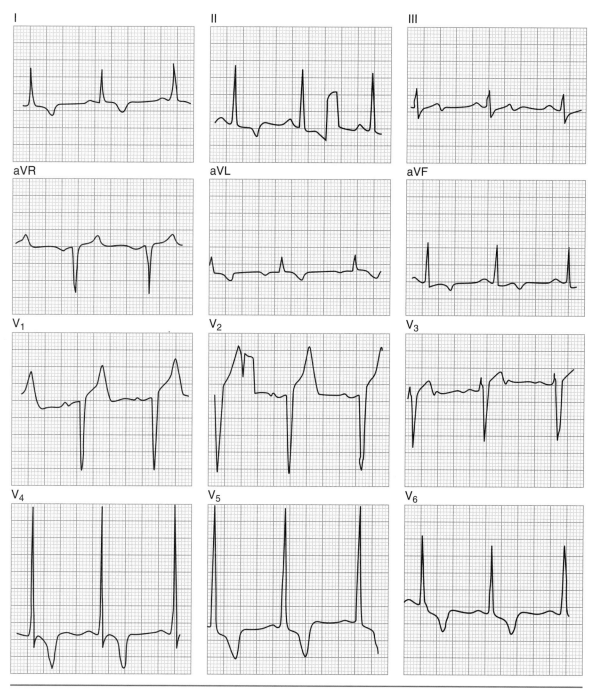

Figure 12.10

1. What is the underlying rhythm? _____

2. What are the acute changes? _____

3. What is your interpretation? _____

4. What can happen next? _____

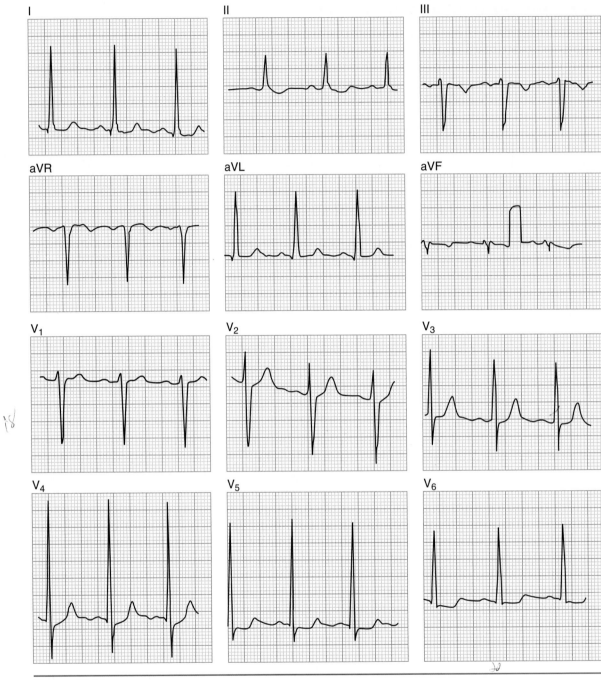

Figure 12.11

1. What is the underlying rhythm? _____

2. What are the acute changes? _____

3. What is your interpretation? _____

4. What can happen next? _____

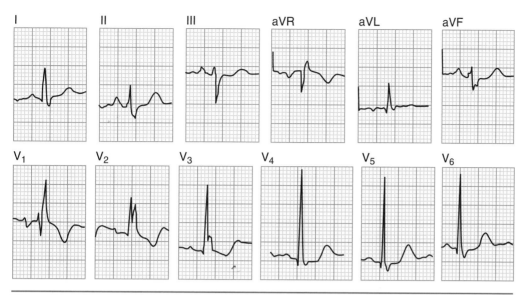

Figure 12.12

1. What is the underlying rhythm? _____

2. What are the acute changes? _____

3. What is your interpretation? _____

4. What can happen next? _____

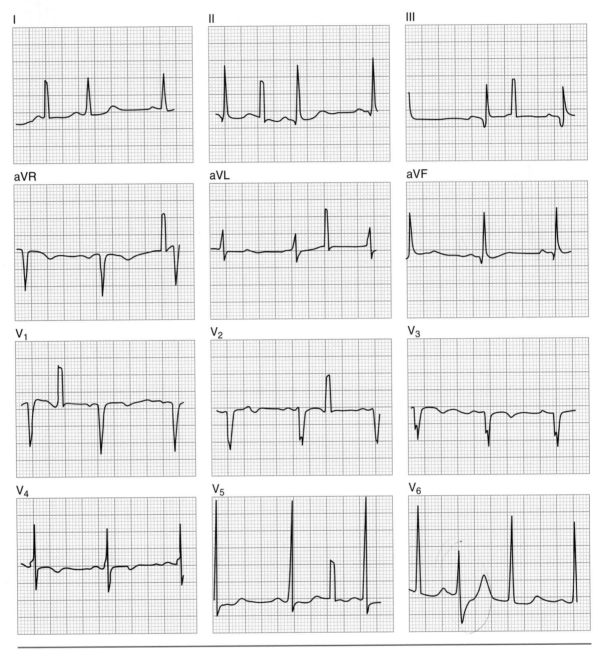

Figure 12.13

1. What is the underlying rhythm? _____

2. What are the acute changes? _____

3. What is your interpretation? _____

4. What can happen next? _____

Arrhythmias due to Abnormal Conduction Pathways

Premise
Widening of the QRS does not always imply bundle branch block.

Objectives

After reading the chapter and completing the Self-Assessment Exercise, the student should be able to

- Define *accessory pathway*.
- Identify the ECG characteristics of presence of an accessory pathway.
- Identify the consequences of arrhythmias that are the result of an accessory pathway (AP).

Key Terms

accessory pathway (AP)	James fibers	orthodromic
antidromic	Kent bundles	Wolff-Parkinson-White
bypass tracts	Lown-Ganong-Levine	(WPW) syndrome
delta wave	(LGL) syndrome	
intranodal bypass tract	Mahaim's fibers	

Introduction

Depolarization from the sinus node travels through atrial tissue and terminates at the crest of the AV node. The PR interval is comprised of the time taken for atrial depolarization, formation of the P wave, and depolarization of the AV node, bundle of His, both bundle branches, and the PR segment. Slow conduction through the AV node accounts for most of the PR segment. If the wave of depolarization can bypass the AV node, then the normal delay that would have been encountered is circumvented, and the PR segment and thus the PR interval will be shortened.

An **accessory pathway (AP)** is an abnormal conduction pathway between an atrium and a ventricle. An AP is a bundle composed of ventricular tissue that exists outside the normal specialized conduction tissue.

Many patients with an AP are not affected nor diagnosed until an episode of supraventricular tachycardia (SVT) has been terminated. Literature review reports males are affected more than females. There is evidence to support that there is a genetic predisposition to APs and the resulting tachycardias.

PREEXCITATION DEFINED

Preexcitation describes early ventricular depolarization, using an accessory pathway rather than the normal AV conduction system. An accessory pathway consists of a myocardial connection at the level of the AV junction. The AV node is "bypassed," thus atrial arrhythmias such as atrial fibrillation can conduct without the normal protective delay in the AV node. Classification by type is not used as much in lieu of naming the anatomic location. Causes of the development of an accessory pathway include, but are not limited to:

- Tumors of the AV ring
- Rhabdomyomas
- Residual connections from the formation of the AV
- An extra muscle bundle composed of ventricular tissue that exists outside the normal, specialized conduction tissue

Preexcitation is of concern since there is a potential for supraventricular tachyarrhythmias. In addition, paroxysmal supraventricular tachycardia (PSVT) and atrial fibrillation that result from an unrecognized preexcitation syndrome can deteriorate into ventricular fibrillation. In some cases of preexcitation, the resulting QRS complex is widened and may be confused with bundle branch block. Also wide QRS complex arrhythmias occurring with preexcitation may be confused with ventricular tachycardia.

PHYSIOLOGY OF ACCESSORY PATHWAY (AP)

As discussed, these extra bundles that exist outside the normal specialized conduction tissue are called APs. There are several of these pathways connecting the atria to the ventricles and common types of preexcitation.

- **Kent bundles** are accessory AV pathways that connect the atrium to the ventricles.
- **James fibers** are atrio-His bundles that connect atrial fibers to the upper part of the AV node. This is also termed as a **bypass tract**.
- **Mahaim's fibers** are APs that connect the AV node and the ventricle (nodoventricular), or those that connect the bundle of His and the bundle branch nodofascicular or from the bundle branch to the ventricles (fascicular ventricular).
- Atriofascicular **bypass tracts** are fibers that connect the atrium to the bundle of His.

Figure 13.1 shows accessory pathways connecting atrial and ventricular tissue.

THE ECG WAVE FORMS AFFECTED BY PREEXCITATION

The ECG pattern of preexcitation consists primarily of a short PR interval because the descending impulse bypasses the normal AV conduction delay. Often, this is the source of AV nodal reentrant tachycardias. During the tachycardia, the QRS can be narrow, wide, and aberrant. If atrial fibrillation occurs with an accessory pathway, the ventricular response is usually very rapid, irregular, and with aberrant ventricular conduction. **Figure 13.2** is the ECG tracing of a patient with atrial fibrillation complicated by the accessory pathway.

In addition, the early depolarization of the ventricles will cause a widened QRS complex called a **delta wave**, a characteristic slurring in the initial wave forms of the QRS. The delta

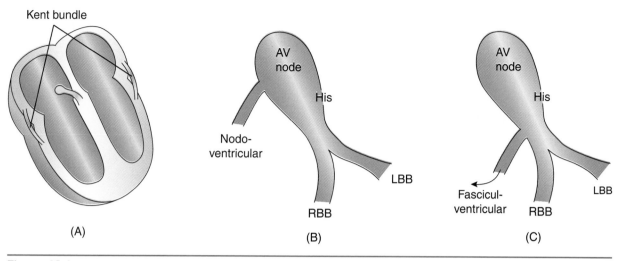

Figure 13.1 (A) The site of the Kent bundles, (B) the James bundle, (C) the Mahaim's fibers. (Adapted from *Understanding Electrocardiography: Arrhythmias and the 12 Lead ECG*, 7th ed., by M. B. Conover, 1996, St. Louis, MO: Mosby-Year Book, Inc.)

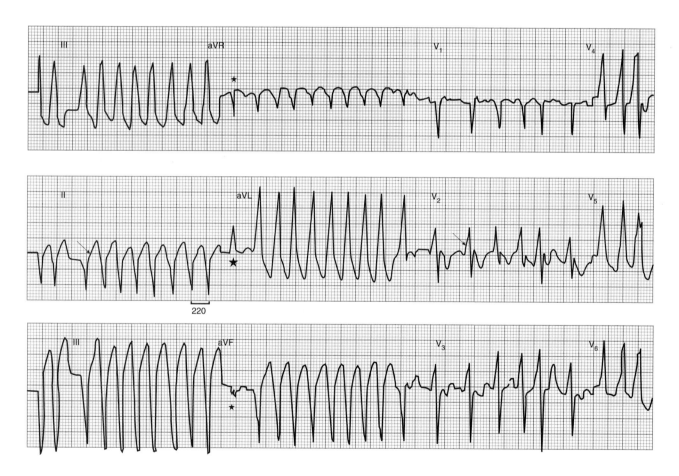

Here she exhibits atrial fibrillation. Note the rapid ventricular rate (about 215) and the irregular RR intervals. Delta waves (arrows) vary in size. Intermittently, the accessory pathway may block—with sole conduction via the AV node—resulting in a narrow-complex beat (stars). Patients with RR intervals under 250 msec have increased risk of progression to ventricular tachycardia or fibrillation. This patient has a 220-msec RR.

Figure 13.2 An ECG tracing of a patient with atrial fibrillation compounded by the use of an accessory pathway. The delta waves are seen in some of the QRS complexes. Note the irregular rhythm, which differentiates this ECG from ventricular tachycardia. The short RR interval reflects the use of the accessory pathway rather than conventional AV node delay.

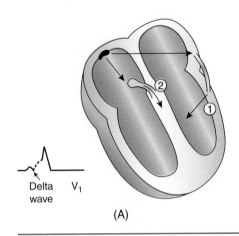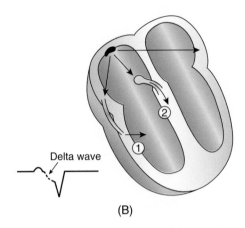

Figure 13.3 The presence of delta waves. Note the distortion on the ascending arm in (A) and on the descending arm in (B) of the QRS complexes as they reflect early activation of ventricular conduction system. (Adapted from *Understanding Electrocardiography: Arrhythmias and the 12 Lead ECG*, 7th ed., by M. B. Conover, 1996, St. Louis, MO: Mosby-Year Book, Inc.)

wave occurs when both the AV node and the accessory pathway participate in ventricular depolarization. The polarity of the delta wave may be positive or negative depending on the direction of conduction as viewed in a specific lead. If the forces of excitation are toward the positive electrode in a lead, the polarity of the delta wave will be positive. Similarly, if the forces of excitation are away from the positive electrode in a lead, the polarity of the delta wave will be negative and produce an abnormal Q wave in leads III and V_1. Finally, if the forces of excitation are perpendicular to the positive electrode in a lead, the polarity will be isoelectric. **Figure 13.3** is a diagram of the conduction from the atria to the ventricles using an accessory pathway and the resulting changes in the QRS complex.

The amplitude of the delta wave depends on several factors, but primarily how quickly the accessory pathway conducts the current ahead of the normal wave of depolarization. If normal and accessory wave fronts arrive simultaneously, there may be no delta wave and the PR interval would be unchanged. However, since there will be sources depolarizing the ventricles, the resulting QRS will be a fusion of both wave fronts.

In summary, the width of the QRS depends on several factors:

- The length of time it takes for conduction through the accessory pathway
- The location of the accessory pathway
- Conduction time between the sinus and AV nodes

Since ventricular depolarization does not follow a normal conduction pathway, repolarization will be out of sequence. The extent of ST segment and T-wave abnormalities occurring with altered ventricular repolarization depends on the source and degree of preexcitation.

Degrees of Preexcitation

There are four degrees of preexcitation:

1. *None.* The patient has a latent accessory pathway and the PR interval and QRS duration are normal. The anatomical source of the pathway is on the lateral side of the left ventricle. This pathway may become active with atrial fibrillation and is capable of antegrade conduction, which can result in a life-threatening arrhythmia.
2. *Minimal,* where the size of the delta wave is very small and not seen in all leads.
3. *Less than maximum,* where the impulse arrives in the ventricle, first using the accessory pathway (short PR interval) and then using the AV node, causing a

fusion beat. The resulting QRS may not have the classic delta wave, but may exhibit an abnormal Q wave, or distortion of the ascending arm of the R wave, or increased QRS voltage. In less than maximum preexcitation, it is difficult to differentiate between ventricular hypertrophy, bundle branch block, and acute myocardial infarction. Clinical presentation, serial ECG, and enzyme studies will facilitate diagnosis.

4. *Maximum preexcitation* is the term used when both ventricles are activated by the accessory pathway. There is almost no PR interval, and the fusing of P to the QRS complex results in the widened QRS.

When preexcitation is suspected, the clinician must assess the PR interval and a delta wave in all leads. The PR may not be obviously shortened and a delta wave may not be visible in all leads taken simultaneously. A 12-lead ECG must be taken during the tachycardia episode and compared with the resting, or normal, ECG to rule out preexitation. **Figure 13.4** is a diagram with corresponding PQRST complexes for the four degrees of preexitation.

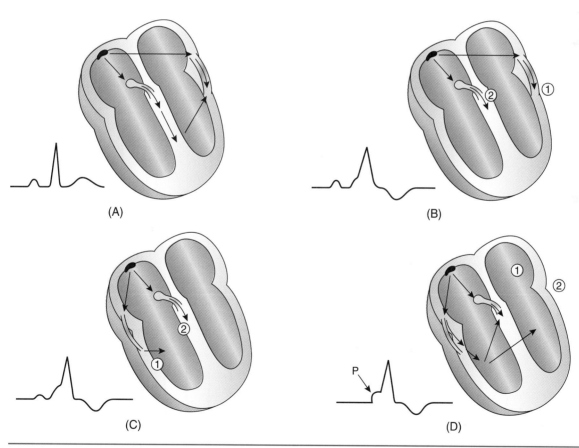

(A)

(B)

(C)

(D)

Figure 13.4 (A) Normal activation: QRS complex showing no visible delta wave, no visible change in the QRS to identify the presence of an accessory pathway. (B) Minimal activation: QRS complex showing positive wave on the ascending arm of the QRS. (C) Less than maximal activation: QRS complex showing positive delta wave in ascending arm of the QRS. Note the short PR interval. Diagram shows the fusion of normal and early forces arriving in the ventricle. The QRS will be a fusion of early and normal depolarizing forces. (D) Maximum activation using an accessory pathway: The PR interval is so minimal as to be nonexistent. The delta wave is obvious as it fuses into the ascending arm of the QRS. (Adapted from *Understanding Electrocardiography: Arrhythmias and the 12 Lead ECG*, 7th ed., by M. B. Conover, 1996, St. Louis, MO: Mosby-Year Book, Inc.)

Concealed Accessory Pathway

When an AP conducts only in a retrograde direction it is concealed. This is because during sinus rhythm, conduction down the AV junction, through, to, and within the ventricles is normal. The PR interval and QRS duration are within normal limits and there is no delta wave.

ARRHYTHMIAS WITH PREEXCITATION

Reciprocating tachycardia occurs when a premature atrial focus conducts down the normal AV conduction system, but uses the accessory pathway to reenter the atria. This is also called circus-movement or reentry tachycardia or **orthodromic** (narrow QRS) reciprocating tachycardia. There are no delta waves because the activation front proceeds in an antegrade direction through the AV node, and in a retrograde direction through the accessory pathway.

The P′ polarity may be negative or positive in lead I and may be seen after the QRS complex. There will be a short PR interval. QRS alternans may be seen. *QRS alternans* is the alteration of the amplitude of the R and S waves of the QRS complex. **Figure 13.5** is an ECG tracing showing QRS alternans.

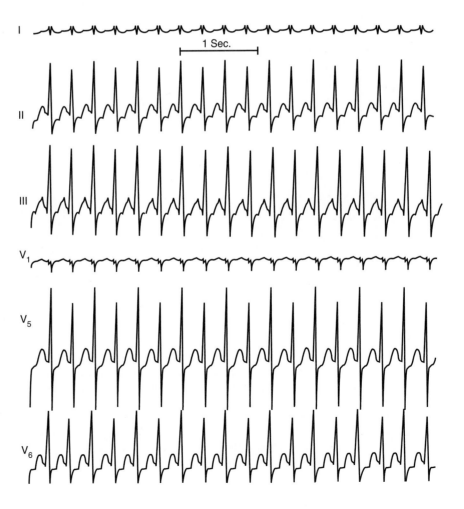

Figure 13.5 QRS alternans. Note the alternating amplitude of the QRS complex in several of the ECG leads in a patient with circus-movement tachycardia. Alternans is not always visible in all the ECG leads. (Adapted from *Understanding Electrocardiography: Arrhythmias and the 12 Lead ECG*, 7th ed., by M. B. Conover, 1996, St. Louis, MO: Mosby-Year Book, Inc.)

A PVC can cause a tachycardia by accessing the atria via the accessory pathway, then traveling down the AV node, His bundle, and into the ventricles. This will result in a narrow QRS tachycardia.

During sinus tachycardia, when a critical rate is reached, the AP is blocked in an antegrade fashion. The impulse may conduct normally, and reenter the atria using the accessory pathway in a retrograde fashion, thus establishing the reentry circuit.

Orthodromic tachycardia can occur using a slower conducting accessory pathway. The reentry circuit uses the AV node in an antegrade direction and a slower conducting AP in the retrograde direction. The slower conduction time from ventricle to atria over the slow AP will produce an RP interval that is long. In fact the P′ will be closer to the QRS that follows it rather than the one that precedes it. The rhythm appears as a junctional tachycardia but the ventricular rate is 130 to 200 beat(s) per minute (bpm). **Figure 13.6** illustrates a 12-lead ECG tracing from a patient with a reciprocating tachycardia. The QRS complexes are narrow, fast, and regular.

Antidromic (wide QRS) tachycardia is a reentry tachycardia that uses the accessory pathway in an antegrade fashion and the AV node in a retrograde direction. The resulting QRS will be wide and the ventricular rhythm may be irregular because of retrograde conduction, though the ventricular pathways may differ. In some cases, a P′ occurs because of the retrograde stimulation of the atria. This P′ may be seen after the QRS, but not in all leads,

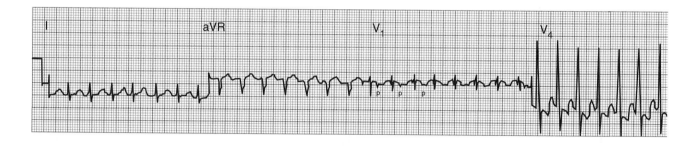

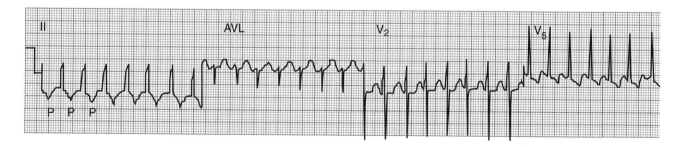

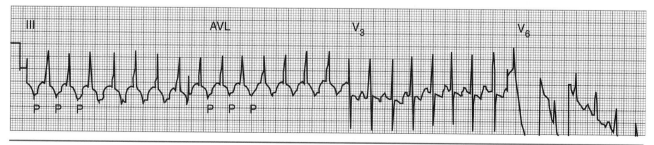

Figure 13.6 A 12-lead ECG from a patient with orthodromic reciprocating tachycardia. Note that the QRS complexes are narrow, PR intervals are short, and delta waves are present in leads III, aVF, and V₂.

since the QRS is so broad. **Figure 13.7** is a 12-lead ECG showing a patient with antidromic reciprocating tachycardia.

Tachycardia can be caused by the use of two APs. There can be antegrade conduction down one AP and retrograde conduction using another AP. In this instance, the QRS will be wide and very difficult to differentiate from ventricular tachycardia.

Atrial fibrillation conducts to the ventricles over an AP in an antegrade fashion. This result is a ventricular rate sometimes greater than 200 bpm, but with irregularity that is characteristic of the atrial fibrillation. Conduction through a rapidly conducting AP can result in an irregular ventricular rate that rapidly deteriorates into ventricular fibrillation.

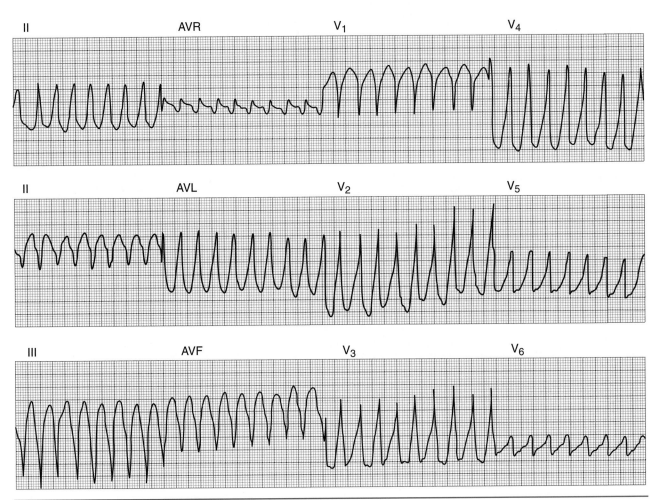

Figure 13.7 A 12-lead ECG showing a patient with antidromic reciprocating tachycardia. Note the broad QRS with opposite T-wave polarity, similar to ventricular tachycardia (v-tach), but it is not v-tach. Concordant negativity is not present in the precordial leads and the QRS in aVR is negative; differential tools in determining if a tachycardia is ventricular or supraventricular in origin. The QRS complex is broad because ventricular depolarization occurs entirely via the accessory pathway.`

LOWN-GANONG-LEVINE (LGL) SYNDROME

The **Lown-Ganong-Levine (LGL) syndrome**, also known as intranodal bypass tract syndrome, was initially described as a combination of a short PR interval, normal QRS configuration, and recurrent supraventricular tachycardias. It was subsequently shown that in patients who exhibit LGL, intranodal fibers bypass the crest of the AV node and one of the intranodal fibers terminates near the bundle of His (**James fibers**). The major conduction delay in the AV node is circumvented and a short PR interval is recorded of less than 0.12 second. Ventricular depolarization will take place via the normal His-Purkinje system, generating a normal QRS complex. **Figure 13.8** illustrates a 12-lead tracing showing the ECG characteristics associated with LGL syndrome.

Many patients will be encountered whose ECG displays a short PR interval and a normal QRS complex, but who have no clinical history of tachycardia. Such tracings probably indicate bypass of the AV node by an intranodal fiber, and should be interpreted as consistent with, but not diagnostic of, the LGL presentation.

In summary the three criteria for diagnosis of the Lown-Ganong-Levine syndrome are:

1. Short PR interval (0.12 second or less)
2. Normal QRS configuration
3. Recurrent paroxysmal tachycardia

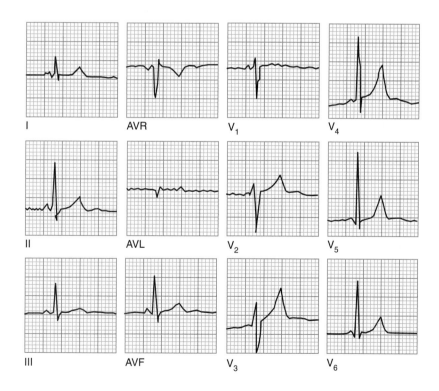

Figure 13.8 A 12-lead ECG showing a short PR interval and narrow QRS complex in a patient with confirmed Lown-Ganong-Levine syndrome.

WOLFF-PARKINSON-WHITE (WPW) SYNDROME

In **Wolff-Parkinson-White (WPW) syndrome**, signs and symptoms of preexcitation occur using accessory AV pathways (Kent bundles) with accompanying tachycardia. WPW occurring without tachycardia is a *WPW pattern*. WPW can occur in healthy hearts. The anatomical presence of the AP may manifest itself later in life or with myocardial infarction or atrial fibrillation.

In WPW, as atrial tissue is depolarized and forms the P wave on the ECG, the depolarizing wave front arrives simultaneously at the crest of the AV node and at the atrial end of the AP. Conduction through the AV node is normally delayed, but the AP is capable of very rapid depolarization. Thus, ventricular tissue is depolarized before the AV node has permitted normal conduction to continue through the His bundle.

If all ventricular tissue is depolarized by the impulse using the AP, the resulting QRS would be different from the sinus-induced QRS. The resulting widened QRS complexes can be confused with bundle branch block or PVCs.

However, as the wave of depolarization slowly spreads out from the prematurely depolarized ventricle, conduction is completed through the AV junction and spreads quickly through the His-Purkinje system.

The result of all of this is a composite of both initial, premature ventricular depolarization (AP) and later activation of the remaining myocardium using the normal conduction system. The initial aberrant activation generates a slurring of the QRS called the delta wave, explained earlier in this chapter.

The changes that occur with myocardial infarction, bundle branch block, and ventricular hypertrophy will be masked by the WPW pattern. Confident diagnosis of the existence of an AP must be made by electrophysiologic testing. Any other conclusion about the electrical conduction system, by simply assessing the QRS, must be discouraged.

The major clinical manifestation of WPW is the recurrent tachycardia. As with LGL syndrome, the AP supports the circulating, reentrant wave of depolarization. However, unlike LGL, the resulting QRS may be normal or widened depending on the direction of the reentrant wave front.

If the AV node is activated in an antegrade fashion, and the bundle of Kent is activated in a retrograde fashion, the QRS complex will be narrow. However, if the bundle of Kent is depolarized in an antegrade fashion, with retrograde depolarization of the AV node, a wide bizarre QRS complex will be recorded. This may mimic ventricular tachycardia.

In summary, the ECG characteristics of a WPW pattern are:

- Short PR interval (0.12 second or less)
- Wide QRS complex
- Delta wave
- Tachycardias with normal QRS
- Tachycardias with wide QRS
- Normal conduction pattern in which the bundle of Kent is not activated and normal pathways of depolarization are followed

Figure 13.9 and **Figure 13.10** are 12-lead ECGs showing classic patterns of early activation.

Wolff-Parkinson-White Pattern

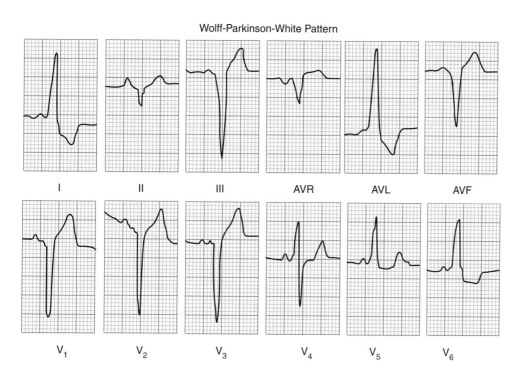

Figure 13.9 A 12-lead ECG showing classic patterns of early activation. Note the short PR interval and the broad QRS complexes. There are positive delta waves in leads I, aVL, V$_4$, V$_5$, and V$_6$. There are negative delta waves in all the other leads.

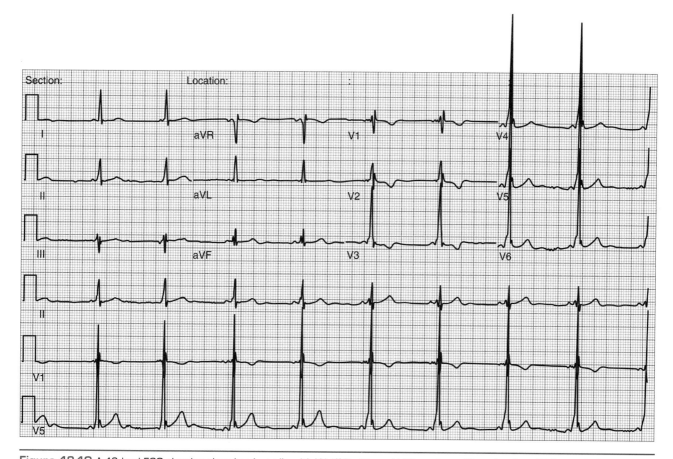

Figure 13.10 A 12-lead ECG showing sinus bradycardia with Wolff-Parkinson-White pattern. Note the short PR interval, distortion in the QRS complex caused by the early activation (delta wave). The shortened PR interval is seen in all leads; the delta waves are most prominent in leads II, aVR, aVL, and V$_3$–V$_6$.

Patients who persist with complaints for paroxysms of tachycardia should be clinically assessed for the possibility of active AP. Surgery or transvenous radio-frequency ablation may be considered in patients who are becoming intolerant of the arrhythmias or have a predilection toward atrial fibrillation. **Table 13.1** summarizes ECG wave forms and characteristics of AP and the mimics with MI and ventricular hypertrophy. **Table 13.2** is a summary of the anatomical sites of the AP and their effects on ECG measurements and configurations.

	Accessory AV Bundle	Intranodal Bypass Tract	Nodofascicular Connection
PR interval	<0.12 sec	<0.10 sec	Normal
QRS duration	>0.11 sec	Normal*	>0.11 sec
Secondary ST-T abnormalities	Present	Absent	Present
Delta waves	Present	Absent	Present
Can mimic myocardial infarction	Yes	No*	Yes
Can mimic ventricular hypertrophy	Yes	No*	Yes

*Must rule out prior pathology within the bundle branch system.

Table 13.1 ECG wave forms, characteristics of accessory pathways, and mimics.

	Pathway	PR Interval	QRS Duration	Delta Wave
Mahaim	Mahaim fibers	0.12–0.20 sec	>0.10 sec Distortion caused by the delta wave	Present
Lown-Ganong-Levine	James bundle from atrium to the bundle of His	<0.12 sec	0.10 sec	None
Wolff-Parkinson-White	Kent bundle from atrium to ventricle	<0.12 sec	>0.10 sec Distortion caused by the delta wave	Present

Table 13.2 Sites of accessory pathways and their effects on ECG measurements and configurations.

SUMMARY

Early activation of the ventricular conduction system outside the normal pathways often results in tachycardias that are confused with ventricular tachycardia. The sudden occurrence of QRS complexes that are different from the patient's normally occurring QRS complexes is highly suspicious of ventricular tachycardia. However, the ECG tracing must be scrupulously examined for abnormalities in the PR interval and QRS complex for signs of the existence of an AP. For example, the delta wave present when the AP is active may be visible only during the tachycardia. In contrast, a patient may exhibit delta waves during bradycardia but not during tachycardia.

The frequent occurrence of tachycardia without any overt cardiac disease may be the first sign of the activation of an AP. Sometimes unexplained tachycardia is the only reported sign heralding pathology in the conduction system. It is important to identify the source of any tachycardia. Conduct diligent and meticulous observation of ECG measurement to ascertain the short PR, delta waves, or other ECG signs of early excitation.

Finally, the ECG in this case can be a valuable tool to be used in conjunction with the available clinical history, and as an evaluation using advanced techniques assessing the electrophysiology of these pathways.

Self-Assessment Exercise
ECG Rhythm Identification Practice

Identify the ECG criteria listed below each ECG, and then compare your answers with those in Appendix A.

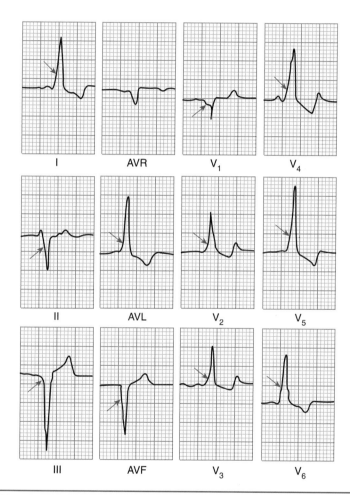

Figure 13.11

1. What is the underlying rhythm? _____

2. What are the abnormalities? _____

    PR interval _____

    QRS _____

3. What is the interpretation? _____

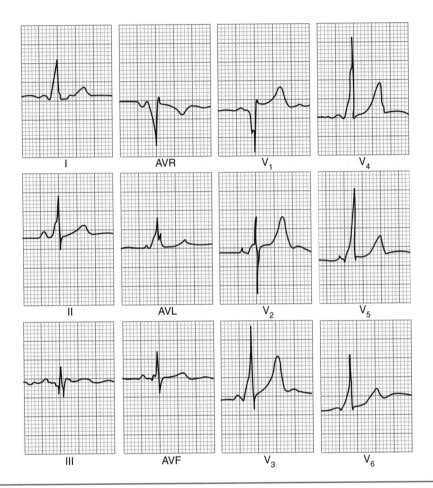

Figure 13.12

1. What is the underlying rhythm? _____

2. What are the abnormalities? _____

    PR interval _____

    QRS _____

3. What is the interpretation? _____

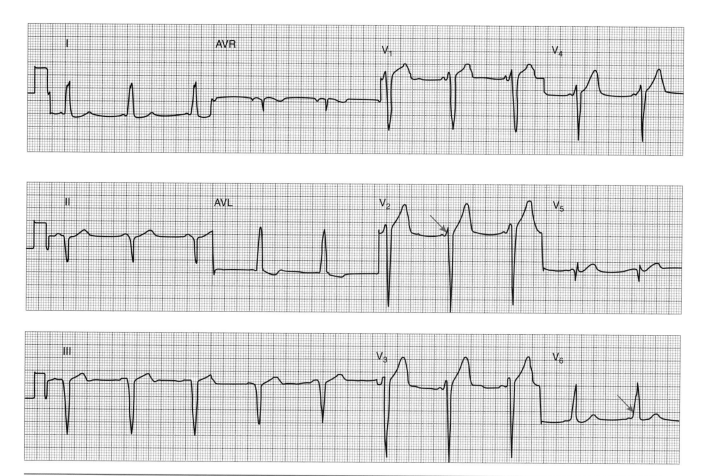

Figure 13.13

1. What is the underlying rhythm? _____

2. What are the abnormalities? _____

   PR interval _____

   QRS _____

3. What is the interpretation? _____

Myocardial Perfusion Deficits and ECG Changes

Premise

Knowledge of the surfaces of the heart, how they are perfused, and how they are viewed by each of the ECG leads provides the basis of a sensible approach to identifying changes that occur with ischemia, injury, and necrosis, as well as the ability to predict possible outcomes.

It is essential that any patient presenting with signs and symptoms of acute coronary syndrome be afforded a multiple lead ECG. Since significant changes may not be seen in some leads, monitoring in one or two leads is simply wrong.

Objectives

After reading the chapter and completing the Self-Assessment Exercises, the student should be able to

- Describe the pathophysiology of acute myocardial ischemia, injury, and infarction.
- Identify the coronary arteries and the structures they perfuse.
- Recognize the ECG changes that occur with ischemia, injury, and necrosis.
- List the complications that can occur with ischemia, injury, and necrosis.
- Identify the ECG leads that are reflective and reciprocal of the area involved.
- Recognize the need for precordial ECG analysis.

Key Terms

acute coronary syndrome (ACS)
akinesis
Brugada syndrome
dyskinesia
fibrinolysis

fixed atherosclerotic obstruction
infarction
injury
ischemia
necrosis

nontransmural (non-Q wave)
positive ST segment coving
reflecting leads
reciprocal leads
trending

Introduction

Myocardial infarction (MI) continues to plague society. Nearly 1.1 million people annually experience acute myocardial infarction (AMI), from which about one-third will die. The pathology of AMI is perfusion deficit attributed to occlusion and/or spasm. Initially the patient may experience pain that reflects ischemia, that is, the lack of perfusion of oxygenated blood. Prolonged insufficiency of oxygenated blood flow results in injury. If the situation persists, necrosis (infarction) will occur. For the purpose of this chapter, the term *perfusion deficit* will encompass conditions resulting in AMI due to infarction or occlusion because of plaque or clot. The pathology of each will be discussed in turn.

The ECG is the most accessible and widely used diagnostic tool for patients experiencing the signs and symptoms suggestive of acute myocardial ischemia. While the prognostic implications of each of the changes seen on the ECG remain a topic of much investigation, some definitions remain constant.

When acute changes are seen in the monitoring and reflecting leads in a patient with suggestive signs and symptoms, they are signals with a high index of suspicion that acute changes are taking place. Those changes must be confirmed by multiple lead ECG analysis and correlated with history, clinical presentation, imaging techniques, and lab value analysis.

Signs of ischemia, injury, and necrosis are often not present or recognized initially on the ECG. **Trending** (repeated ECG recordings with comparison) the patient at specific, frequent intervals, using the multiple lead ECG, lab values, and clinical findings, contributes to early diagnosis and the treatment plan. Trending also monitors the effects of the selected interventions.

Time is a critical factor for successful reperfusion. Therefore, early recognition of the classic signs of ischemia, injury, and necrosis using multiple lead ECG analysis is vital for successful patient outcomes.

It is critical for all health care professionals to know how to interpret the ECG as soon as possible to identify patients at high risk for myocardial ischemia, injury, and infarction. Early identification of ECG signs, substantiated with patient history and assessment, are essential in order to initiate the most appropriate interventions in the least amount of time to provide for effective reperfusion.

CORONARY ARTERY PERFUSION

Recall that the two primary arteries that supply blood to the myocardium are the left and right coronary arteries. They originate at the sinuses of Valsalva, which are located in the aorta just above the cusps of the aortic valve (Chapter 1).

As their names imply, the left coronary artery (LCA) supplies blood to the anterior and left side of the heart while the right coronary artery (RCA) supplies blood to the right side. The LCA divides almost immediately into two primary branches, the left anterior descending (LAD) and the left circumflex artery. Some hearts have a variant artery with a third branch called the ramus intermedius, which is located between the LAD and circumflex. The LAD delivers blood to the left ventricular free wall. In addition, several branches of the LAD called septal perforating arteries supply the proximal portion of the intraventricular septum and the main trunk of the right bundle branch. The LAD also is responsible for perfusing both major fascicles of the left bundle branch system.

There are arteries and branches of the LAD that furnish blood to the high lateral, lateral, and anterolateral walls of the left ventricle. The left circumflex artery (LCx) supplies blood to the lateral and posterior-lateral walls of the left ventricle. In a left-dominant system, the circumflex winds around the heart and gives rise to the posterior descending artery (PDA). In a right-dominant system, the PDA originates from the dominant RCA and supplies blood to the inferior and posterior walls of the left ventricle.

Recall that the RCA supplies blood to the right atrium and the right ventricle. In approximately half of human hearts, a branch of the RCA forms the sinus node artery that supplies the sinus node. In the remaining hearts, the sinus node artery is a branch of the left circumflex. In most hearts (90 percent), the RCA will branch into the AV node artery that supplies

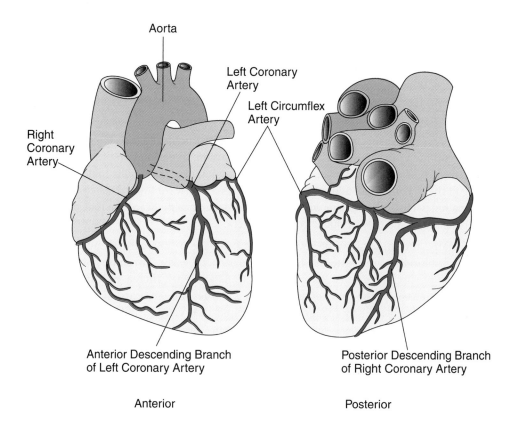

Aorta

Left Coronary
Artery

Left Circumflex
Artery

Right
Coronary
Artery

Anterior Descending Branch
of Left Coronary Artery

Posterior Descending Branch
of Right Coronary Artery

Anterior   Posterior

Figure 14.1 Coronary
artery perfusion, anterior
view and posterior view.

the AV node, as the name implies. In the remaining 10 percent, this artery is a branch of
the left circumflex. In 90 percent of hearts, the RCA gives rise to the PDA (right-dominant
system). The septal perforating branches of the PDA profuse the posterior intraventricular
septum. Right and left septal perforating arteries often anastomose and provide collateral
circulation.

Figure 14.1 is an illustration of the heart's coronary perfusion, anterior, and posterior
views.

PATHOPHYSIOLOGY OF ACUTE MYOCARDIAL INFARCTION

While myocardial infarction is an acute process, it may occur because of a chronic
accumulation of atheromatous plaque formation in the coronary arteries. Simply put,
the bulging and/or rupture of the plaque may significantly obstruct blood flow. In most
cases, without total occlusion, stenosis of a coronary artery can lead to MI. The fibrous
cap of the atheromatous plaque can fracture or rupture. Subsequently, ulceration of the
plaque frequently results in the development of an obstructive thrombus or spasm of the
artery. This can cause acute, total occlusion and subsequent MI. Thrombus formation
resulting from ulceration of the atherosclerotic plaque is stimulated by the exposure of
underlying collagen and other thrombogenic substances to blood flow and the subsequent release of thromboplastic elements from the plaque's necrotic core. This exposure
is followed by:

- Platelet adhesion and aggregation
- Release of thromboplastin, which initiates the coagulation cascade

- Formation of platelet plugs
- Incorporation of fibrins, red blood cells, and plasminogen into the final clot

Coronary artery spasm can occur in nonoccluded coronary arteries, **fixed atherosclerotic obstruction** (the term that describes a lesion in a vessel with an atheromatous plaque), and the grafts used in coronary bypass surgery. Coronary artery spasm can also result in MI due to restriction of blood flow distal to the spasm.

The process of myocardial injury in an acute MI is time-dependent. Necrosis develops over several hours in the presence of coronary occlusion. The evolution of MI follows the "wave front" phenomenon of myocardial ischemia and injury. This results in necrosis originating in the ischemic subendocardium that progresses outward toward the epicardium. If the situation persists, the damage will involve an entire area of myocardium that should have been perfused by the now-occluded coronary artery.

Initially, the injury may be reversible and salvage of myocardial muscle mass is possible if blood flow is restored, but this must occur early. Thromboembolic occlusion is the precipitating cause of most infarctions and with increased duration of the occlusion (necrosis), the area of injury will enlarge and myocardial damage often becomes irreversible. Early recognition and rapid intervention reduce mortality and may improve long-term left ventricular function. The opportunity for reperfusion increases as time-to-treatment decreases. For instance, one intervention, percutaneous transluminal coronary angioplasty (PTCA), may yield the best outcomes when performed within 1 hour after onset of signs and symptoms of the acute event. If there is any delay, **fibrinolysis** (use of medication to dissolve components of the occlusion) may be considered.

Current therapy is directed at preventing thrombosis and dissolving the platelet-rich clot with fibrinolytics. Evaluation and research continue to determine the optimal doses of fibrinolytic agents. Ultimately, GP IIb/IIIa inhibition (with aspirin and heparin) in combination with other fibrinolytic agents may become first-line intervention in all patients. Precise therapies and interventions continue to be the subject of intense clinical research.

Consequences of Coronary Artery Occlusion

Occlusion of the LAD results in anterior wall MI. If the occlusion occurs sufficiently high in the vessel at a point where blood flow to the entire bundle branch system is affected, intraventricular conduction disturbances also occur. In addition, loss of a great deal of myocardial wall motion occurs and ventricular failure can ensue. Occlusion of the left circumflex artery will result in lateral wall MI. With a left-dominant system, occlusion may result in inferoposterior wall MI.

Occlusion of the RCA will result in inferior and/or posterior wall MI. Proximal occlusion will result in right ventricular wall MI and may affect the electrical conduction system. A major consequence of right ventricular infarction is hemodynamic in nature.

The distinction between MI and unstable angina (USA) is at best semantic in most patients. The distinction can rarely be made with confidence early on in presentation. The term **acute coronary syndrome (ACS)** is therefore preferred because it refers to the constellation of symptoms manifesting as the result of acute myocardial ischemia and infarction. The therapy of ACS is divided into patients with persistent ST segment elevation (STEMI), generally greater than 20 to 30 minutes, and those without ST segment elevation (NSTEMI).

Unstable angina presenting with non–ST segment elevation (NSTEMI) comprises a clinical syndrome that presents with chest pain or its anginal equivalent, for example, dyspnea, jaw pain, arm pain, and indigestion, which may be manifestations of decreased coronary artery perfusion. Patient presentation is difficult to differentiate from other forms of ACS and from noncardiac chest pain. They will have atypical patterns, varying ages, and a higher likelihood of renal insufficiency, and it will be difficult to accurately interpret biomarkers.

In patients with chest pain and ST segment elevation, the possibility of acute evolving MI is very high and they are candidates for fibrinolytic-revascularization therapy. If there is no ST segment elevation, patients are unlikely to benefit from fibrinolytic therapy, with few exceptions. In fact, outcomes may be worse. Patients without ST segment elevation in leads I and aVL generally get the same initial therapy whether they are ultimately diagnosed with MI or unstable angina.

For the purposes of this text, chest pain describes a wide range of subjective terms that patients may use. These include but are not limited to:

- Abdominal or stomach discomfort
- Aching belly pain
- Agida
- A pencil stuck up under my jaw
- Burning
- Difficulty getting one's breath
- Fullness in the chest
- Grasping pain
- Hard to breathe
- Heaviness
- It woke me up
- It's different
- Point tenderness over an area of the chest or epigastrium
- Pressure
- Shoulder aches
- The worst pain ever
- Tightness and tingling or pain in the arm or jaw

Some patients who are clinically confirmed as having AMI present with nondiagnostic changes on ECG. Classically, these include nonspecific ST-T changes are scattered among various leads but do not show a pattern that can readily be equated with a specific focus.

Through alterations in wave forms, the ECG allows for visualization of the myocardial disease continuum. Impaired blood flow through coronary arteries results in varying degrees of myocardial damage, depending on the duration and extent of flow reduction. Acute interruption of blood supply to the myocardium is followed by depletion of the myocardial metabolic reserve, when the process of necrosis or infarction begins. This process is seen in the leads that explore the damaged area.

Techniques used to identify myocardial ischemia and necrosis include but are not limited to serum biomarkers, ST segment changes reflecting ischemia, and Q waves reflecting loss of electrically functioning myocardial tissue.

Serum biomarkers include creatinine kinase isoenzyme (CK-MB), troponins, and I and T myoglobin. Troponins are superior in sensitivity and specificity for myocardial cell destruction. The is no normal range of troponin; it is either present or not. By the time any of the cardiac markers becomes positive, some form of myocardial cellular damage has occurred.

The ECG changes include ST segment elevation at the J point in two or more contiguous leads (new or presumed new to the patient):

- 0.2 mV or more in leads V_1, V_2, or V_3 and
- 0.1 mV or more in other contiguous leads

In transmural cardiac injury the duration of ECG manifestations vary. Those observed during coronary angioplasty or in patients with coronary spasm may change or disappear rapidly when the coronary occlusion is removed. Transmural injury secondary to coronary thrombosis resolves gradually following spontaneous or therapeutic restoration of flow. It is critical for rapid restoration of perfusion to salvage myocardium and minimize irreversible injury.

Reflecting and Reciprocal Leads

ECG signs of ischemia, injury, and necrosis are best seen in the leads facing the affected surface of the heart. These leads are called the **reflecting leads**. **Reciprocal leads** are those that are in the same plane but the event is a reflection, or mirror image. Events that reflect the inferior surface are leads II, III, and aVF and the reciprocal leads are I and aVL. Similarly, leads I, aVL, and V_6 reflect the lateral surface, and leads II, III, and aVF are the reciprocal leads.

The standard 12-lead ECG is limited in that it neither monitors the true posterior surface nor provides much information about the right ventricle. It is clinically necessary to do additional leads on the right side of the heart, because inferior wall MI may be complicated by extension to the right ventricle or to the posterior wall.

Lead V_{4R} is very informative. ST elevation in V_{4R} is 90 percent predictive of right ventricular wall MI. This lead will also help the clinician identify:

- The site of coronary occlusion
  - ST elevation and positive T waves indicate proximal occlusion of the RCA.
  - Normal ST segments and positive T waves may indicate distal RCA occlusion.
  - Normal ST segment and negative T waves implicate the occlusion of the circumflex artery.
- Patients at risk for AV conduction defects
- Patients who would benefit most by aggressive reperfusion techniques

In a normal heart, V_{4R} through V_{6R} resemble the ECG complexes seen in lead V_1, but are lower in amplitude. The posterior leads resemble V_6, but are also of lower amplitude. Remember, posterior infarction accompanies inferior wall MI in perhaps 30 percent of the patients. Right ventricular involvement may occur in as many as one-third of inferior wall MI.

In any patient where STE in present in leads II and III with lead III greater than lead II, the 15-lead ECG is highly recommended to detect an otherwise elusive right ventricular and posterior disease. When a multiple lead ECG is not available, a modified V_{4R} should be taken and evaluated (see Chapter 3).

Modified V_{4R}

- Prepare as for MCL:
- Place one electrode on right chest in the V_4 position.
- Place another electrode on the left shoulder.
- Attach the right chest electrode to the positive lead wire.
- Attach the left shoulder electrode to the negative lead wire of the same lead pair (in this case, lead I).
- Turn the ECG recorder to the lead number of the wire pair you used.

The posterior surface is reflected by leads V_7 and V_8; the reciprocal leads are V_1–V_4. **Table 14.1** summarizes the reflecting leads. **Figure 14.2** provides illustrations of the surfaces of the heart as seen by the reflecting and reciprocal leads. **Figure 14.3A** and **Figure 14.3B** are graphic illustrations of reflecting and reciprocal changes on the ECG.

Surface of the Heart	Reflecting Leads
Inferior	II, III, aVF
Inferolateral	II, III, aVF; I, aVL, V_5
Inferior and right ventricular	II, III, aVF, V_{4R}
Anterior	V_3, V_4
Anteroseptal	V_1–V_4
Lateral	I, aVL; V_3–V_6
Extensive anterior	I, aVL; V_1–V_6
High lateral	I, aVL
Posterior	V_1, V_2, V_3 (reciprocal)

Table 14.1 The surface of the heart as seen by the reflecting leads.

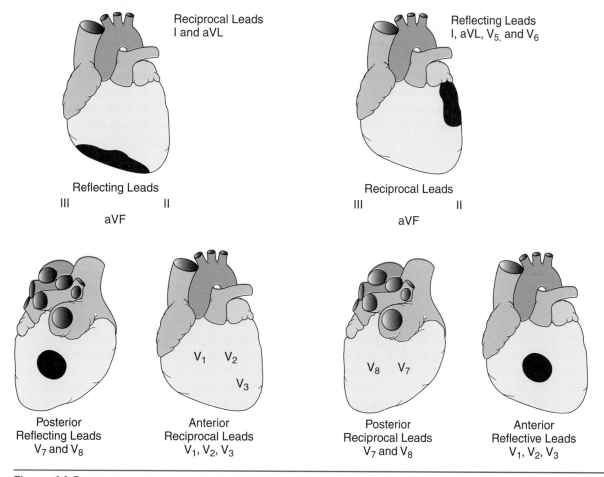

Figure 14.2 Reflecting and reciprocal leads highlighting the area of the heart the lead sees: (A) inferior surface reflecting leads II, III, and aVF and the reciprocal leads I and aVL; (B) high lateral surface reflecting leads I, aVL, V_5, and V_6 and the reciprocal leads II, III, and aVF; (C) posterior reflecting leads V_7–V_9 and the reciprocal leads V_1–V_3; and (D) anterior reflecting leads V_1–V_3 and the reciprocal leads V_7 and V_8.

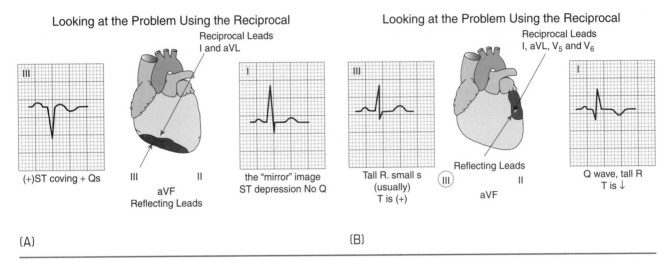

Looking at the Problem Using the Reciprocal

Reciprocal Leads
I and aVL

(+)ST coving + Qs

III   II
aVF
Reflecting Leads

the "mirror" image
ST depression No Q

Looking at the Problem Using the Reciprocal

Reciprocal Leads
I, aVL, V₅ and V₆

Tall R. small s
(usually)
T is (+)

Reflecting Leads
III   II
aVF

Q wave, tall R
T is ↓

(A)   (B)

Figure 14.3 (A) Graphic representation of inferior reflecting leads with the ECG as compared to the reciprocal changes—anatomical and on the ECG. (B) The same approach to the reflecting leads and reciprocal changes with the ECG seen from the point of view of lateral wall changes.

MONITORING MYOCARDIAL ISCHEMIA, INJURY, AND NECROSIS ON THE ECG

The phrase *time is muscle* seems trite and overused, but the concept of time is crucial. The term implies that early recognition and early intervention are critical to minimizing cardiac deficits. The prudent practitioner will develop a sense of urgency based upon collection of observations, assessments, and diagnostic tools to prepare for appropriate intervention to affect reperfusion.

When blood flow is compromised, the affected area of the heart is unable to conduct electrical impulses normally and contractility is impaired. The characteristic changes on the ECG will represent the degree of functional insult in the lead system facing that insult. Direct patient assessment will provide insight into deficits in cardiac output.

In ischemia the ECG changes include T-wave inversion and ST segment depression in the lead facing or reflecting the ischemic tissue. With injury the ECG changes include ST segment elevation in the lead reflecting the injured muscle. In necrosis the significant ECG change is the development of Q waves greater than 0.04 second in the lead reflecting the necrotic tissue.

Changes in Wave Forms

The process of ischemia, injury, and infarction is represented by ST segment elevation, T-wave inversion, or the presence of Q waves in the leads facing the surface of the heart that is affected.

ST Segment Depression. ST segment depression may be nonspecific, as well as an important index of myocardial ischemia. ST segment depression may indicate subendocardial (non-Q wave) infarction or may be present as a reciprocal change in leads opposite the area of acute injury. ST segment depression can be seen during anginal attacks or during a positive stress test. Identical ST segment alteration in the lateral as well as inferior leads can be produced by the effects of antiarrhythmic medications, such as digitalis and quinidine. Other conditions such as hypothermia and electrolyte imbalances—principally hyperkalemia or hypokalemia—affect wave forms and segments.

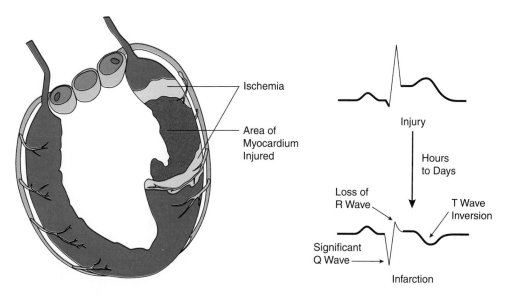

Figure 14.4 The injured myocardium and the accompanying acute changes: the Q wave and ST-T changes initially and after time has passed.

Left ventricular hypertrophy is seen on the lateral leads of the 12-lead ECG as ST segment depression. Such changes over the right precordial leads are slightly more reliable for specific pathologic conditions, present with right ventricular hypertrophy and infarction of the true posterior wall.

ST segment abnormalities may also be a normal variant in up to 20 percent of otherwise healthy females.

ST Segment Elevation.

ST segment elevation (J point elevation) is also a normal variant, but new ST segment elevation in a lead facing a surface of the heart greater than 1 mm is an acute sign. ST segment elevation is also known as the current of injury pattern. Again, ST segment elevation greater than 1 mm in the limb leads and greater than 2 mm in the precordial leads indicates an evolving AMI until proven otherwise. ST segment elevation is usually evident soon after transmural injury is recognized so that steps in reperfusion can be implemented as quickly as possible.

The ST segment elevation associated with infarction usually encompasses the T wave in its contour. This is to be contrasted with other minor causes for alterations in ST segment contour. One such change, called early repolarization, is a normal variant to the ST segment often seen in about 1 to 2 percent of younger, male patients. Elevated, concave ST segments are commonly located in the precordial leads. **Figure 14.4** is a representation of the injured myocardium and the accompanying ECG changes in the lead reflecting the injury.

Recall that myocardial ischemia may be indicated by ST depression in a reciprocal lead. It is critical to assess clinical presentation and the ECG is one of the valuable tools in making the diagnosis of ischemia, injury, and infarction. The clinician must be vigilant and maintain a high index of suspicion for any patient who presents with chest pain of any description. ST elevation in contiguous leads *points* to the *problem*. Reciprocal (mirror image) ST depression in a lead *opposite* the surface *helps* confirm the problem. True reciprocals may not always be present.

Figure 14.5A is a generic illustration of normal ST-T waves, nonspecific ST-T changes, and a 12-lead ECG with nonspecific ST-T changes. Later, it was confirmed that the changes were an early manifestation of an infarction. The patient reportedly described a "feeling of agida low in the belly." This is further evidence that ECG confirmation of an MI requires 12-lead ECG analysis and trending the patient from baseline. ECG analysis at the time of chest pain is critical.

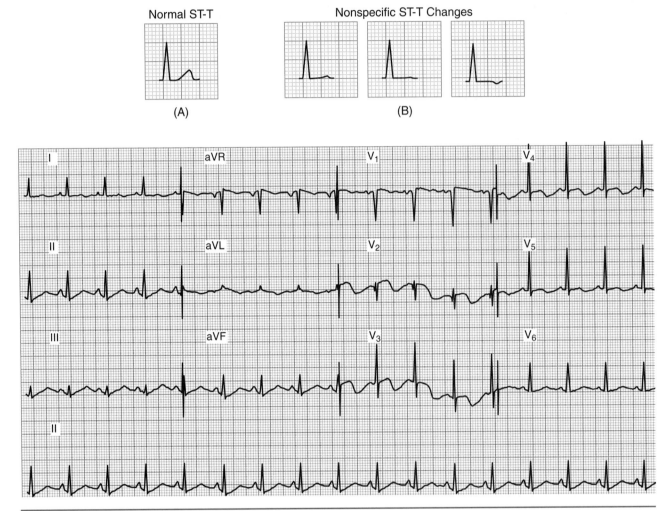

Normal ST-T

Nonspecific ST-T Changes

(A)

(B)

Figure 14.5 Illustrations of (A) normal and (B) nonspecific ST-T. (C) is a 12-lead ECG showing nonspecific ST-T changes on a 12-lead tracing that was later confirmed as an early manifestation of MI. The patient reportedly described a "feeling of agida low in the belly."

Figure 14.6 is an ECG tracing from a patient who presented with substernal chest pain radiating to the left arm, shortness of breath, pallor, and diaphoresis. Changes in ST segments occurred from the time of the initial encounter to 14 minutes after oxygen therapy and nitroglycerin.

ST segment elevations related to myocardial injury usually appear convex or curved. Sometimes this is referred to as a **positive ST segment coving**. Following acute infarction, or when resolution of ischemia has taken place, the ST segment usually returns toward baseline; this usually occurs in the first 72 to 96 hours after damage.

To summarize, one of the following criteria is necessary to make the diagnosis of transmural injury:

- Elevation of the origin of the ST segment at 0.04 second past the J point and of greater than or equal to 1 mm in two or more limb leads or precordial leads V_4–V_6, or greater than or equal to 2 mm in two or more precordial leads V_1–V_3.

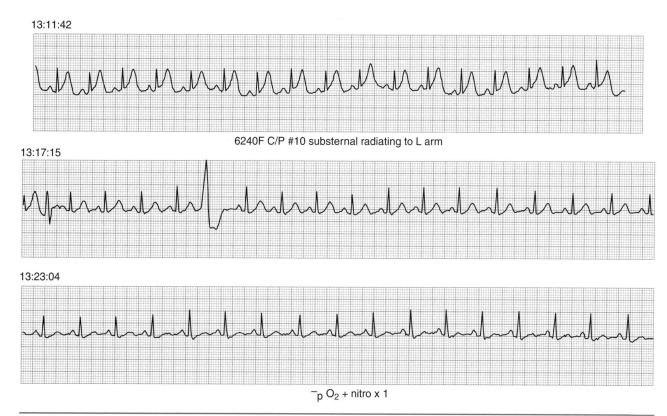

13:11:42

6240F C/P #10 substernal radiating to L arm

13:17:15

13:23:04

⁻p O₂ + nitro x 1

Figure 14.6 Prehospital ECG tracings from a patient who presented with substernal chest pain reported as 10 (on a scale of 1–10, 10 being the worst), radiating to the left arm, shortness of breath, pallor, and diaphoresis. In the first tracing (13:11:42), the ECG shows sinus at 100 beat(s) per minute (bpm) with 2 mm ST segment elevation. At 13:17:15, ST segment is at baseline and the rate is 93 bpm; pain was reported as a 7. At 13:23:04, ST segment shows 1 mm depression. The patient reported relief from pain (a 3), color improved, respiratory effort was unimpaired. The patient was later successfully reperfused.

- Depression of the origin of the ST segment at the J point of greater than or equal to 1 mm in two or more leads V_1–V_3, with ST segment elevation greater than 1 mm in two or more leads V_7–V_9.

Other cardiac conditions that cause ST segment elevation include:

- *Pericarditis* ST elevation is marked by a flat or concave ST segment and usually accompanied by T-wave elevation and depressed PR segments.
- *Ventricular Aneurysm* ST segment elevation that does not return to baseline over time.

Ventricular aneurysm is a condition where a portion of infarcted myocardial tissue does not contract or expand normally. During ventricular systole, that portion of the myocardium bulges outward instead of contracting. This major wall motion disorder is usually seen on the ECG as the persistent ST segment elevation that continues well after the infarction, lasting for months or even years. However, it should be noted that wall motion disorders can be present without ECG changes. Left ventricular aneurysm following extensive infarction may show persistent ST segment inversion over the damaged muscle. This ST segment elevation may be present for years and may be confused with acute necrosis or may mask future ischemic episodes.

Akinesis describes the lack of motion, and **dyskinesia** the paradoxical bulging during ventricular systole. Patients with suspected wall motion disorders are chronically fatigued due to the low cardiac output.

ST elevation associated with ventricular aneurysm also exhibits an upward convex form that is usually seen with accompanying deep Q waves. Clinical presentation and matching of ECG changes over time are necessary. Remember that ECG signs that support a diagnosis of AMI are ST elevation in the presence of reciprocal ST depression and/or Q waves in leads opposite the suspected surface.

Minor ST-T Abnormalities. Daviglus, Liao, and Greenland completed a long-term study of trending the 12-lead ECG of men without overt cardiac disease. They found that those with persistent nonspecific minor ST-T abnormalities had an increased long-term risk of mortality due to MI, coronary heart disease (CHD), and cardiovascular disease (CVD). This study underscores the potential value of including nonspecific ECG findings, especially ST-T abnormalities, in the overall assessment of cardiovascular risk.

Criteria for minor ST-segment depression are *either* of the following:

- No ST-J depression as much as 0.5 mm. ST segment downward sloping and segment or T-wave nadir at least 0.5 mm below PR baseline, in any of leads I, II, aV_L, or V_2–V_6.
- ST-J depression of 1 mm or greater and ST segment upward sloping or U-shaped, in any of leads I, II, aVL, or V_1–V_6.

T-Wave Changes. The T-wave contour is susceptible to many extracardiac factors. T-wave inversion or flattening is nonspecific for ischemic heart disease, but the presence of deep, symmetric T-wave inversion is somewhat more suggestive of the diagnosis of ischemia. T-wave contour is not only affected by many pathologic cardiac conditions but may also be altered by exercise, hyperventilation, food ingestion, smoking, or significant electrolyte disturbance.

The normal amplitude for T-wave excursion has never been firmly established. In precordial T waves that are greater than 10 mm in deflection, however, hyperkalemia should be highly suspected. They may also be seen in the right precordial leads in patients with left ventricular hypertrophy. It is because of these considerations that ST segments and T waves should be interpreted only after the QRS has been carefully analyzed.

Symmetrical T-wave inversion in a lead that normally has an upright T wave is an acute sign and may be clinically associated with ischemia. T-wave inversion that is symmetrical and greater than 5 mm in depth is called nadir T waves. **Figure 14.7** is a graphic illustration of the nadir T waves and an ECG tracing showing both ST segment elevation and nadir T waves.

Because T-wave inversion may be due to other causes, it is vital that the clinician compare clinical history and patient presentation to the changes as they are noted. Cardiac causes of T-wave inversion include:

- Bundle branch block
- Ventricular hypertrophy
- Pericarditis

Noncardiac causes of T-wave inversion include:

- Electrolyte disorders
- Shock
- Positional changes such as posturing with dyspnea, or the patient is seated in the upright rather than supine position
- Central nervous system disorders such as subarachnoid hemorrhage and stroke

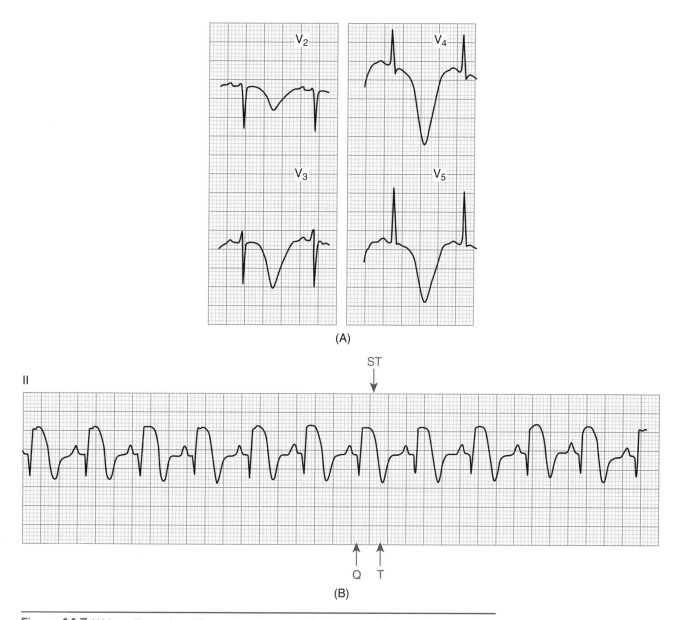

Figure 14.7 (A) is an illustration of T-wave inversion and nadir T waves. (B) is an ECG tracing of sinus at 100 bpm with acute changes reflecting inferior myocardial infarction: Q waves 5 mm, 6 mm ST segment elevation, and nadir T waves.

Minor T-Wave Abnormalities. Minor T-wave abnormalities may be associated with occult cardiac events. They may accompany other minor wave form abnormalities such as changes in ST segments. Accepted criteria for minor T-wave abnormality are either of the following:

- T-wave amplitude zero (flat), negative, or diphasic (negative-positive type only) with less than 1 mm negative phase in leads I, II, V_3–V_6 or in lead aV_L when R-wave amplitude is 5.0 mm or greater

- T-wave amplitude positive and T- to R-wave amplitude ratio of less than 1:20 in any leads I, II, aVL, or V_3–V_6 when R-wave amplitude in the corresponding leads was 10 mm or greater

Abnormal U Waves. An abnormal U wave is a frequent mark of ischemic heart disease. It is most often recorded in leads I and II, and in precordial leads V_5 and V_6. A negative U wave is seen in from 10 to 60 percent of patients with AMI, and in up to 30 percent of patients with inferior MI. Appearance of a negative U wave may precede other ECG changes of infarction by up to several hours.

Q Waves. Q waves are absent in most leads in the normal ECG. A word of caution, however; there are small Q waves commonly present in leads I, aVL, aVF, V_5, and V_6. Significant, pathologic Q waves are wide, greater than 0.04 second in duration, and at least one-quarter of the amplitude of the entire QRS.

In AMI the foremost change of the QRS complex is the development of a Q wave. The new Q waves will be seen in those leads that explore the particular area of infarction. Necrotic tissue has no polarity; thus with acute myocardial necrosis, the forces of depolarization are no longer generated in the damaged areas. The remaining forces of ventricular depolarization are accentuated, displacing the mean QRS vector in each lead system away from the zone of necrosis. The forces of depolarization will be seen moving away, and a Q wave or negative deflection will be recorded. The lead system closest to the infarcted tissue will record the most significant Q waves. At the same time, the reciprocal leads will show initial positive deflection. While the necrotic area is no longer capable of depolarization, contraction, or repolarization, it is still surrounded by an area of ischemic myocardium, incompletely depolarized with each ventricular activation.

Figure 14.8 illustrates the flow of current as it is affected by necrosis.

In the patient who presents with chest pain, a detailed clinical history including history of present illness, past medical conditions, and a family history of risk factors and accurate reporting of the ECG to include ST-T and QRS configuration is necessary. Prompt application of the 12-lead ECG on any patient with chest pain is necessary to ensure that transmission of data, accurate reporting, and diagnosis are available for rapid intervention.

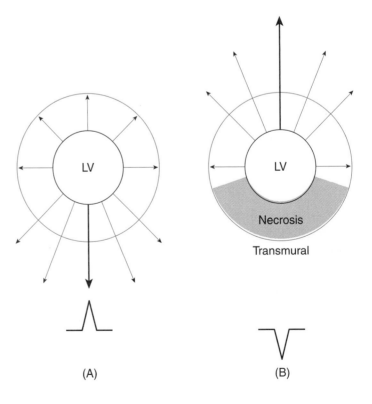

Figure 14.8 Illustrations showing (A) the flow of current toward the reflecting lead and the resulting positive deflection; and (B) transmural necrosis and the deflection away from the necrotic area and the subsequent negative deflection.

Transmural infarctions (full thickness infarction) produce Q waves. While the presence of Q waves is the hallmark of infarction, there is no way to determine whether Q waves represent an evolving event, a recent event, or are a historical sign of old infarction. Thus, a detailed clinical history and accurate reporting of the QRS configuration are critical. A request for previous ECGs for comparison is always advisable.

Q waves will persist over time. While they occasionally decrease in size, rarely do they resolve completely. Other conditions can produce pathologic Q waves, including ventricular hypertrophy, diffuse myocardial disease, and the fascicular blocks.

Absence of Q waves does not rule out MI. MI that does not involve all three layers of the heart is called **nontransmural** and often Q waves are not present in the leads reflecting the infarction.

ECG Indicators of Perfusion Deficits

ST segment elevation and Q waves are reliable indicators of the anatomic location of injury and infarction in the heart. The depth of ST depression and the number of leads demonstrating ST segment depression and/or T-wave inversion reflect the amount of heart muscle that is ischemic. Q waves are the hallmark of infarction; however, Q waves may not appear on the ECG until late in the course of infarction indicating necrosis has occurred. Early in the course of MI, the most prominent ECG finding is ST segment elevation in the lead reflecting the injured tissue. A confirming feature is ST depression (reciprocal changes) in the lead opposite the injury.

Presence or absence of reciprocal changes helps differentiate between conditions with diverse etiologies for chest pain such as pericarditis, ischemia, aneurysm, and gastrointestinal problems. ST segment elevation, with reciprocal changes, indicates the myocardium is in immediate danger. Without intervention, necrosis, that is, irreversible loss of functioning muscle, will occur. Therefore, when evaluating a suspected MI patient, the clinician must observe for ST segment elevation in all leads to establish the correct diagnosis.

INFERIOR WALL (DIAPHRAGMATIC) MYOCARDIAL INFARCTION

Inferior wall myocardial infarction (IWMI, or inferior wall MI) usually results from occlusion of the RCA. In the acute phase ST segment elevation and/or Q waves are seen in contiguous leads II, III, and aVF. There is reciprocal ST segment depression in leads I and aVL, and the lateral precordial leads V_5 and V_6. For any patient in whom ST segment elevation is present in leads II and III, with lead III greater than lead II, the 15-lead ECG is highly recommended to detect otherwise elusive right ventricular and posterior disease. Again, when a multiple lead ECG is not available, a modified V_{4R} should be taken and evaluated.

With further evolution, the ST depression resolves, the T wave is less inverted, but the Q waves persist. Eventually, the T waves return to normal, and the fibrotic scar on the inferior wall is represented by Q waves. There are two aspects of inferior wall myocardial infarction that deserve emphasis at this point:

1. With Q waves in leads II, III, and aVF, the mean axis of depolarization may be shifted to the left, more negative than −30 degrees. In the setting of inferior wall infarction with leftward shift of axis, left anterior fascicular block (hemiblock) cannot be diagnosed.

2. A Q wave in standard lead III may be entirely normal and thus must always be interpreted in light of ECG changes seen in standard leads II and aVF. The Q wave

in these two leads must be 0.04 second in duration, and 25 percent of the amplitude of the R wave to be considered diagnostic for myocardial damage.

Figure 14.9 is an illustration of the surface of the heart affected by inferior wall MI. The accompanying ECG patterns reflect the Q waves and ST segment elevation in limb leads II, III, and aVF. Note the reciprocal changes in lead I.

Approximately half of all inferior wall MIs may lose criteria for significant Q waves in about 6 months following necrosis. Therefore, small Q waves in the inferior leads that do not fulfill criteria for significant Q waves must still be interpreted with caution and should alert the observer that an acute inferior MI pattern might once have been present.

Occlusion of a dominant circumflex artery can cause inferior wall MI. In this case, ST segment elevation is present in one or more of the lateral leads aVL, V_5 and V_6. Also, conduction defects secondary to inferior wall MI are transient and include first-degree AV block and Type I second-degree AV block.

Although inferior infarction typically involves a small amount of left ventricular myocardium, these infarctions should be taken just as seriously in terms of diagnosis and treatment. Inferior wall MIs may extend to the posterior left ventricular wall particularly in a right-dominant coronary artery system. Right ventricular involvement occurs in one-third of inferior wall MIs. Unfortunately, right ventricular wall MI is recognized infrequently.

All abnormal inferior wall ECG tracings require the analysis of the right precordial leads. Of critical importance is the analysis of lead V_{4R}, which identifies:

- The affected coronary artery
- Presence of right ventricular wall infarction
- Presence of AV nodal conduction defect

ECG changes are specific for the level of vascular occlusion. ST segment elevation in the inferior leads occurs only when proximal right coronary disease exists. Elevated T waves in the inferior leads are seen in distal right coronary disease. Inverted T waves appear in inferior leads with distal left circumflex disease. **Table 14.2** summarizes the characteristics of inferior wall MI using V_{4R}.

Clinical Implications

Once inferior wall MI has been confirmed, the clinician must be vigilant for changes in sinus rate and AV conduction defects, especially complete AV block. Parasympathetic activity is common with inferior wall MI and bradycardia. Further potential complications are hypotension and hypoperfusion, so much so that administration of vasodilating medications is at risk for grave complications. In addition, leads V_2–V_4 and V_{4R} should be monitored for anterior involvement and reciprocal changes reflecting extension to the posterior surface.

Proximal right coronary artery	ST segment elevation 1 mm or more
Distal right coronary artery	ST segment may not be elevated; coves into a positive T wave
Circumflex coronary artery	T wave is inverted

Table 14.2 Summary of the ECG characteristics found in inferior wall MI as seen in V_{4R}.

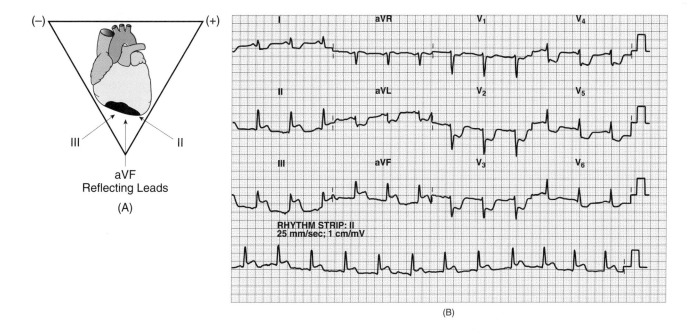

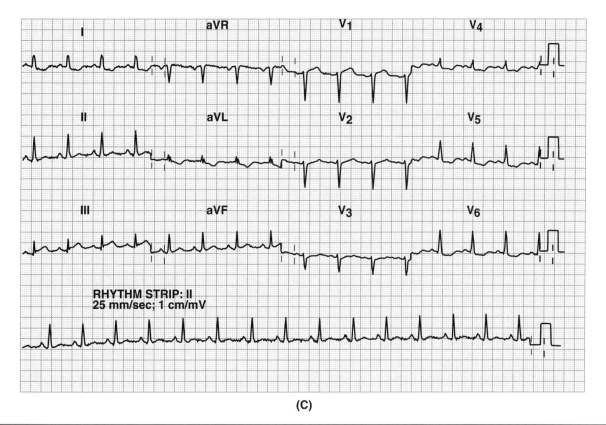

Figure 14.9 (A) is an illustration of the leads that face the inferior surface of the heart. (B) is a 12-lead ECG showing the changes in the injury pattern in the limb leads. Note the changes in leads II, III, and aVF that include ST segment elevation. (C) is the 12-lead ECG on the same patient, after reperfusion. Note in this case the return of the ST segment to baseline 6 minutes after treatment.

ANTERIOR WALL MYOCARDIAL INFARCTION

A QS or QR complex in leads V_1–V_4 is diagnostic of an acute anterior wall myocardial infarction (AWMI, or anterior wall MI). A decrease in the R-wave height (excursion) over the anterior precordial leads is also consistent with acute anterior necrosis. Reversed R-wave progression, the R wave diminishing from V_1 to V_4, is often overlooked as a criterion for anterior wall damage. In addition, absent or poor R-wave progression over the anterior precordial leads may be seen in left ventricular hypertrophy or right ventricular hypertrophy (see Chapter 8). It is important to remember that T-wave inversion over the anterior precordial leads may be a normal variant, most often seen in younger females under 30 years of age.

In acute non-Q-wave anterior wall MI, there is ST segment depression with T-wave inversion in leads I, aVL, and V_6 but no significant alteration of the QRS configuration. These changes slowly return to baseline as acute necrosis resolves. **Figure 14.10** is a 12-lead ECG of anterior wall MI.

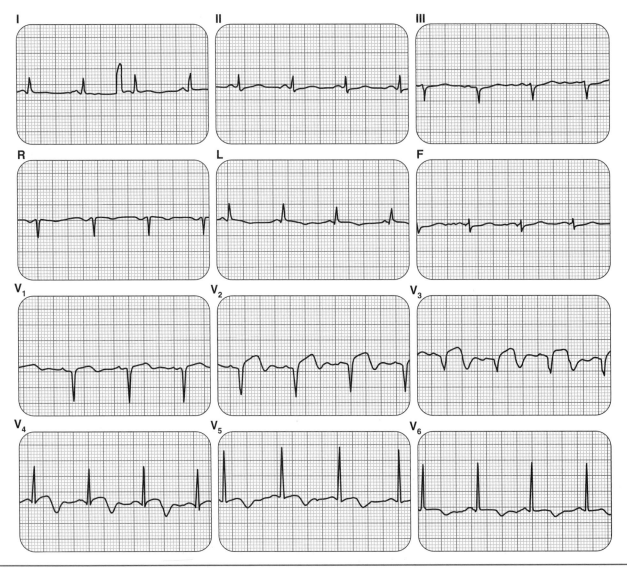

Figure 14.10 The 12-lead evidence of anterior wall MI. There are no significant changes in lead II, other leads demonstrate acute changes: Q waves, ST elevation, and inverted T waves in the precordial leads V_2–V_4. V_4 and V_5 show ST elevation and inverted T waves; V_6 shows horizontal ST segments with inverted T waves. Interpretation: sinus rhythm at 78 bpm with acute signs supporting the interpretation of anteroseptal wall MI and anterolateral ischemia.

ECG wave forms	ECG changes
ST Segment	↑V_1–V_4, I and aVL
T wave	Symmetric inversion from ST↑
Q wave	V_1–V_4
QS complex	V_1–V_4
R wave	Loss or R wave progression

Table 14.3 ECG changes with anterior wall MI.

In summary, the magnitude of anteroseptal or anterior myocardial infarction may be judged by the extent of the precordial leads involved. Sequential ECGs should be carefully scrutinized for evidence of an altered and unstable conduction system.

Acute obstruction of the LAD will result in anterior wall MI. ST segment elevation and/or Q waves in one or more leads from V_1 through V_4 are are significant signs. There may be small Q waves in V_5 and V_6 that were there normally; however, reciprocal changes will be found in leads II, III, and aVF. **Table 14.3** summarizes the characteristics of anterior wall MI.

Clinical Implications

Because anterior infarctions frequently involve a large area of myocardium, cardiogenic shock is very common in the acute phase of this infarction area. Some patients may have sympathetic hyperactivity resulting in sinus tachycardia and hypertension.

Once anterior wall MI has been diagnosed, the clinician must also be vigilant for changes in AV conduction defects such as Type II second-degree AV block or complete AV block. Signs of left anterior fascicular block may be visible in leads II, III, and aVF. In addition, leads V_5 and V_6 should be carefully monitored for signs of extension to the left lateral wall.

ANTEROSEPTAL WALL MYOCARDIAL INFARCTION

Anteroseptal wall MI is sometimes called midanterior myocardial infarction. Specific ECG changes are ST elevation, circumscribed to aVL and V_2, with ST segment depression in leads III, aVF, and V_4. **Figure 14.11** is a 12-lead ECG with evidence of anteroseptal wall MI.

ANTEROLATERAL WALL MYOCARDIAL INFARCTION

There may be instances when there is ECG evidence of acute necrosis in leads I and aVL, but none in V_5 or V_6. This represents an infarction on the high lateral wall of the left ventricle (high lateral infarction) not seen in conventional leads V_5 and V_6. In such instances, all precordial leads should be moved up one intercostal space (high lateral leads). This simple manipulation may unmask acute infarction changes in V_5 and V_6 that would otherwise be

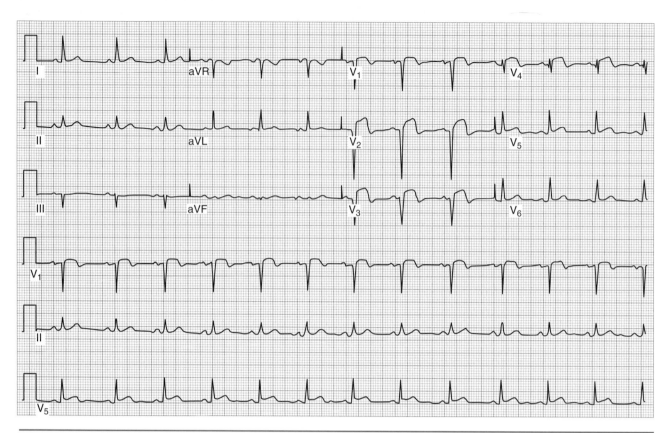

Figure 14.11 A 12-lead ECG with evidence of anteroseptal wall MI. The QRS in lead V_1 is essentially negative; deep Q waves in V_1–V_3 with ST segment elevation from V_1 to V_5. Interpretation: sinus at 75 bpm with acute signs supporting the anteroseptal wall MI and anterolateral ischemia.

missed. These criteria are important because small, insignificant Q waves may be generated in the normal lateral precordial leads, representing septal depolarization in a left-to-right direction. Significant Q waves in the lateral precordial leads V_2–V_5 are at least 25 percent of the total amplitude of the QRS complex.

Figure 14.12 is an illustration of the surface of the heart affected by anterolateral wall MI. The accompanying ECG patterns reflect the Q waves and ST segment elevation in precordial leads V_5 and V_6.

Clinical Implications

Patients may be more prone to ventricular ectopics and arrhythmias. In addition, limb leads should be observed for fascicular block.

LATERAL WALL MYOCARDIAL INFARCTION

Lateral wall myocardial infarction (LWMI, or lateral wall MI) most often results from occlusion of the circumflex artery. ST segment elevation and Q waves are seen in leads I, aVL, V_5, and V_6. A drop in QRS amplitude in these leads may indicate lateral wall MI. Reciprocal ST segment depression may be seen in V_1. Lateral wall MI usually results from extensions of

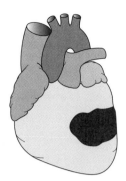

Reflecting Leads
V_2, V_3, V_4,
V_5, V_6, I, aVL (lateral)

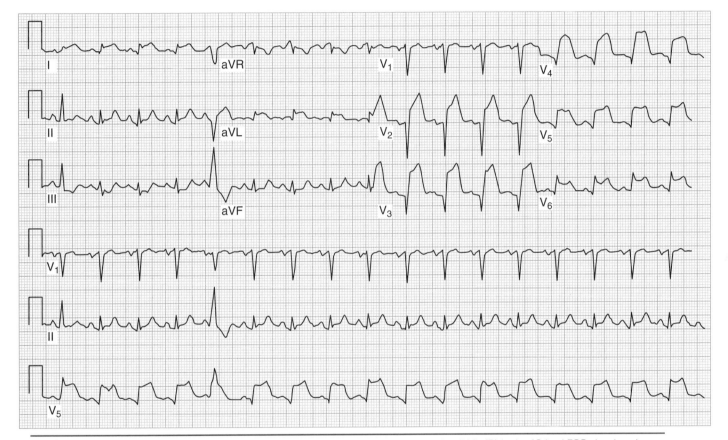

Figure 14.12 (A) is an illustration of the surface of the heart affected by anterolateral wall MI. (B) is the 12-lead ECG showing sinus at 100 bpm with 2 mm ST segment elevation at I and aVL, with reciprocal ST depression in III and perhaps aVF. There are Q waves in V_2–V_6. There is progressive ST elevation in V_2–V_4; 5 mm ST elevation in V_5, and 4 mm ST elevation in V_6. Interpretation: sinus at 100 bpm with acute signs supporting the anterolateral wall MI.`

anterior or inferior wall MI. Conduction defects are rare. **Figure 14.13** is an illustration of lateral wall MI and the resulting ECG changes. **Table 14.4** summarizes the characteristics of lateral wall MI.

Clinical Implications

Once lateral wall MI has been diagnosed, the clinician should be vigilant for changes that indicate cardiogenic shock or congestive heart failure.

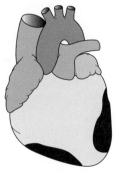

Reflecting leads
V₄, V₅, V₆
I, aVL

Reflecting leads
III, aVF, II

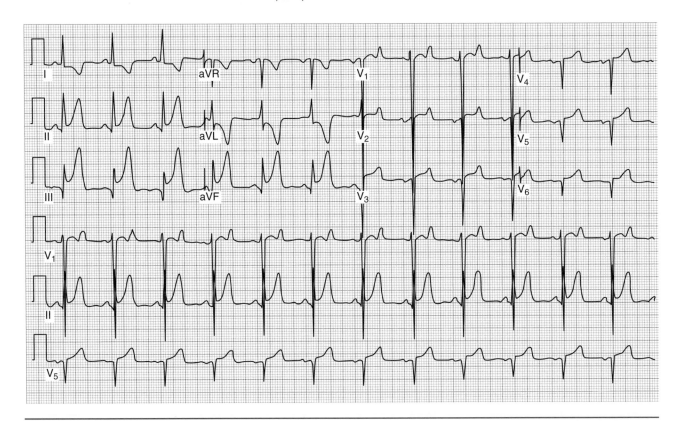

Figure 14.13 (A) is an illustration of lateral wall MI and, in this patient, inferior wall MI. Sinus rhythm at 76 bpm with Q waves and ST elevation in V_4–V_6, significant for lateral wall MI. There are Q waves and ST elevation in the inferior leads II, III, and aVF indicating inferior MI. Interpretation: sinus rhythm at 76 bpm with acute signs supporting the lateral and inferior wall MI.

ECG Changes	Early (Ischemia)	Late (Necrosis)
ST segment	Elevated in I, aVL, V_5–V_6	
T wave	Inverted I, aVL, V_5	
Q wave		I, aVL, V_5–V_6
QS complex		I, aVL, V_5–V_6

Table 14.4 Summary of the ECG characteristics found in lateral wall MI.

POSTERIOR WALL MYOCARDIAL INFARCTION

Posterior wall MI are caused by occlusion of the dominant RCA or the circumflex artery. As explained earlier, posterior wall MIs are particularly common in conjunction with inferior wall MI. Characteristic ECG changes are tall R waves and ST segment depression in leads V_1 or V_2, with R-wave height greater than S-wave depth in lead V_1. In posterior MI, there are tall R waves in leads V_1 and V_2.

While there is ST segment depression in leads V_1 and V_2, a true posterior lead will display ST elevation. These are considered reciprocal changes because the lead directly reflecting the posterior wall is not commonly monitored.

The posterior ventricular leads, V_7–V_9, are true views of the posterior surface and should be recorded in clinically suspect patients without 12-lead ECG changes. However, since criteria for reperfusion therapy require ST segment elevation in two contiguous leads, the value of a posterior ECG can be significant. If acute changes are documented in the posterior leads, there is justification for reperfusion intervention. Be aware that positioning the patient for these leads may be uncomfortable, and resulting artifact and patient movement may complicate the tracing. **Figure 14.14** contains two ECGs illustrating inferoposterior wall MI and the resulting ECG changes. **Table 14.5** summarizes ECG changes associated with posterior wall MI.

Clinical Implications

Because the RCA supplies the sinus and AV nodes in most hearts, posterior infarctions are frequently identified with AV conduction disturbances and changes in sinus rate and rhythm. Also, since a posterior wall MI may result in papillary muscle dysfunction, the clinician must observe for signs and symptoms of cardiogenic shock, heart failure, and signs of AV conduction defects.

RIGHT VENTRICULAR MYOCARDIAL INFARCTION

Right ventricular myocardial infarction (RVMI, or right ventricular MI) is caused by proximal occlusion of the RCA. Although a true right ventricular wall MI can occur independently, it is more commonly associated with inferior wall MI because the right ventricle is not well represented on a standard ECG. It is critical to perform and interpret right-side precordial leads in all suspected inferior wall MIs. In a right ventricular wall MI, ST segment elevation will present in right-sided chest leads. A useful ECG indicating right ventricular involvement shows 1 mm or greater ST elevation in lead V_{4R} which is the mirror image of lead V_4 but it is obtained from the right chest.

A right-side set of precordial leads (the mirror image of the left-side leads) is very useful in diagnosing inferior wall MIs because right ventricular infarction may be life-threatening and is treated differently from the more common left ventricular wall MI. **Figure 14.15** is an illustration of a right ventricular wall MI from right coronary artery disease. **Table 14.6** summarizes the characteristics found in right ventricular wall MI.

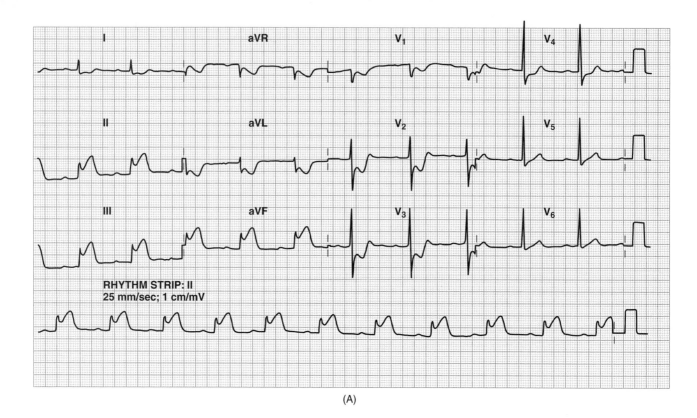

(A)

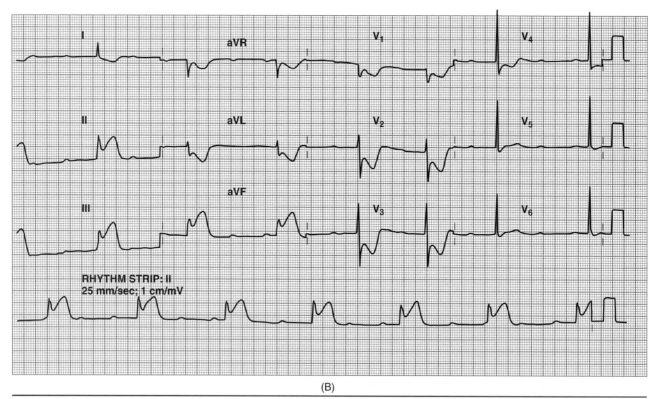

(B)

Figure 14.14 (A) Two 12-lead ECGs from a patient with acute inferoposterior MI. Note the acute changes in the limb leads II, III, and aVF (inferior). Note the R waves, ST depression in V_2 and V_3, and the reciprocal of the posterior surface. Interpretation: sinus rhythm at 67 bpm with first-degree AV block (50 bpm). (B) Acute signs supporting inferoposterior MI complete AV block. Since 12 lead transmission was not available, after relaying the chief complaint and patient presentation, the prehospital description to the physician was "Sinus with complete AV block; atrial rate 100 ventricular rate 37. ST segment elevation 4–7 mm in the inferior leads (II, III, aVF); reciprocal ST depression in leads I and aVL; tall R waves in V_3–V_4; ST depression in precordial leads V_2–V_4. Right precordial leads unavailable at this time." The patient was reperfused within 17 minutes on arrival to the hospital.

ECG Changes	Early (Ischemia)	Late (Necrosis)
R wave		Tall in V_1, V_2
		$R > S$ in V_1
ST segment	Depressed in V_1, V_2	
T wave	Up in V_1, V_2	
Q wave		V_7, V_8
QS complex		V_7, V_8

Table 14.5 Summary of ECG changes with posterior wall MI.

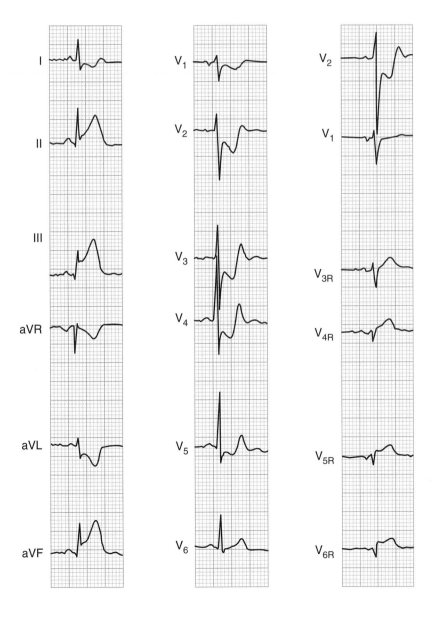

Figure 14.15 Acute inferoposterior wall MI and right ventricular wall MI. Note the elevated ST segment in lead V_{3R} indicating an occlusion in the proximal right coronary artery and right ventricular involvement. (From *The ECG in Emergency Decision Making*, by H. J. J. Wellens and M. B. Conover, 1992, Philadelphia: W.B. Saunders Co.)

ECG Changes	Early (Ischemia)	Late (Necrosis)
R wave		
ST segment	Elevated in V_1, V_2	
	Elevated in II, III, aVF	
T wave		
Q wave		V_1–V_{4R}
QS complex		V_1–V_{4R}

Table 14.6 Summary of ECG changes with right ventricular wall MI.

Clinical Implications

Complications of right ventricular wall MI include hypotension, decreased cardiac output, and cardiogenic shock. Patients are sensitive to drugs with a side effect of hypotension. Signs and symptoms of right ventricular wall MI include:

- Hypotension
- Jugular venous neck distenstion
- Ventricular gallop: S_3
- Summation gallop: $S_3 + S_4$
- Diminished urine output

It is critical to note that these signs may be present without evidence of pulmonary congestion.

NON-Q-WAVE MYOCARDIAL INFARCTION

Absence of Q waves does not rule out MI. Subendocardial infarction may occur without Q waves on the ECG. The designation of nontransmural is made when all three layers of the myocardium are not involved; this is also called non-Q-wave MI. Non-Q-wave infarctions clinically are smaller than Q-wave infarctions as measured by cardiac serum enzyme markers (CPK criteria). They may be associated with a higher frequency of postinfarction angina and recurrent ischemic events. (At this printing, the literature makes conflicting distinctions in this regard.)

Angiographies of patients often show a recanalized vessel. Subendocardial injury causes ST-T-wave changes. Specifically ST segment depression drags down the T wave or the T wave becomes inverted as a result of delayed repolarization in the ischemic myocardium. In some cases only small Q waves (less than 5 mm in depth) or diminished R-wave amplitude (less than 10 mm) may appear.

The characteristic changes seen in non-Q-wave MI involve repolarization abnormalities. Patients may present with ST segment elevation, depression, or both, with isolated T-wave inversion. No early ECG changes can predict the evolution of a non-Q-wave MI.

In non-Q-wave MI, the location of the ST segment depression is not always an accurate indicator of the specific site of the ischemia. Recall that ST segment depression seen in one lead can reflect the mirror-image (reciprocal) sign of ischemia occurring elsewhere in the heart.

In approximately 9 percent of non-Q-wave infarctions there is transmural injury to the inferoposterior wall of the left ventricle. These patients will present with isolated ST segment depression in leads V_1 to V_4. A representative ECG finding of anterior non-Q-wave infarction is a down-sloping ST depression, not the typical horizontal ST segment depression seen with posterior MI. There is also an accompanying T-wave inversion.

Patients who present with only T-wave changes have a lower mortality rate than those who present with ST segment depression and T-wave changes.

To estimate the timing of the infarction, the clinician must assess all changes and trending at specific intervals. The prognosis of non-Q-wave infarction among patients with fibrinolysis is better than that of a diagnosed Q-wave infarction; therefore a high index of suspicion should prevail. There should be close observation for ST segment elevation or depression, T-wave inversion, changes in heart rate, rhythm, QRS duration, and changes in the PR interval. ECG changes must be weighed in conjunction with patient history, clinical presentation, and cardiac enzyme analysis.

To summarize, ECG changes suspicious of non-Q-wave MI include:

- *Inferior wall* leads II, III, and aVF; symmetrical convex ST segment depression.
- *Anterior wall* leads V_1–V_4; ST elevation in V_1 with ST depression in V_2–V_4 without associated posterior wall MI. Inverted or diphasic T waves with a terminal inverted segment in V_2 and V_3.
- *Lateral wall* leads I, aVL, V_5, and V_6; symmetrical convex ST segment depression; inverted or diphasic T waves.

PSEUDO-INFARCTION PATTERNS

Left ventricular hypertrophy generates poor R-wave progression over the anterior precordial leads, suggesting an anterior wall MI. Such poor R-wave progression is due to enhanced forces of ventricular depolarization over the lateral wall of the left ventricle. This pseudo-infarction pattern is of particular importance in a patient with aortic valve disease, whose initial clinical presentation may include significant anginal pain.

Pulmonary embolus, emphysema, and chronic obstructive pulmonary disease with right ventricular hypertrophy may also present with poor precordial R-wave progression. In this instance, the right axis deviation, if present, may be adequate to differentiate anterior wall MI from right ventricular hypertrophy.

Pneumothorax is another common etiology of a pseudo-infarction pattern on ECG. Because of displacement of the heart and mediastinum, the QRS voltage is reduced and the QRS axis significantly shifted, generating what is interpreted as pathologic-appearing Q waves.

As noted earlier, hyperkalemia classically causes peaked T waves, which may incorporate some ST segment elevation. This is easily confused with the acute current of myocardial injury.

Wolff-Parkinson-White (WPW) preexcitation can cause what may appear to be pathologic Q waves in both the inferior and anterior leads due to initial aberrant forces of depolarization through the accessory bypass tract. In patients with WPW, conduction down the accessory tract often creates a delta wave on many of the ECG leads. This makes further conclusions regarding the QRS morphology as it relates to infarction difficult and at times impossible.

Patients with hypertrophic cardiomyopathy (HCM) often have significant Q waves on their ECG. Rather than infarction, these Q waves represent hypertrophied asymmetric ventricular muscle with distortion of the normal patterns of depolarization. Always suspect a pseudo-infarction pattern when the clinical setting and laboratory data do not correlate with ECG suggestion of infarction.

There may also be dramatic alterations to the T waves and ST segments with sudden increases in intracranial pressure. In these patients, changes do not reflect a primary myocardial problem, but rather changes in repolarization due to enhanced sympathetic nervous system activity.

Early Repolarization

Early repolarization with ST segment elevation in the anterior leads can be a normal variant. More pronounced in some, a 1 to 2 mm ST segment elevation can lead to the erroneous diagnosis of either pericarditis or acute myocardial necrosis. In instances of early repolarization, there is usually a notch at the end of the R wave with an upward concavity to the ST segment. In addition, the T-wave morphology remains distinct and separated from the ST segment.

NONCLASSIC ECG PRESENTATION OF ACUTE MYOCARDIAL INFARCTION

In older patients suffering an AMI, the classic ECG changes of ST elevation and reciprocal depression may not be evident early on. New-onset atrial fibrillation, with or without chest pain, may herald the infarction. If there is any suspicion following the acute rhythm disturbance, classic changes such as ST elevation on 12-lead ECG and associated elevated enzyme studies should be initiated to help confirm the diagnosis.

ECG complications such as left bundle branch block may mask the ability of the 12-lead ECG to confirm an MI. In left bundle branch block, the initial forces of left-to-right septal activation are no longer intact. So, when anterior wall MI occurs, the resulting Q wave and ST elevation are not visible in the precordial leads. The left current of flow overshadows the Q waves seen with inferior and anterior wall MI. Correlation of clinical presentation with current and previous 12-lead ECG tracings is vital in making this diagnosis.

CONTINUOUS ST SEGMENT MONITORING

As stated previously, there are limitations to the absolute diagnostic value of the standard 12-lead ECG in initially confirming an acute or recent infarction. In fact, the initial ECG that is diagnostic of acute injury is seen only in approximately a quarter of the patients who have a final diagnosis of an AMI. Trending or taking subsequent ECGs can assist in establishing the diagnosis of MI, but valuable time may be lost in the process because serial ECGs are frequently not performed for several hours unless the patient's condition changes. Occasionally, ST segment changes go undetected until late in the course of infarction after the opportunity for optimal treatment and reperfusion has passed. Continuous ST segment monitoring is thus an important tool for detecting early signs of injury and infarction. Continuous ST segment monitoring can be done noninvasively to detect reperfusion in patients who receive fibrinolytic therapy.

Continuous ECG monitoring using a single-lead system should never be used to confirm or rule out infarction. Trending the patient using 12-lead ECG is valuable to confirming other ECG changes suggestive of AMI, such as loss of R-wave progression and the presence of T-wave inversion. Some facilities employ a computerized 12-lead ECG that is updated every 20 seconds. The ECGs are simultaneously analyzed and compared with previous readings. If four sequential tracings meet predetermined threshold criteria an alarm will sound alerting the clinician to new changes. Changes in the 12-lead may indicate a cardiac event in advance of patient complaint. In lieu of such a system, it may be advisable to perform 12-lead ECG every 30 minutes and whenever the patient has:

- Recurrent pain
- Signs and symptoms of heart failure
- Any new ectopy

Figure 14.16 is a quick reference to the surfaces of the heart as seen in the leads reflecting those surfaces. Table 14.7 is a basic review of one method of assessing ST segment changes in a systematic manner. Table 14.8 outlines the most effective lead systems for observation and anticipated complications.

Look at all three limb leads
- ST ↑ in lead II; look at lead III
- ST ↑ in lead III; look for reciprocal changes in lead I
- ST ↑ in lead III >lead II; immediately go to right-sided precordial leads
- ST OK in lead II; look at lead I
- ST ↑ in lead I; look at reciprocal changes in lead III; go to precordial leads

Table 14.7 How to initially assess the ECG for acute changes.

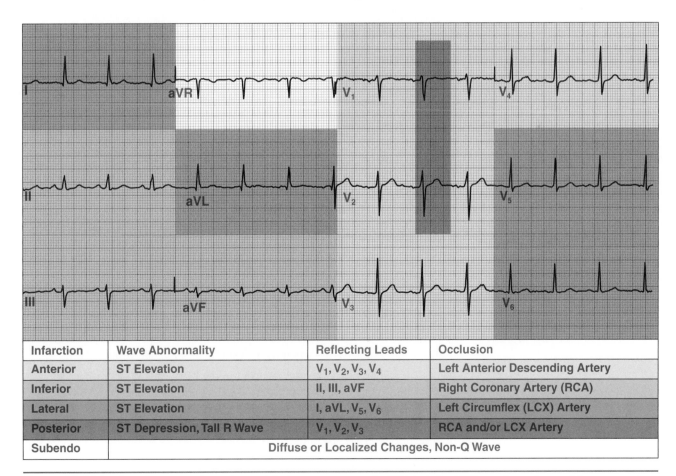

Infarction	Wave Abnormality	Reflecting Leads	Occlusion
Anterior	ST Elevation	V_1, V_2, V_3, V_4	Left Anterior Descending Artery
Inferior	ST Elevation	II, III, aVF	Right Coronary Artery (RCA)
Lateral	ST Elevation	I, aVL, V_5, V_6	Left Circumflex (LCX) Artery
Posterior	ST Depression, Tall R Wave	V_1, V_2, V_3	RCA and/or LCX Artery
Subendo	Diffuse or Localized Changes, Non-Q Wave		

Figure 14.16 A quick reference to the surfaces of the heart as seen on the ECG, including ECG wave form abnormalities common to coronary artery occlusion.

Coronary Artery	Primary Area of Distribution	Site of Infarction and Anticipated Lead System Visualization	Complications
Right Coronary Artery	1. 55% of the SA node	Inferior wall MI	1. Sinus bradycardia, blocks, and arrest
	2. 90% of the AV node		2. AV junctional rhythm
	3. Penetrating portion of the bundle of His	Leads II, III, aVF	3. First-degree AV block
	4. Right atrium and ventricle		4. Second-degree AV block, Type I, Wenckebach
	5. Left inferior, diaphragmatic surface		5. Complete AV block
	6. Posterior IV septum		6. Papillary dysfunction
	7. Left inferoposterior fascicle		
Left Anterior	1. Left anterior wall	Left anterior wall MI	1. Bundle branch blocks and/or fascicular block
Descending Artery	2. Anterior two-thirds of the IV septum	Precordial leads to demonstrate MI process	2. Type II AV block
	3. Bundle of His		3. Complete AV block
	4. Right bundle branch	V_1 for right bundle branch block	4. Septal defect
	5. Left anterosuperior fascicle	Limb leads to observe for conduction defects	
Left Circumflex Artery	1. 45% of the SA node	Left lateral wall MI	1. As in inferior wall MIs
	2. 10% of the AV node		2. Rupture of the left ventricular free wall
	3. Left infero diaphragmatic surface	Leads I, aVL, V_6	3. Ventricular aneurysm
	4. Left lateral wall		4. Papillary dysfunction
	5. Left infero posterior fascicle		

Table 14.8 The relationship of coronary artery perfusion to the sites of MI—the most reflective lead systems for observation.

BRUGADA SYNDROME

The **Brugada syndrome** is a group of signs and symptoms that reflect a genetic structural abnormality that is characterized by specific abnormal ECG findings and an increased risk of sudden cardiac death. It is also known as sudden unexpected death syndrome (SUDS). Although the ECG findings of Brugada syndrome were first reported among survivors of cardiac arrest in 1989, it was only in 1992 that the Brugada brothers recognized it as a distinct clinical entity, causing sudden death by causing ventricular fibrillation.

The Burgada sign is a pattern seen on the ECG to include the following:

- Persistent and unique ST elevations occur in the ECG leads V_1–V_3 with a right bundle branch block (RBBB) appearance with or without the terminal S waves in the lateral leads that are associated with a typical RBBB.

- A prolongation of the PR interval (a conduction disturbance in the heart) is also frequently seen.

- The ECG can fluctuate over time, depending on the autonomic balance and the administration of antiarrhythmic drugs. Adrenergic stimulation decreases the ST segment elevation, while vagal stimulation worsens it.

- An exaggerated J wave occurs—the precise place where the QRS complex and the ST meet is called the J point. When the J point is elevated it is called a J wave. It is also called the Osborne wave as seen in hypothermia and hypocalcermia.
- The administration of Class Ia, Ic, and III drugs increases the ST segment elevation, and also fever. Exercise decreases ST segment elevation in some patients but increases it in others (after exercise when the body temperature has risen). The changes in heart rate induced by atrial pacing are accompanied by changes in the degree of ST segment elevation. When the heart rate decreases, the ST segment elevation increases and when the heart rate increases the ST segment elevation decreases. However, the contrary can also be observed.
- There is an increased frequency of coupled PVCs preceeding the onset of ventricular tachycardia and fibrillation. Syncope is present and caused by the fast polymorphic ventricular tachycardia and ventricular fibrillation.

The cause of death in Brugada syndrome is ventricular fibrillation. These arrhythmias appear with no warning. While there is no exact treatment modality that reliably and totally prevents ventricular fibrillation from occurring in this syndrome, treatment lies in termination of this lethal arrhythmia before it causes death. This requires an implantable cardioverter-defibrillator (ICD), which continuously monitors the heart rhythm and will defibrillate an individual if ventricular fibrillation is noted.

COCAINE-INDUCED CHEST PAIN AND INFARCTION

Of the many complications that are associated with cocaine use, the most frequent complaint is chest pain. The incidence among cocaine users who present to the hospital has been reported to be as high as 40 percent. Ischemia, including acute coronary syndrome (ACS), is the most common cocaine-associated cardiac disorder.

Other cocaine-related cardiac complications include coronary artery spasm, AMI, atherosclerosis, myocarditis, endocarditis, cardiomyopathy, arrhythmias, and hypertension. Of all patients presenting with cocaine-associated chest pain, approximately 6 percent are experiencing MI and 15 percent have ACS.

The risk of MI is 24-fold higher in the first hour after cocaine use, but has been documented for up to 6 weeks following cocaine withdrawal. Demographic and historical factors are not reliable for predicting cocaine-associated MI, but most patients are young, male cigarette smokers without other risk factors for atherosclerosis. Young patients should be questioned about cocaine use if they present with chest pain, and anyone with potential cocaine toxicity should receive a complete evaluation.

The pathophysiology of cocaine-induced myocardial ischemia is multifactorial, and the extent to which the mechanisms may interact is unknown. Coronary thrombosis can develop in the presence of normal or diseased coronary arteries, possibly as a result of alterations in platelet and endothelial functions. Studies have provend that cocaine increases human platelet activation and aggregation. Additionally, vascular spasm may cause damage to the endothelium, creating a nidus for platelet aggregation and fibrin deposition and resulting in thrombus formation. Patients who are treated for cocaine use and/or abuse should be assessed for possible ischemic changes. Verily, patients presenting with signs and symptoms of angina or myocardial infarction should be assessed for history of cocaine use.

SUMMARY

By current estimates, millions of people in the United States have a new or recurrent AMI each year, one-third of which prove fatal. Among patients with nonfatal MI, many experience debilitating loss of cardiac muscle because of delay in recognition, diagnosis, and successful reperfusion.

Despite decades of pharmacologic and percutaneous reperfusion, supported by advances in resuscitation technology, the principal cause of MI morbidity and mortality is still delay from onset of signs and symptoms to recognition and treatment.

There has been considerable progress in the mastery of prehospital recognition acute changes using multiple lead ECG analysis. Twelve-lead transmission is becoming the standard, the goal being to recognize the acute changes significant for myocardial ischemia, injury, and necrosis in a timely fashion and intervene to prevent cardiac death. Since 1990 it is suggested that paramedics, nurses, and physicians be educated to recognize candidates who would benefit from any intervention to limit cell death and reestablish and maintain perfusion. The U.S. National Heart Attack Alert Program recommends that emergency medical services (EMS) systems provide out-of-hospital 12-lead ECGs to facilitate early identification of AMI and that all advanced lifesaving vehicles be able to transmit a 12-lead ECG to a hospital.

When transmission is not possible, prehospital providers should be able to describe the ECG to the physician in an organized manner. In any clinical setting a vital aspect of patient survival is the correct reporting of the ECG changes that reflect arrhythmias, ischemia, injury, and infarction. This ability involves knowledge and organization of data to provide the physician with insight into the patient's circumstance in order to prepare for prompt intervention.

The multiple lead ECG continues to be a valuable tool in the hands of an educated and discriminating medical professional. As with any other diagnostic tool, the 12-lead ECG is a beneficial adjunct to thorough history taking, physical examination, and monitoring the clinical course. Serial multiple lead ECGs are vital in tracking the course of the infarction. The clinician must always remember that the patient and the ECG are a package and should take effort not to treat one without the other.

Self-Assessment Exercises

Matching

Match the term in the left column with the definition in the right column, and then compare your answers with those in Appendix A.

Term	Definition
_____ 1. Anterior wall MI	A. ST elevation 3–4 weeks post-MI
_____ 2. Current of injury	B. ST elevation
_____ 3. Inferior wall MI	C. Q, ST ↑ II, III, aVF
_____ 4. Transmural MI	D. Q, ST ↑ V_3, V_4, V_5, V_6
_____ 5. Ventricular aneurysm	E. Q, ST ↑, hyperacute T waves

ECG Rhythm Identification Practice

Identify the ECG criteria listed below each ECG, and then compare your answers with those in Appendix A.

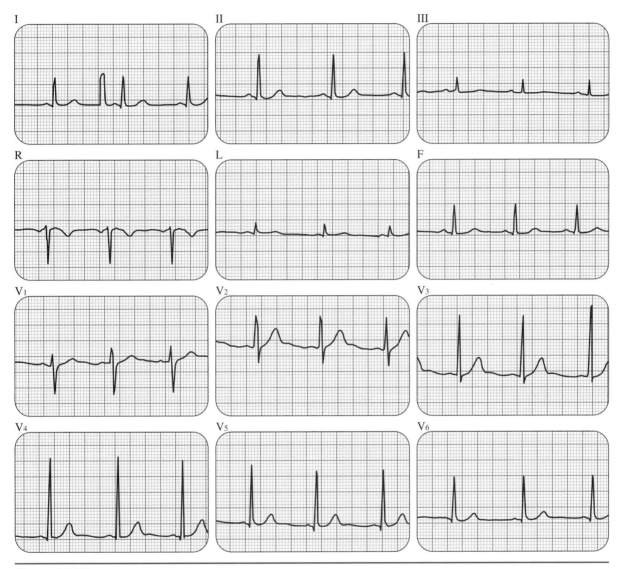

Figure 14.17

1. What is the underlying rhythm? _____

2. What are the acute changes? _____

3. What is your interpretation? _____

4. What can happen next? _____

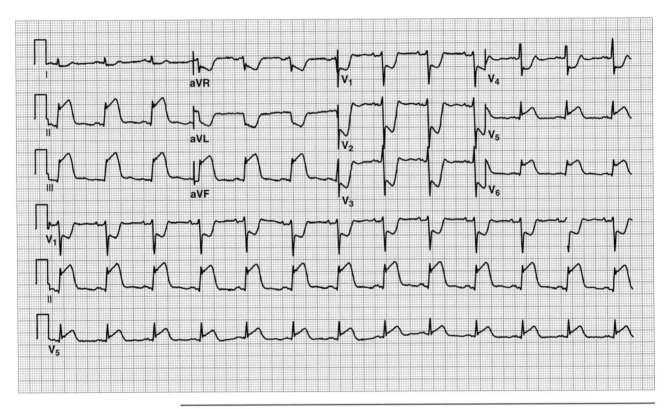

Figure 14.18

1. What is the underlying rhythm? _____

2. What are the acute changes? _____

3. What is your interpretation? _____

4. What can happen next? _____

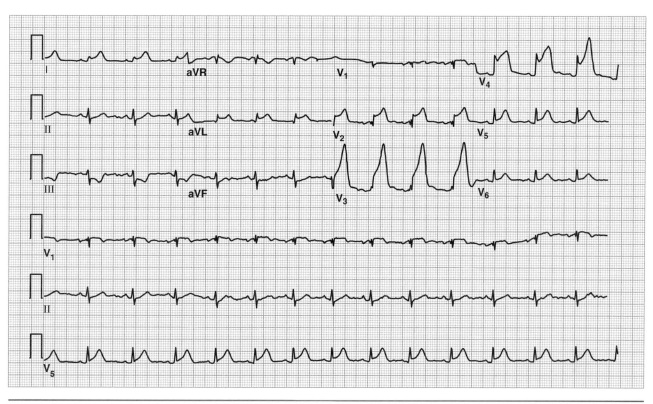

Figure 14.19

1. What is the underlying rhythm? _____

2. What are the acute changes? _____

3. What is your interpretation? _____

4. What can happen next? _____

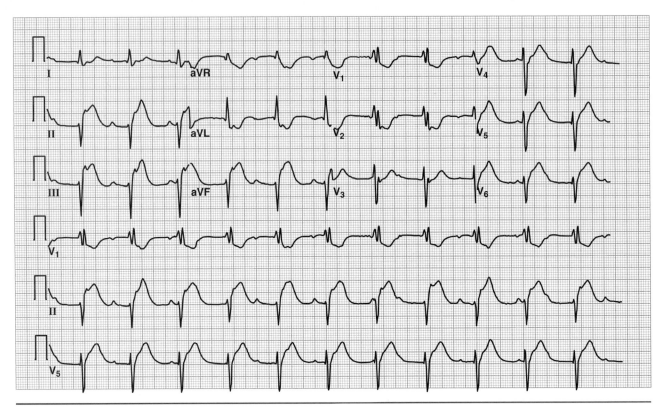

Figure 14.20

1. What is the underlying rhythm? _____

2. What are the acute changes? _____

3. What is your interpretation? _____

4. What can happen next? _____

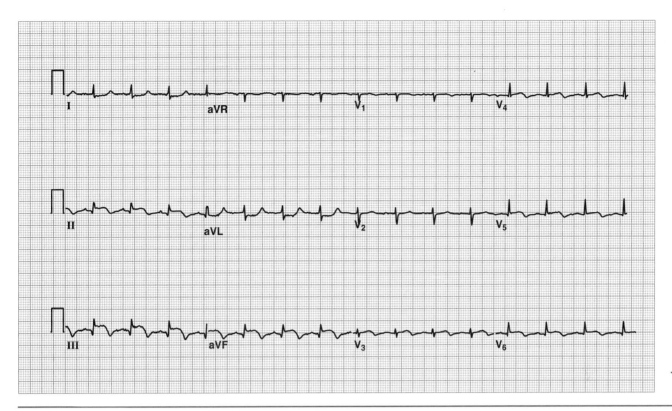

Figure 14.21

1. What is the underlying rhythm? _____

2. What are the acute changes? _____

3. What is your interpretation? _____

4. What can happen next? _____

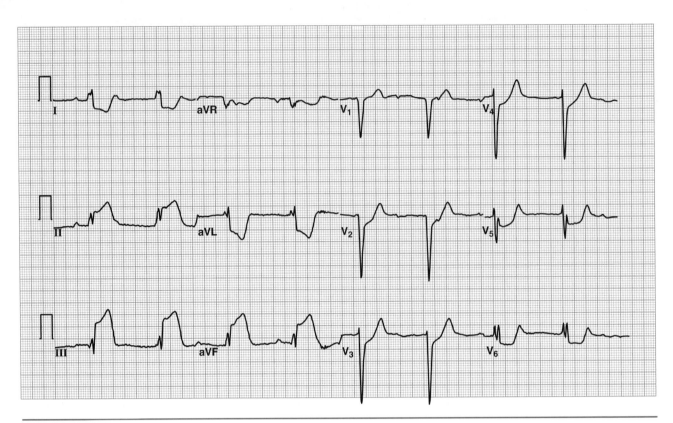

Figure 14.22

1. What is the underlying rhythm? _____

2. What are the acute changes? _____

3. What is your interpretation? _____

4. What can happen next? _____

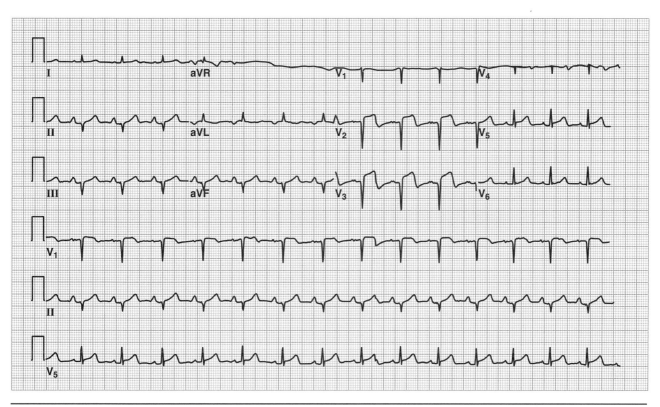

Figure 14.23

1. What is the underlying rhythm? _____

2. What are the acute changes? _____

3. What is your interpretation? _____

4. What can happen next? _____

Electronic Pacemakers

Premise

The purpose for electronic pacing is to provide an energy source that will guarantee a minimum ventricular rate when the heart's conduction system cannot. Electronic pacing does not guarantee myocardial tissue response.

Objectives

After reading the chapter and completing the Self-Assessment Exercises, the student should be able to

- Identify pacemaker artifact, and calculate its rate and the escape interval.
- Identify the chambers of the heart that are being paced.
- Identify the mechanism by which the pacemaker is being activated or inhibited.
- Recognize ECG signs of pacemaker malfunction.

Key Terms

AV interval	inhibited	programmed upper rate
asynchronous	mode of pacemaker	limit (PURL)
demand	response	rate-adaptive or
electronic capture	overdrive suppression	physiologic
escape interval	oversensing	sensitivity
failure to capture	pacemaker	threshold
failure to sense	pacemaker identification	undersensing
fusion	code	
hysteresis		

Introduction

The heart has an intrinsic system that provides for the source and conduction system of electrical energy in an organized fashion. Disturbances in the source or within the conduction system can cause life-threatening arrhythmias. These may be drug induced or due to intrinsic conduction defects.

Electronic pacemakers are used primarily in the management of bradycardia resulting from the heart's inability to stimulate or conduct electrical impulses. They are also used to suppress ectopics and the onset of certain tachycardias.

PACEMAKER CODES

To better understand, more easily evaluate, and document ECG characteristics of **pacemakers**, additional language should be added to the ECG vocabulary, to clarify intrinsic function from pacemaker function. The five-letter **pacemaker identification code** of the Intersociety Committee on Heart Disease (ICHD) was designed in an effort to explain how a pacemaker operates.

The *first* letter of the code indicates the chamber being paced:

A = atrial

V = ventricular

D = dual, indicating both right atrium and right ventricle being paced

The *second* letter indicates which chamber's activity is being sensed:

A = atrial

V = ventricular

D = dual, indicating both chambers' activities are being sensed

O = neither chamber is sensed

The *third* letter indicates the **mode of pacemaker response**:

I = inhibited

T = triggered

D = dual, indicating the pacer is capable of both functions

O = not applicable

The *fourth* letter stands for the type of changes or the programmability that can be made by noninvasive means:

P = programmability of rate and/or output

R = rate modulation

C = communicating

M = multiprogrammable

These settings include rate, energy output, ability to sense, refractory period, and other variables as technology increases.

The *fifth* letter stands for the response of the pulse generator to sensing tachycardias and reflects the antitachycardia function.

Commonly, the first three letters of the code are used to describe pacemaker activity. For example, in a demand, single-chamber (ventricular) pacer, both sensing and pacing circuits are in use. Thus, this pacer would be called a VVI pacer: *V* for the ventricular chamber being paced, *V* for the intrinsic ventricular activity being sensed, and *I* for the ventricular function inhibited by the sensed intrinsic QRS.

Another example would be the DDD pacemaker. The first *D* means dual pacing activity; both atrial and ventricular chambers are paced. The second *D* means dual sensing activity; both atrial and ventricular intrinsic activity is being sensed. The third *D* identifies what the pacer will do (pace or not) based on sensed event.

For example, a sensed event in the atrium inhibits atrial pacing and triggers a ventricular pacing stimulus after the programmed **AV interval**. A sensed beat in the ventricle inhibits the pacer's output in the ventricle.

THE LANGUAGE OF PACEMAKER FUNCTION

In addition, the names given to pacemaker-generated wave forms and intervals differentiate them from the patient's intrinsic wave forms and intervals.

Committed is a term used in dual-chamber pacing, when ventricular stimulation will occur after atrial stimulation at a preset interval. If ventricular stimulation is programmed to occur always after atrial stimulation, this is termed fully committed. When normal or paced atrial excitation occurs and normal (intrinsic) AV conduction results, ventricular pacing will be inhibited.

Partially committed refers to pacemakers that have safety pacing. For example, after the atrial spike occurs, the pacemaker looks for any sensed event within 110 milliseconds (ms). If a ventricular event is sensed during that time, the pacemaker forces a ventricular spike at the end of 110 ms. If nothing is sensed during the first 110 ms following the atrial spike, the pacer will inhibit on any ventricular sensed event after 110 ms or it will pace at the end of the AV interval.

A refers to pacer-induced atrial depolarization.

AV interval is the time between paced atrial and paced ventricular activity.

VA interval is the time between paced ventricular and paced atrial activity.

VV interval is the distance measured between two paced ventricular events.

RV interval is the distance from the intrinsic ventricular event and the paced ventricular event that follows the pacemaker's escape interval.

Notation is a set of numbers indicating pacer mode and programmed timing parameters, seen on patient identification cards. For example, a notation may be 60/160/150. The 60 is the lowest rate limit. The pacemaker is programmed to track spontaneous rate, and if this intrinsic rate falls below 60 per minute, the pacer is programmed to provide the stimulus. The 160 is because in dual-chamber pacing, the AV interval is measured in milliseconds; for example, 160 ms equals 0.16 second. The 150 is the pacemaker's programmed maximum rate of delivery. In this example, the paced rate should never exceed 150 beat(s) per minute (bpm).

Table 15.1 is a summary of the intrinsic ECG terms and correlating pacemaker terminology.

When referring to the intervals between intrinsic function and pacing function, the terminology will afford an easy explanation. For example, in atrial pacing, the interval between the intrinsic P wave and the paced atrial beat would be the PA interval. Similarly, the interval between the intrinsic QRS and the paced QRS, would be the RV interval. **Figure 15.1** is an ECG tracing indicating the RV and VV intervals.

Intrinsic Wave Form	Pacemaker Term
P wave	A
PR interval	AV interval
PP interval	AA interval
QRS complex	V
RR interval	VV interval

Table 15.1 Analogous terminology for intrinsic and pacemaker wave forms.

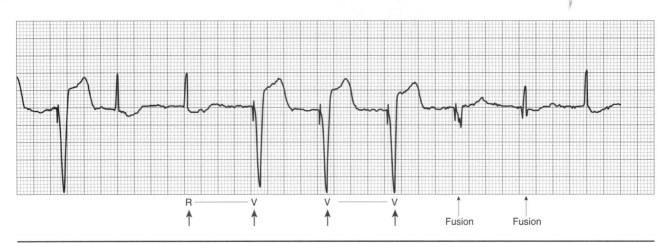

Figure 15.1 An ECG tracing indicating the RV and VV intervals. Note the distance between the second, intrinsic QRS (R) and the first paced QRS (V), the distance between two paced QRS complexes (RR). The RV = the VV interval. There are two paced QRS complexes that are a merging of paced and normal forces depolarizing the ventricles. The VV interval remains constant as the supraventricular source had not yet accelerated beyond the pacer's preset rate. Note the combination or fusion of the pacer spike and the intrinsic QRS complex. The pacer fires on time, and there is a combination of paced and intrinsic forces.

PACEMAKER COMPONENTS

Pulse Generator

An electronic pacemaker consists of two primary components: the pulse generator, which is the energy source, and the pacing electrode, which delivers the electrical stimulus. External pacemakers that deliver a current through the skin from one electrode to another are called transcutaneous (*trans*–through, *cutaneous*–the skin). The pulse generator of the transvenous pacemaker can be external or implanted. A transvenous pacemaker (*trans*–through, *venous*–the vein) uses a pacing catheter that is connected to the pacemaker and threaded into the right ventricle so that it comes in contact with the right ventricular endocardial tissue.

Pacemaker generators are frequently of the built-in cardiac monitor/defibrillator type or handheld devices. Implanted pacemaker generators are encased in titanium or stainless steel housing that is hermetically sealed to protect the circuitry.

Pacemaker circuitry changes constantly. It has evolved from transistorized circuits, and their sizes have decreased appreciably. Newer pacemakers are very small and programmable, sometimes using telephone transmission. **Figure 15.2** is a drawing of the torso with anterior and posterior (AP) transcutaneous pads superimposed.

Transcutaneous pacemakers (TCPs) are external devices manufactured separately or incorporated into defibrillators/monitors. Some are designed with a pacing cassette to be inserted into the defibrillator console, and others have pacing controls integrated into the system. In a TCP, the electrodes are attached to the patient and to the pacemaker by a special multifunction pad/electrodes. ECG leads also are attached to the patient as the intrinsic ECG signal must be monitored constantly. The pacemaker must be able to read the patient's ECG to know when to pace and when not to pace. The pacemaker's internal timing mechanisms will sense and recognize the patient's QRS complex. If the pacemaker is set for 50 bpm, and the patient's pulse rate drops below 50, the pacer will discharge a current to guarantee a minimum rate of 50 bpm. All TCP are demand pacemakers and will discharge a current at whatever rate is chosen for that patient.

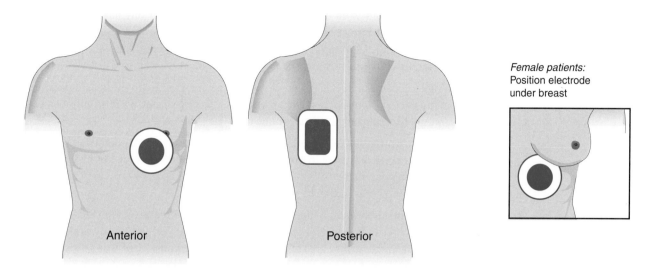

Female patients:
Position electrode
under breast

Anterior

Posterior

Figure 15.2 A torso with anterior and posterior (AP) transcutaneous pads, indicating their placement. The insert shows the position of the anterior pad for female patients.

Pacemaker Catheters and Electrodes

Transvenous pacing is relatively new, beginning in 1959. A pacemaker catheter is inserted using a venous approach so that the distal tip is in the right ventricle. The pacemaker catheter is attached to a pulse generator.

Pacemaker catheters, often referred to as the lead or the electrode, are the link between the pacemaker and the heart. These catheters transmit an impulse to the heart, and in some pacemakers, transmit the heart's intrinsic electrical activity back to the pacemaker.

Pacemaker catheters are either bipolar or unipolar. Bipolar catheters have positive and negative electrodes, which come in contact with heart tissue. The distal, negative electrode is the stimulating electrode.

Unipolar electrodes have only the negative electrode at the distal tip of the catheter. The positive or indifferent electrode is part of the pulse generator. Unipolar systems are very sensitive to intracardiac as well as extracardiac signals.

Noninvasive, transcutaneous pacing electrodes (multifunction pads/electrodes) are large, pregelled patches that can be anterior-posterior (AP) or anterior-left lateral (AL). The AP placement is common and does not interfere with defibrillation if needed. The landmarks for placement of the TCP pacing electrodes are well defined by the manufacturer, and the polarity should not be reversed. If the electrodes are reversed, failure to capture may occur. Defibrillation can be performed through the same multifunction pads/electrodes.

External pacing electrodes may be multifunctional (ECG monitoring, defibrillation/synchronized cardioversion, and pacing) or single function (pacing only). Whatever the manufacture capabilities, during demand pacing the patient's ECG must be monitored through ECG electrodes.

Pacemaker Energy

The current output from the pacemaker is measured in terms of milliamperes (mA). The amount of mAs, or signal, must be of such an amplitude to cause capture but not so strong as to cause diaphragmatic pacing. The minimum amount of current required to elicit electronic and mechanical capture is **threshold**.

Sensitivity is the ability of the pacemaker to process the heart's intrinsic signals and is programmed in millivolts (mV). When the sensitivity is set at its smallest number, the pacemaker senses all intrinsic signals. As the sensitivity is set at larger numbers, the pacemaker progressively ignores intrinsic signals.

For example, pacemakers set at zero or low numbers are sensitive to the heart's function as with demand pacing. Conversely, if the pacemaker sensitivity is set at a large number, the pacemaker would function at a fixed-rate mode or asynchronously.

When depolarization is not sensed, the pacemaker is said to be **undersensing**. Some ectopic intrinsic activity may vary in amplitude, and the pacemaker may not be sensed by a normally operating pacemaker. When interference is sensed as if it were a depolarization wave form, the pacemaker is said to be **oversensing**.

In a transcutaneous system, a higher current of output is required to overcome chest wall resistance. The result is a painful procedure to the patient. The possibility of skin burn is minimized by the large surface area of the pregelled pacing pads.

Pacemaker Artifact and Pacer-Induced QRS Complexes

When a pacemaker stimulus is delivered, a sharp, perfectly vertical artifact is seen on the ECG. This is the pacer artifact, or spike. On the ECG, the pacemaker spike of a unipolar system usually generates a signal (the pacer spike) that is larger than the stimulus from a bipolar signal. Sometimes bipolar spikes are difficult to see, and some may not be seen at all.

Each pacer spike will be seen on the ECG in direct association with the wave form of the chamber being paced. This association is called **electronic capture**. When a pacer spike occurs at the appropriate time, and there is no QRS complex associated with it, this is called **failure to capture**.

The QRS from a unipolar system is usually seen as a large QS complex with the T wave in the opposite direction. The QRS from a bipolar system is primarily negative but may not be greater than 0.12 second. Regardless of the amplitude and direction of every pacer-induced QRS, every captured QRS should result in mechanical capture, that is, a palpable carotid pulse. **Figure 15.3** is an ECG tracing showing a rhythm with a paced QRS.

Pacemaker Fusion

Occasionally, the pacemaker fires at the same time a supraventricular impulse reaches the ventricles and the two forces will collide or fuse and simultaneously depolarize the

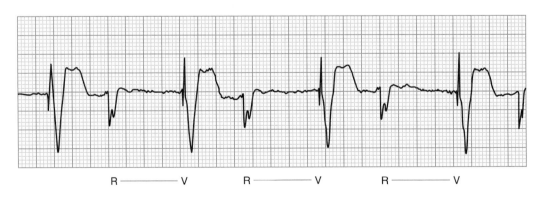

Figure 15.3 An ECG tracing showing the intrinsic QRS (0.12 second) followed by a paced QRS. The rhythm takes on a bigeminal pattern; the RV intervals are consistent.

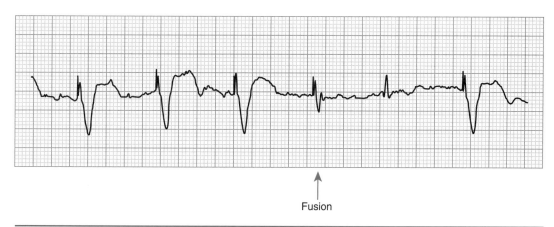

Fusion

Figure 15.4 An ECG tracing showing four paced QRS complexes. The fourth complex is a combination of pacer and normal QRS activation. This is pacemaker fusion. The RV and VV intervals are consistent.

ventricles. This collision of forces, **fusion,** will cause a change in the pacer-induced QRS. The pacer-induced fusion beat will take on the characteristics of both energy sources, causing a decreased amplitude and duration. **Figure 15.4** is an ECG tracing showing evidence of pacemaker fusion. Note the decreased amplitude of the QRS.

TEMPORARY AND PERMANENT PACING

The word *temporary* in electronic pacing varies in interpretation and is relative to the purpose and goal desired for the patient. For instance, temporary pacing can be noninvasive (transcutaneous) for a short period of time, minutes for example, or transvenous, yet externally controlled, and used for only a few days. If the problem is corrected, the pacing electrode is easily removed.

Implanted pacemaker generators can be a temporary solution for a patient and can be utilized for months or even years. The pacemaker is designed to manage the heart rate until a definitive operative procedure can be performed. For instance, in a child whose weight is slight, and in whom pulmonary function would improve with age, the use of temporary transvenous implanted pacing would provide a satisfactory ventricular rate until such time as the corrective procedure could be accomplished. **Figure 15.5** shows an implanted pacemaker generator.

Classification

Pacemakers are classified according to their activity as either asynchronous or demand pacemakers.

Asynchronous Pacemakers (VOO). Asynchronous pacemakers are also called fixed-rate or continuous pacemakers and generate a current at a fixed, preset rate. These pacemakers may be used in cases of congenital AV block or other conditions where there is no functional (natural) intrinsic rhythm. A fixed-rate or continuous pacemaker fires continuously, regardless of the patient's intrinsic rhythm. The possibility of a pacing stimulus firing during the heart's vulnerable period is great, and the patient could suffer pacer-induced ventricular tachycardia or fibrillation. There is no sensing mechanism in a fixed-rate pacemaker.

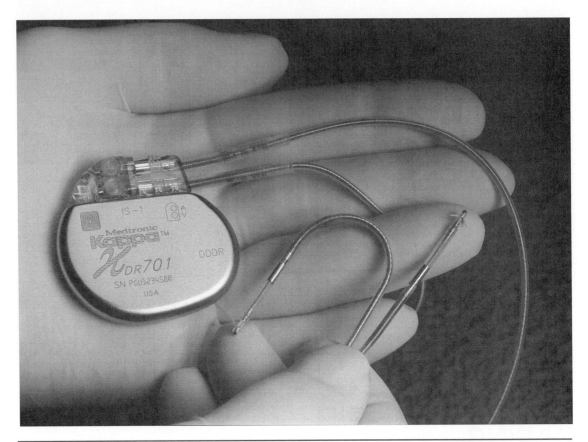

Figure 15.5 An implantable pulse generator (pacemaker) and the platinized pacemaker electrodes. Note the relative size of the pacemaker. It generates the electrical impulse that is transmitted through the electrodes to the endocardium. These implantable, flexible electrodes have soft plastic tines or phlanges that are compressed during implantation. Once inserted, these tines deploy to hold the pacemaker in place and limit the chance of dislodgement. (Courtesy Medtronic, Inc.).

Demand Pacemakers (VVI/AAI). Demand or inhibited pacemakers fire only when needed, or on **demand**. Demand or synchronous pacemakers have a sensing device and a timer that is preset for a specific rate, or *escape interval*. The sensing mechanism interprets the signal received from the patient's rhythm, allowing for intrinsic function. If an impulse is sensed within the pacemaker's preset rate, the pacemaker is inhibited, does not pace, and the timer is reset. If an impulse is not generated after the appropriate interval, the pacer fires, and the timer is again reset. Usually, the distance between the intrinsic QRS and the first paced QRS (*RV interval*) is the same as the distance between two consecutive paced beats (*VV interval)*; that is, RV should equal VV.

The **escape interval** is the time from the last sensed beat to the first pacer spike. The duration of the escape interval is preset according to the desired rate. For example, if the preset rate is 60 bpm, the escape interval is 1 second, or five large blocks on ECG paper. A pacer-induced QRS should occur within 1 second of the previously sensed QRS complex.

Similarly, if the preset rate is 75 bpm, the escape interval is 0.8 second, or four large blocks on the ECG paper. If the patient rate drops below the preset rate, the pacemaker will guarantee the minimal preset rate. In most demand pacemakers, the escape interval is programmed to be constant.

If the sensing electrodes are located in the atrium, the pacemaker senses the patient's intrinsic atrial depolarization. If the sensing electrodes are located in the ventricle, the pacemaker senses the patient's intrinsic ventricular depolarization.

If a demand pacemaker fires prematurely, this is **failure to sense**. This is dangerous to the patient since the premature pacer energy can occur during the vulnerable phase of the intrinsic T wave, and pacemaker-induced tachycardia or fibrillation may result.

Sensing failure can be oversensing or undersensing. Undersensing would cause the pacemaker to behave like an asynchronous device. Oversensing could cause long pauses beyond the escape interval.

Hysteresis

Hysteresis is a feature of some permanent pacemakers that allows for programming of a longer escape interval between the intrinsic complex and the first paced event. It is a delay mechanism that allows a little more time for the intrinsic pacemaker to generate a natural impulse. This prolonged interval should be the same every time it occurs and should occur only between the intrinsic and first paced event.

The advantage to hysteresis is to allow for intrinsic function within a safe and reasonable rate range, thus promoting normal function as long as possible. The problem is that some pacemakers are programmed with long periods of hysteresis, and on the ECG, this feature may be mistaken for pacemaker malfunction. Differences in escape and pacing intervals should cause concern for pacer malfunction until proven otherwise. **Figure 15.6**

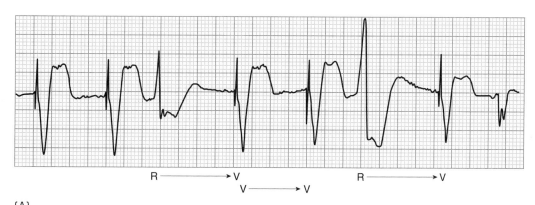

(A)

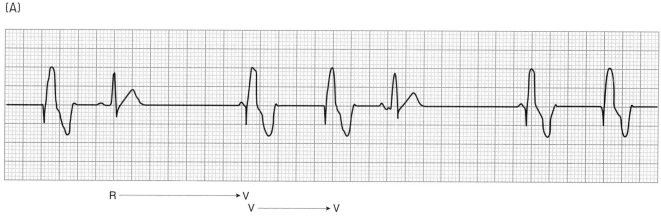

(B)

Figure 15.6 Example of hysteresis. In (A), note the difference in the measurements between the RV and VV intervals; the first RV interval is 0.12 second longer than the VV interval. This is consistent, even when the next intrinsic QRS is a PVC. In (B), note the long RV which is clearly longer than the VV interval. This would be interpreted as pacemaker malfunction unless the clinician knew the patient was programmed with hysteresis. (ECG courtesy John Stasic, Medtronic Inc.)

shows examples of hysteresis. Note the difference in the measurements between the RV and VV intervals. This is a documented ECG from a patient with hysteresis programmed into the pacemaker function. The observer would interpret this as pacemaker malfunction, and without documentation about this patient's pacemaker specifications, the operator would be correct.

Atrial Pacemakers

Atrial pacemakers are often used in conditions of sinus (SA) arrest and when conduction through the AV node is intact. The pacing catheter is threaded transvenously so that the electrode is located in the right atrium and acts as an artificial SA node and senses the patient's intrinsic P wave.

Atrial pacemakers also are used in bradycardia; they drive the heart at a rate faster than the intrinsic rate. When a pacemaker is stimulating the atrium, each pacing spike should produce a P wave. Atrial pacemakers are not used in patients with atrial arrhythmias.

VENTRICULAR PACEMAKERS

The earliest and most common mode of pacing is ventricular. Ventricular pacing can be external (transcutaneous or transvenous) or implanted. In ventricular pacing, the impulse stimulates the ventricles. The paced QRS will be preceded by a pacing spike and the pacer-induced QRS should result in a palpable carotid pulse (mechanical capture).

Fixed-rate ventricular pacing is seldom used. Recall that fixed-rate pacing is not sensitive to the intrinsic QRS and fires continuously without regard for the patient's own heart rhythm. The fixed-rate pacing current could fall during the vulnerable phase of the cardiac cycle and cause repetitive firing, pacer-induced ventricular tachycardia, or fibrillation.

When an ECG tracing shows only ventricular pacing, the observer will be unable to determine if the pacemaker is an asynchronous pacer or a demand pacer functioning 100 percent of the time. Sometimes the patient knows the type of pacemaker, and sometimes the patient will carry an identification card explaining the name and type of pacer implanted. **Figure 15.7** is an ECG tracing of a ventricular pacer. There are no intrinsic QRS complexes.

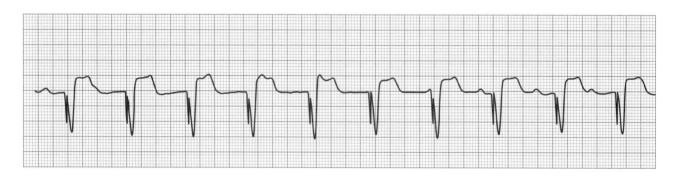

Figure 15.7 An ECG tracing of a ventricular pacer. There are no intrinsic QRS complexes. It is not vital that the clinician determine the underlying rhythm. It is not possible to determine if this is a demand or an asynchronous pacemaker as there are no intrinsic beats. The ECG is interpreted as a ventricular pacer at 75 bpm.

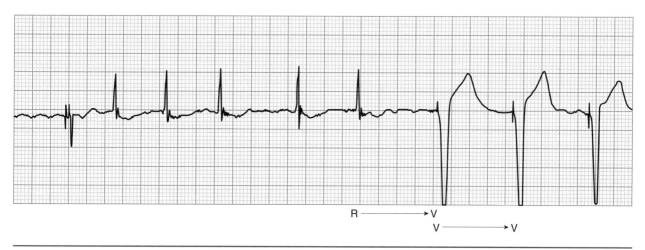

R ——————→V

V ——————→ V

Figure 15.8 An ECG tracing of atrial fibrillation with an ventricular demand pacemaker. Note that the RV and VV intervals are similar.

Ventricular Demand Pacemakers

Ventricular demand or QRS-inhibited pacemakers are used frequently and are the only type used for transcutaneous pacing at this time. This pacemaker has both sensing and pacing mechanisms. Both mechanisms are situated in the ventricle and thus sensitive to the patient's intrinsic QRS complex. The pacemaker is programmed not to fire; thus, the pacemaker is **inhibited** by the patient's own QRS complex. The demand ventricular pacemaker is ideal in the use of any bradycardia because of these two unique features:

1. sensing the patient's intrinsic QRS
2. ability to fire only when needed

Figure 15.8 is an ECG tracing showing the escape intervals with a demand ventricular pacemaker.

Noninvasive TCP are ventricular demand pacemakers and are a temporary solution to a bradycardia. A TCP provides quick and safe, although uncomfortable, application of a pacing device. With TCP, the external electrodes and lead wires are attached to the monitor/defib/pacer apparatus. The advantages are that the application is very quickly done and the operator can control the rate and amplitude of impulses. The major disadvantage is that it is uncomfortable for the patient. As soon as possible, a transvenous catheter is inserted and attached to the external pacemaker during the definitive stage of patient care.

Triggered Ventricular Pacemakers

Like a ventricular-inhibited pacemaker, the triggered ventricular pacemaker has both sensing and pacing capabilities. This pacemaker fires when the patient's intrinsic rate falls below a preset limit but differs from a QRS-inhibited pacer in the manner in which it is programmed to respond. A demand ventricular pacemaker will be inhibited by the QRS and not issue a stimulus; the triggered pacemaker does issue a stimulus. In fact, the pacemaker spike is seen in the middle of the QRS. The spike does alter the QRS morphology, making it difficult to assess for pacemaker malfunction.

Dual-Chamber Pacemakers. Dual-chamber pacing is when transvenous catheters are implanted into the right atrium and the right ventricle. The advantage to this mode of pacing is that the atria and ventricles are paced in sequence, allowing for atrial contribution to cardiac output. Dual-chamber pacemakers depend on a stable atrial rhythm for proper function.

The dual-chamber pacemaker can be preset with variations:

- Atrial inhibited
- Ventricular inhibited
- Atrial synchronous ventricular inhibited

In each of these settings, the pacer AV interval is programmed to a specific duration. The dual-chamber pacemaker can be used for problems with sinus node function, firing in the atria and allowing normal progress through the AV conduction system, and ultimately causing ventricular depolarization. If AV block occurs, the ventricular pacer will fire at the end of the programmed AV interval, thus guaranteeing a minimum ventricular rate.

Regardless of the mode of pacing, if all the components are functioning, the pacing stimulus will be released as designed, each pacemaker stimulus will result in myocardial response or capture, and the escape interval will be constant. Finally, for every captured QRS complex, there should be a mechanical capture, that is, a palpable carotid pulse. **Figure 15.9A** is a drawing of an implanted dual-chamber pacemaker. **Figure 15.9B** is an ECG tracing of a dual-chamber pacer. Note the pacer spike before A and V wave form.

If the intrinsic arrhythmia is atrial fibrillation or flutter, or frequent episodes of atrial tachycardia occur, this pacemaker may not be suitable. In patients whose atrial arrhythmias may preclude them from the use of the DDD or VDD pacemakers, but would benefit from an increase in paced atrial and ventricular function, the physician might consider the use of a biosensor to reflect physiologic needs and alter pacing function accordingly. These are the **rate-adaptive or physiologic** pacers.

There are pacemakers with a feature that will give a **programmed upper rate limit (PURL)** at which the pacemaker can pace the ventricle. In instances where the atrial rate exceeds the ventricular rate, each ventricular pace is delayed until the PURL is reached. In other words, if the PURL is 100 bpm, the ventricular pacer will not fire at an interval less than 600 ms.

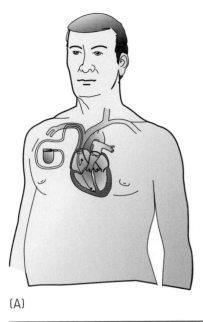

(A)

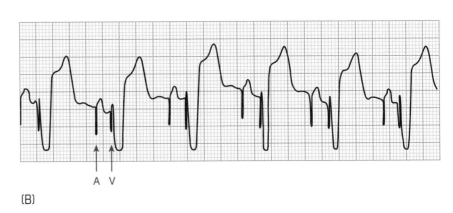

A V

(B)

Figure 15.9 (A) An implanted dual-chamber pacemaker. Note the position of the atrial and ventricular pacemaker catheters. (B) is an ECG tracing of a dual-chamber pacemaker. Note the fixed AV intervals.

Rate-Responsive Pacemakers

As technology accelerates, pacemakers are being designed that support the patient's quality of life and respond to the body's demands. For instance, there are demand pacemakers that can be programmed to respond to a change in physiologic demand. These pacemakers are sensitive to the patient's activity and respiratory rate and blood temperature. There are other parameters under investigation, such as metabolic status and blood pH. Once the sensing mechanism processes the information, the pacemaker determines what the desired rate should be and increases or decreases accordingly.

Since these pacemakers are sensor-controlled, rate determination changes to match patient activity moment-to-moment. These pacemakers are rate-responsive, rate-adaptive, or rate-modulating.

Overdrive Suppression

Overdrive suppression is physiologically defined as inhibitory effect of an ectopic on a slow underlying rhythm. This is how ectopics take over in the tachycardias. That is, overly excitable myocardial tissue can result in unwelcome tachycardias that recur and may render the patient unstable. Electronic overdrive suppression, that is, the delivery of continuous rapid pacing, has been used to control recurrent sustained supraventricular tachycardia and atrial fibrillation, and well as in torsades de pointes (TdP). For example, in the case of TdP, this arrhythmia may be suppressed with defibrillation, but it recurs, requiring the patient to be defibrillated frequently. Despite the good intention, the frequent shocks cause damage to the myocardium.

Another example is refractory bouts of atrial tachycardia. In either of these situations, the application of transvenous or transcutaneous pacing at an RV interval less than the intrinsic normal QRS-to-ectopic interval may prevent recurrence of the tachycardia until such time as other therapies can be invoked.

During the temporary pacing at high rates, the voltage and rate can be lowered slowly until a reasonable rate range is reached. If the ectopic recurs, the rate and voltage can be increased to regain control.

PACEMAKER MALFUNCTION

Demand pacers should never be late, nor should they ever be premature.

Failure to Function

Problems with pacemaker function are related to timing and the ability to fire, sense, and capture. If the patient's implanted pacemaker fails to function or fire the stimulus, there will be no pacer spike, and the ECG will show what remains of the patient's intrinsic rhythm. In cases of suspected pacemaker malfunction, a transvenous or transcutaneous pacer can be applied as soon as possible and set to a reasonable rate. There is no danger of competition to the suspected defunct implanted pacemaker. **Figure 15.10** is an example of failure to function. There is a paced rhythm and, suddenly, no pacing artifact; the patient is in complete AV block.

A timing problem exists when the escape interval alters or takes too long. This could be a problem with the timing mechanism or indicate end of life (EOL) for the pacemaker. It should be noted that the least likely problem is timing mechanism failure. Interval changes

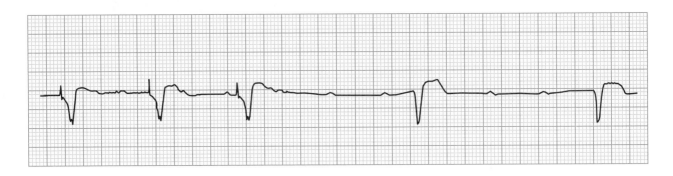

Figure 15.10 ECG showing failure to function. The first four complexes are paced beats. Following is a visible sinus at 100 bpm with complete AV block with a ventricular rhythm at 30 bpm.

are usually due to oversensing. An abrupt change in an interval, but consistent over time, would indicate EOL. The danger here is the resulting inappropriate bradycardia.

Failure to Sense

Failure to sense is the occurrence of premature pacing. The chamber involved may respond to the pacing stimulus or not, depending on the state of refractoriness of the tissue involved. The pacemaker fires without regard to the patient's intrinsic function and competes with the patient for control of heart rate. The danger here is that the pacing spike may fall during the vulnerable period of the cardiac cycle, causing repetitive firing, ventricular tachycardia, or fibrillation.

Occasionally, the patient rate and the pacemaker rate are so similar that it appears that there is failure to sense. Plot out the VV intervals and then the RV intervals. If they are the same, the pacemaker is said to be isorhythmic (the same rhythm). **Figure 15.11A** is an example of failure to sense.

Failure to Capture

When a pacemaker is stimulating adequately, each pacer spike would produce a wave form indicating electronic capture. An atrial pacer should produce a pacer-induced P wave; a ventricular pacer should produce a pacer-induced QRS. When a pacer spike fails to produce the paced complex or the pacer-induced QRS fails to produce a pulse, the problem is a failure to capture. This may be a problem with the position of the catheter or inadequate voltage. Failure to capture also may reflect the inability of the heart to respond to the stimulus.

If failure to capture persists, occurs frequently, or results in bradycardia, application of a transcutaneous or transvenous pacer is in order. **Figure 15.11B** is an ECG tracing showing failure to capture.

ASSESSING THE PACEMAKER ECG

Approach the ECG in a stepwise fashion:

- Whenever possible, identify the patient's underlying rhythm.
- Identify the mode of pacing: demand versus asynchronous.

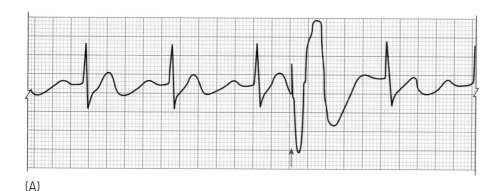

(A)

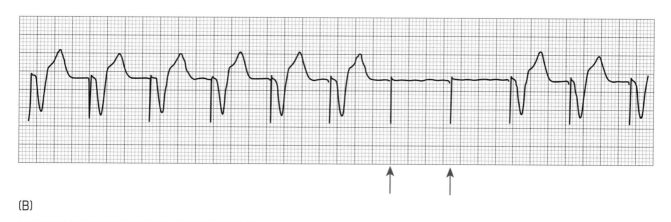

(B)

Figure 15.11 (A) Ventricular pacer with failure to sense. The pacer spike is too early and dangerously close to the T wave. Pacers should never be premature as they may cause pacer-induced tachycardia. (B) is an ECG showing two episodes of failure to capture (arrows).

- Evaluate the pacemaker function. To identify a pacer in the demand mode, you must see the patient's own intrinsic QRS.
  - Measure the distance between two paced beats (the pacing interval).
  - Compare the distance between the patient's last normal beat and the first paced beat (the escape interval—sometimes called the demand interval). These measurements should be the same. In other words, the paced interval equals the escape interval. The documentation will include identification of the patient's rhythm and rate and an assessment of the pacer. For example, "atrial fib at 70 to 85 bpm, a ventricular demand pacer at 72 bpm. The escape and paced intervals are constant." Recall that the demand pacer is set or timed to function within the escape interval. That interval should not change. If the interval is measured to be longer or shorter than what is expected, this is reportable as the pacer may not be functioning properly.
- Assess the patient's pulse and perfusion. Assess for dizziness, episodes of fainting, edema, dyspnea, chest pain, and hiccough.

Assessing the Dual-Chamber Pacemaker on ECG

The dual-chamber pacer is programmed to provide both atrial and ventricular function in sequence. This is to provide as near normal perfusion as possible. It is important to determine how the pacer functions in terms of its sensing capabilities.

- Identify the patient's underlying rhythm.
- Evaluate the escape interval.
  - Measure the distance between the first of the pacer artifacts for two paced beats.
  - Plot back in time and determine which wave forms match this interval, that is, the patient's P wave or the QRS complex. This will give an indication of which complex is being sensed by the pacer.
  - Assess the patient's pulse and perfusion. Assess for dizziness, episodes of fainting, edema, dyspnea, chest pain, and hiccough.

COMPLICATIONS OF PACING

Catheter Dislodgement

Dislodgement of the catheter electrode is a problem that occurs 1 percent of the time. Dislodgement of the transvenous catheter can result in failure to capture or in inappropriate stimulation. If there is a change in the position of the catheter, the paced ECG pattern will change. One complication is perforation of the ventricular septum. In this instance, the catheter electrode may penetrate the ventricular septum and pace from the left ventricle. While the pacer stimulus (spike) may be seen on the ECG, there may not be a captured QRS complex. An indication of perforated septum is a positive pacer-induced QRS.

Perforation

The pacemaker catheter can perforate the right ventricular septum or the right ventricular wall. If the catheter perforates the right ventricular wall and stimulates the diaphragm, the patient will hiccough to the ventricular paced rate. If a pacemaker catheter perforates the myocardium, pacemaker capture will stop. In addition, a perforated myocardium can lead to cardiac tamponade.

When an electrode perforates the septum, this will cause a sudden change in the polarity of the paced QRS complex. Recall that the paced right ventricle elicits a broad negative (QS) deflection on leads II and V_1. If the left ventricle is stimulated by the pacer, the pacing spike will be followed by a broad positive (QS) deflection on leads II and V_1. In addition, the pacer catheter may not come in contact with ventricular tissue, which will result in failure to capture. **Figure 15.12** is an example of positive paced QRSs in a patient with documented perforated septum.

Skeletal Muscle Inhibition

Newer pacemakers have better filtering devices and are less susceptible to interference. Some pacemakers are more interactive and sensitive to intrinsic cardiac activity and may be more susceptible to interference. Unipolar pacemakers are more susceptible to interference than bipolar pacemakers. In either of these situations, the pacemaker may sense the activity, and being unable to discriminate the source, become inhibited from its programmed function. On ECG, this will be interpreted as failure to function.

This should not be confused with skeletal muscle movement seen with transcutaneous pacing. As the pacing current passes through skin and skeletal muscle, a predictable twitching will occur. As current is increased until electronic capture is achieved, the intensity of muscle twitching also will increase. This does not interfere with transcutaneous pacing function.

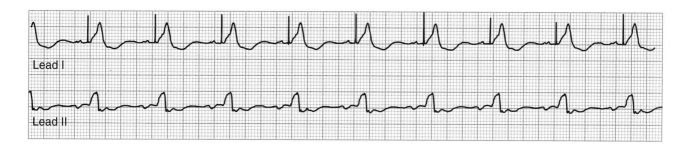

Figure 15.12 An example of positive paced QRSs in a patient with documented perforated septum. Note the positive paced complexes.

Interference. Depending on the type and amplitude of an external source of energy, a demand pacer may be unable to discriminate between intrinsic electrical forces and the unknown source. Interference of pacemaker function is of concern especially by electronic devices held close to the patient's chest, and the implanted device. The rule of thumb is to maintain a 6 inch distance from the item. Magnets should be avoided as contact between the pacemaker and the magnet may force the pacemaker into fixed function.

SUMMARY

The purpose of the electronic pacemaker is to provide an artificial stimulus when the heart's own electrical system is failing. With the increase in variability of pacer applications comes an increase in complexity. The rapid progress in research and technology has provided an increase in pacer applications for a wider variety of problems. Recently the design of a wireless pacemaker allows a patient's heart condition to be monitored remotely allowing an immediate response if something goes wrong within the heart or the device.

Another innovation is cardiac resynchronization therapy (CRT) also known as a biventricular pacing. This device involves positioning pacer wires in the atrium and both ventricles to facilitate synchronous ventricular function. CRT is a consideration for patients with moderate to severe heart failure and for those whose symptoms persist despite a medication regimen. CRT is also used to treat certain conduction problems and some ventricular arrhythmias.

Assessing pacemaker function to determine problems with failure to function, sense, and capture are consistent with all pacing devices. The use of a consistent approach to ECG rhythm analysis will help detect problems with any of these functions.

Self-Assessment Exercises
Matching

Match the term in the left column with the definition in the right column, and then compare your answers to those in Appendix A.

Term	Definition
Term	**Definition**
____ 1. AA interval	A. Ability of the pacemaker to process the heart's intrinsic signals
____ 2. AV interval	B. Ability to allow a longer escape interval for the first paced event
____ 3. Asynchronous	C. A pacer spike and no paced QRS or P wave
____ 4. Capture	D. A pacer functions prematurely
____ 5. Committed	E. A pacer that recognizes intrinsic function and paces only when necessary
____ 6. Demand pacer	F. A series of letters to describe pacemaker function
____ 7. Failure to capture	G. Distance between the intrinsic beat and the first paced event; also known as the pacer escape interval
____ 8. Failure to sense	H. Distance between two paced atrial events
____ 9. Hyteresis	I. Distance between two paced ventricular events
____ 10. Inhibited	J. Fixed-rate pacing; no sensing mechanism
____ 11. Milliampere (mA)	K. In dual-chamber pacing, when the AV interval is preset
____ 12. Millivolt (mV)	L. May indicate septal perforation on the ECG
____ 13. Overdrive suppression	M. Minimum amount of current required to elicit electronic capture
____ 14. Pacemaker code	N. Pacer spike plus a P or broad, negative QRS
____ 15. Pacer spike plus a positive broad QRS	O. Pacemaker ability to increase or decrease pacing rates in response to biosensors
____ 16. Programmed upper rate limit (PURL)	P. Preset time between paced atrial and paced ventricular activity
____ 17. Rate-adaptive	Q. Rapid rate pacing to deter tachycardias
____ 18. RV interval	R. Rate limit for pacemakers
____ 19. Sensing	S. Sensitivity
____ 20. Threshold	T. The ability for the pacer to sense a P and/or QRS and not fire
____ 21. VV interval	U. Unit of measurement for electrical sensitivity
	V. Unit of energy in pacemakers

ECG Rhythm Identification Practice

For the following rhythms, fill in the blanks and then compare your answers with those in Appendix A.

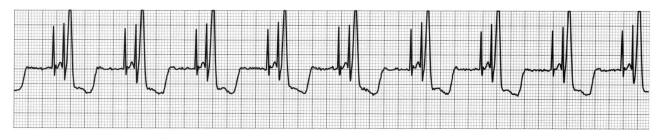

Figure 15.13

1. QRS duration _____
2. QT interval _____
3. Ventricular rate/rhythm _____
4. Atrial rate/rhythm _____
5. PR interval _____
6. Identification _____
7. Symptoms _____
8. Treatment _____

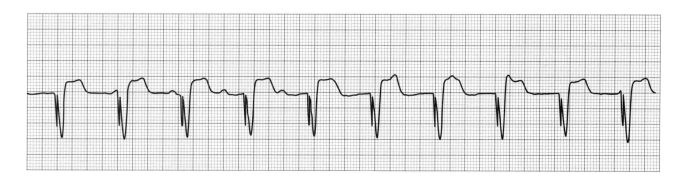

Figure 15.14

1. QRS duration _____
2. QT interval _____
3. Ventricular rate/rhythm _____
4. Atrial rate/rhythm _____
5. PR interval _____
6. Identification _____
7. Symptoms _____
8. Treatment _____

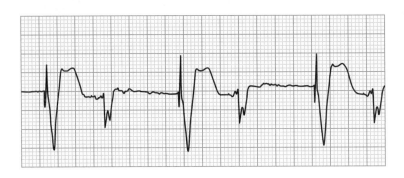

Figure 15.15

1. QRS duration _____
2. QT interval _____
3. Ventricular rate/rhythm _____
4. Atrial rate/rhythm _____
5. PR interval _____
6. Identification _____
7. Symptoms _____
8. Treatment _____

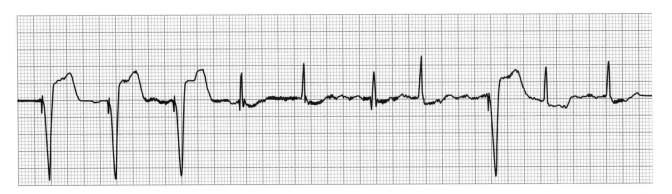

Figure 15.16

1. QRS duration _____
2. QT interval _____
3. Ventricular rate/rhythm _____
4. Atrial rate/rhythm _____
5. PR interval _____
6. Identification _____
7. Symptoms _____
8. Treatment _____

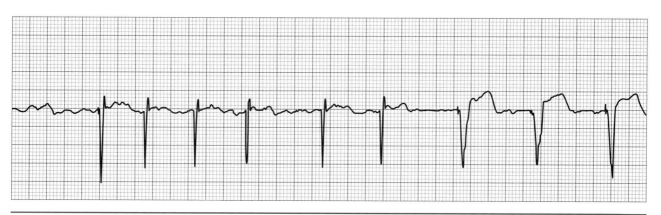

Figure 15.17

1. QRS duration _____
2. QT interval _____
3. Ventricular rate/rhythm _____
4. Atrial rate/rhythm _____
5. PR interval _____
6. Identification _____
7. Symptoms _____
8. Treatment _____

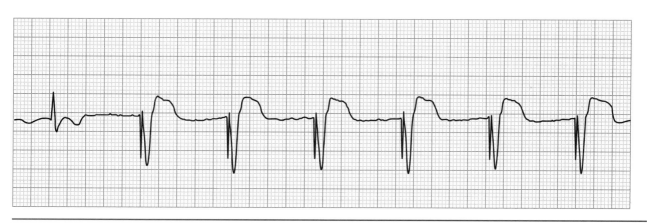

Figure 15.18

1. QRS duration _____
2. QT interval _____
3. Ventricular rate/rhythm _____
4. Atrial rate/rhythm _____
5. PR interval _____
6. Identification _____
7. Symptoms _____
8. Treatment _____

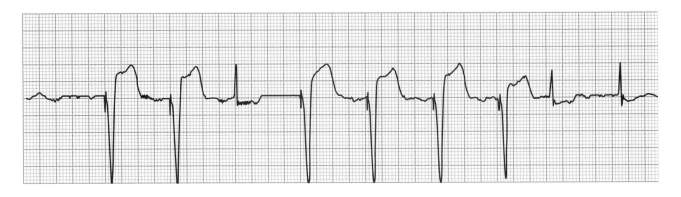

Figure 15.19

1. QRS duration _____
2. QT interval _____
3. Ventricular rate/rhythm _____
4. Atrial rate/rhythm _____
5. PR interval _____
6. Identification _____
7. Symptoms _____
8. Treatment _____

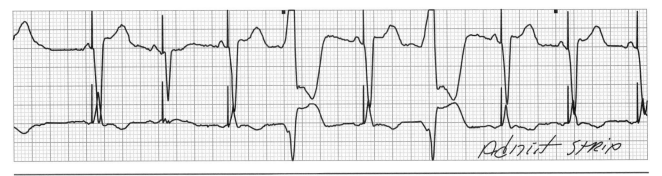

Figure 15.20

1. QRS duration _____
2. QT interval _____
3. Ventricular rate/rhythm _____
4. Atrial rate/rhythm _____
5. PR interval _____
6. Identification _____
7. Symptoms _____
8. Treatment _____

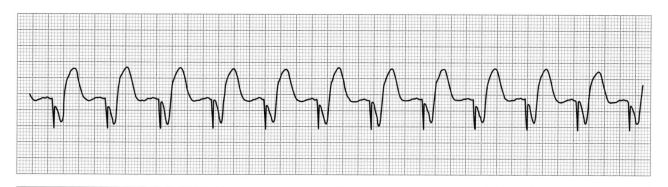

Figure 15.21

1. QRS duration _____
2. QT interval _____
3. Ventricular rate/rhythm _____
4. Atrial rate/rhythm _____
5. PR interval _____
6. Identification _____
7. Symptoms _____
8. Treatment _____

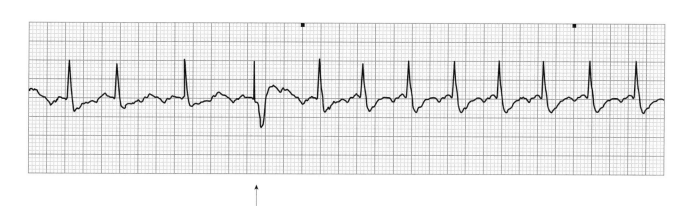

Figure 15.22

1. QRS duration _____
2. QT interval _____
3. Ventricular rate/rhythm _____
4. Atrial rate/rhythm _____
5. PR interval _____
6. Identification _____
7. Symptoms _____
8. Treatment _____

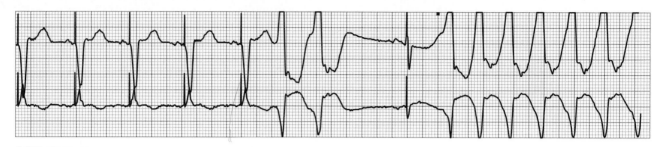

Figure 15.23

1. QRS duration _____
2. QT interval _____
3. Ventricular rate/rhythm _____
4. Atrial rate/rhythm _____
5. PR interval _____
6. Identification _____
7. Symptoms _____
8. Treatment _____

General Review and Assessment Exercises

ECG Rhythm Identification Practice

For the following rhythms, fill in the blanks and then compare your answers with those in Appendix A.

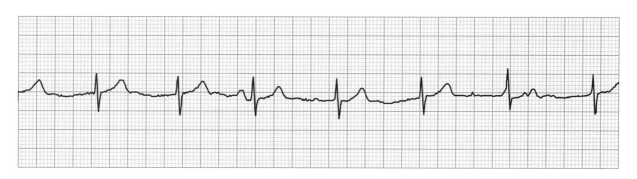

Figure 16.1

1. QRS duration _____
2. QT interval _____
3. Ventricular rate/rhythm _____
4. Atrial rate/rhythm _____
5. PR interval _____
6. Identification _____
7. Symptoms _____
8. Treatment _____

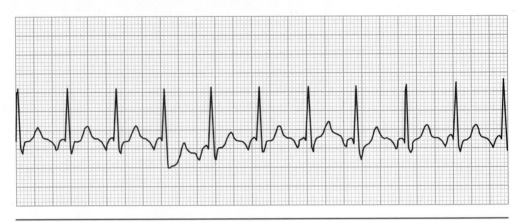

Figure 16.2

1. QRS duration _____
2. QT interval _____
3. Ventricular rate/rhythm _____
4. Atrial rate/rhythm _____
5. PR interval _____
6. Identification _____
7. Symptoms _____
8. Treatment _____

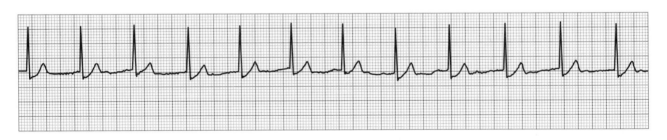

Figure 16.3

1. QRS duration _____
2. QT interval _____
3. Ventricular rate/rhythm _____
4. Atrial rate/rhythm _____
5. PR interval _____
6. Identification _____
7. Symptoms _____
8. Treatment _____

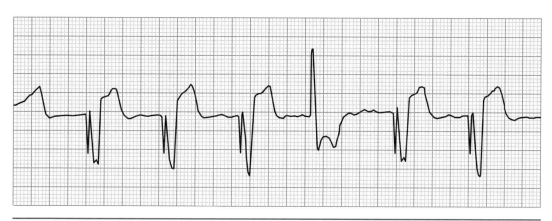

Figure 16.4

1. QRS duration _____
2. QT interval _____
3. Ventricular rate/rhythm _____
4. Atrial rate/rhythm _____
5. PR interval _____
6. Identification _____
7. Symptoms _____
8. Treatment _____

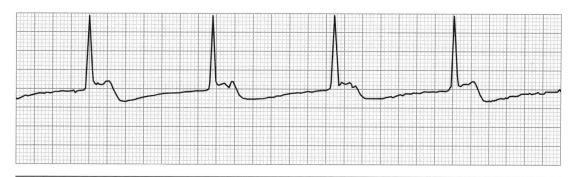

Figure 16.5

1. QRS duration _____
2. QT interval _____
3. Ventricular rate/rhythm _____
4. Atrial rate/rhythm _____
5. PR interval _____
6. Identification _____
7. Symptoms _____
8. Treatment _____

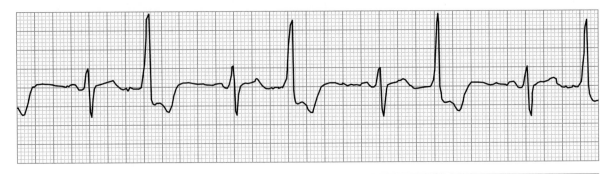

Figure 16.6

1. QRS duration _____
2. QT interval _____
3. Ventricular rate/rhythm _____
4. Atrial rate/rhythm _____
5. PR interval _____
6. Identification _____
7. Symptoms _____
8. Treatment _____

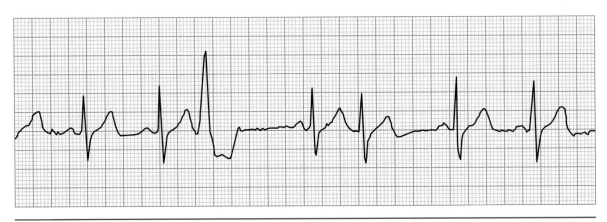

Figure 16.7

1. QRS duration _____
2. QT interval _____
3. Ventricular rate/rhythm _____
4. Atrial rate/rhythm _____
5. PR interval _____
6. Identification _____
7. Symptoms _____
8. Treatment _____

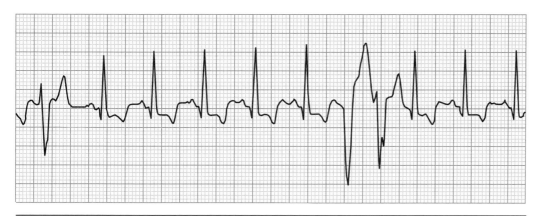

Figure 16.8

1. QRS duration _____
2. QT interval _____
3. Ventricular rate/rhythm _____
4. Atrial rate/rhythm _____
5. PR interval _____
6. Identification _____
7. Symptoms _____
8. Treatment _____

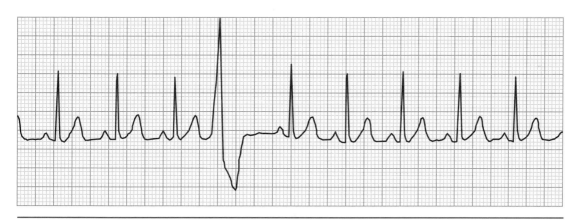

Figure 16.9

1. QRS duration _____
2. QT interval _____
3. Ventricular rate/rhythm _____
4. Atrial rate/rhythm _____
5. PR interval _____
6. Identification _____
7. Symptoms _____
8. Treatment _____

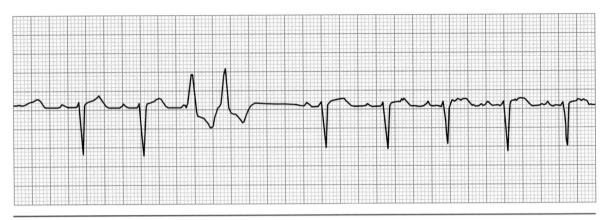

Figure 16.10

1. QRS duration _____
2. QT interval _____
3. Ventricular rate/rhythm _____
4. Atrial rate/rhythm _____
5. PR interval _____
6. Identification _____
7. Symptoms _____
8. Treatment _____

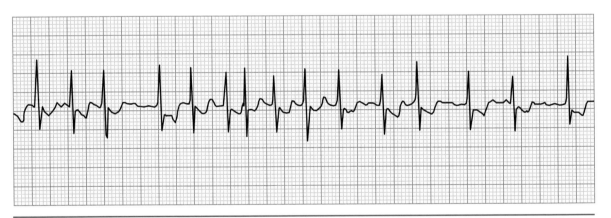

Figure 16.11

1. QRS duration _____
2. QT interval _____
3. Ventricular rate/rhythm _____
4. Atrial rate/rhythm _____
5. PR interval _____
6. Identification _____
7. Symptoms _____
8. Treatment _____

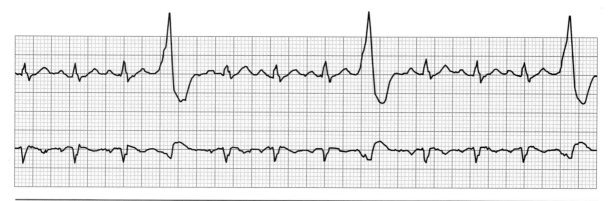

Figure 16.12

1. QRS duration _____
2. QT interval _____
3. Ventricular rate/rhythm _____
4. Atrial rate/rhythm _____
5. PR interval _____
6. Identification _____
7. Symptoms _____
8. Treatment _____

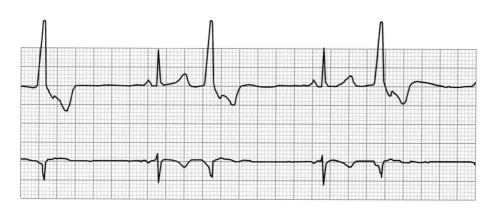

Figure 16.13

1. QRS duration _____
2. QT interval _____
3. Ventricular rate/rhythm _____
4. Atrial rate/rhythm _____
5. PR interval _____
6. Identification _____
7. Symptoms _____
8. Treatment _____

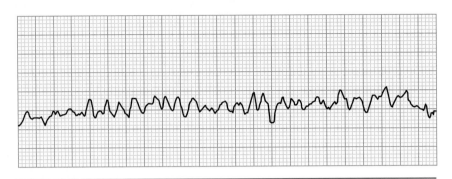

Figure 16.14

1. QRS duration _____
2. QT interval _____
3. Ventricular rate/rhythm _____
4. Atrial rate/rhythm _____
5. PR interval _____
6. Identification _____
7. Symptoms _____
8. Treatment _____

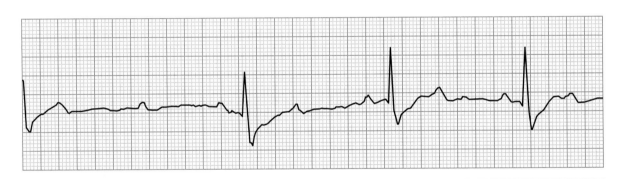

Figure 16.15

1. QRS duration _____
2. QT interval _____
3. Ventricular rate/rhythm _____
4. Atrial rate/rhythm _____
5. PR interval _____
6. Identification _____
7. Symptoms _____
8. Treatment _____

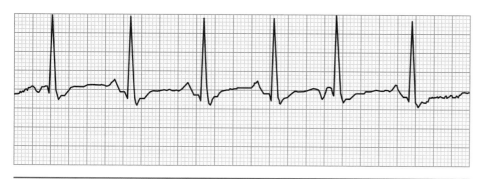

Figure 16.16

1. QRS duration _____
2. QT interval _____
3. Ventricular rate/rhythm _____
4. Atrial rate/rhythm _____
5. PR interval _____
6. Identification _____
7. Symptoms _____
8. Treatment _____

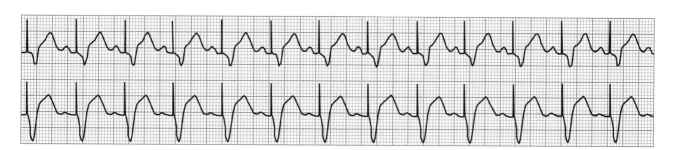

Figure 16.17

1. QRS duration _____
2. QT interval _____
3. Ventricular rate/rhythm _____
4. Atrial rate/rhythm _____
5. PR interval _____
6. Identification _____
7. Symptoms _____
8. Treatment _____

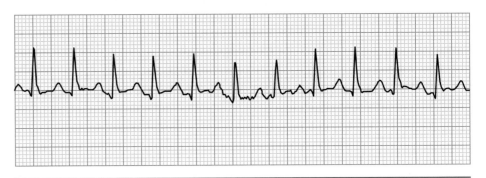

Figure 16.18

1. QRS duration _____
2. QT interval _____
3. Ventricular rate/rhythm _____
4. Atrial rate/rhythm _____
5. PR interval _____
6. Identification _____
7. Symptoms _____
8. Treatment _____

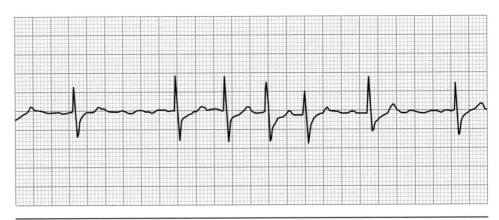

Figure 16.19

1. QRS duration _____
2. QT interval _____
3. Ventricular rate/rhythm _____
4. Atrial rate/rhythm _____
5. PR interval _____
6. Identification _____
7. Symptoms _____
8. Treatment _____

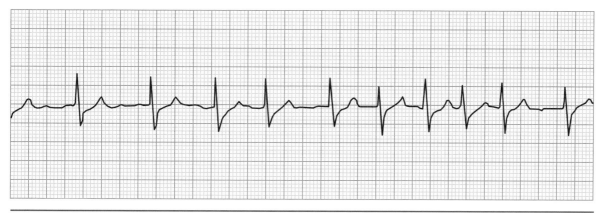

Figure 16.20

1. QRS duration _____
2. QT interval _____
3. Ventricular rate/rhythm _____
4. Atrial rate/rhythm _____
5. PR interval _____
6. Identification _____
7. Symptoms _____
8. Treatment _____

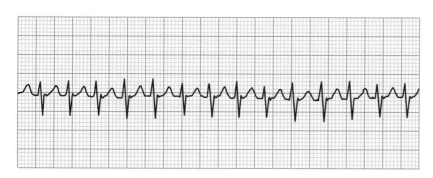

Figure 16.21

1. QRS duration _____
2. QT interval _____
3. Ventricular rate/rhythm _____
4. Atrial rate/rhythm _____
5. PR interval _____
6. Identification _____
7. Symptoms _____
8. Treatment _____

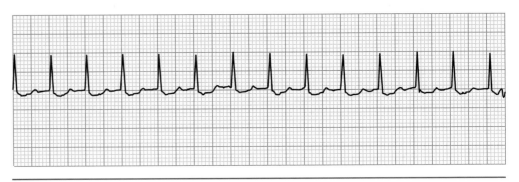

Figure 16.22

1. QRS duration _____
2. QT interval _____
3. Ventricular rate/rhythm _____
4. Atrial rate/rhythm _____
5. PR interval _____
6. Identification _____
7. Symptoms _____
8. Treatment _____

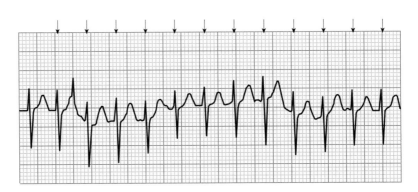

Figure 16.23

1. QRS duration _____
2. QT interval _____
3. Ventricular rate/rhythm _____
4. Atrial rate/rhythm _____
5. PR interval _____
6. Identification _____
7. Symptoms _____
8. Treatment _____

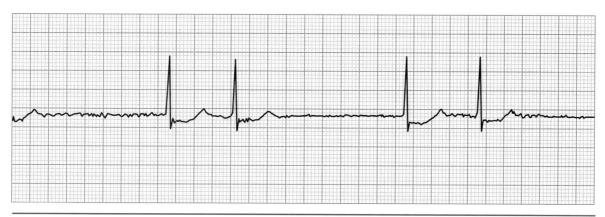

Figure 16.24

1. QRS duration _____
2. QT interval _____
3. Ventricular rate/rhythm _____
4. Atrial rate/rhythm _____
5. PR interval _____
6. Identification _____
7. Symptoms _____
8. Treatment _____

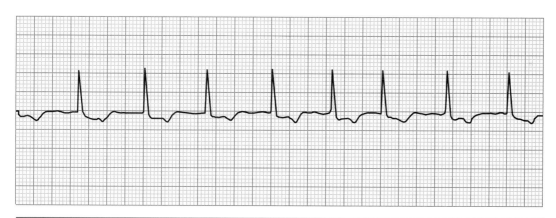

Figure 16.25

1. QRS duration _____
2. QT interval _____
3. Ventricular rate/rhythm _____
4. Atrial rate/rhythm _____
5. PR interval _____
6. Identification _____
7. Symptoms _____
8. Treatment _____

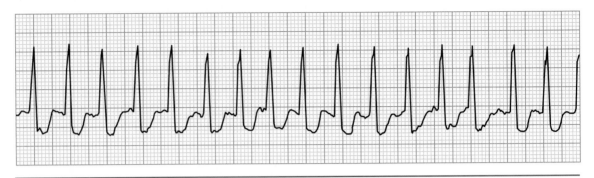

Figure 16.26

1. QRS duration _____
2. QT interval _____
3. Ventricular rate/rhythm _____
4. Atrial rate/rhythm _____
5. PR interval _____
6. Identification _____
7. Symptoms _____
8. Treatment _____

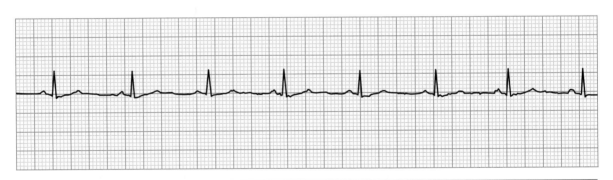

Figure 16.27

1. QRS duration _____
2. QT interval _____
3. Ventricular rate/rhythm _____
4. Atrial rate/rhythm _____
5. PR interval _____
6. Identification _____
7. Symptoms _____
8. Treatment _____

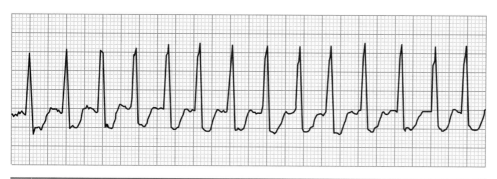

Figure 16.28

1. QRS duration _____
2. QT interval _____
3. Ventricular rate/rhythm _____
4. Atrial rate/rhythm _____
5. PR interval _____
6. Identification _____
7. Symptoms _____
8. Treatment _____

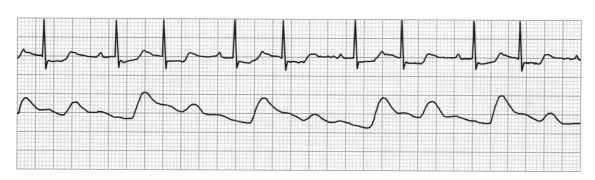

Figure 16.29

1. QRS duration _____
2. QT interval _____
3. Ventricular rate/rhythm _____
4. Atrial rate/rhythm _____
5. PR interval _____
6. Identification _____
7. Symptoms _____
8. Treatment _____

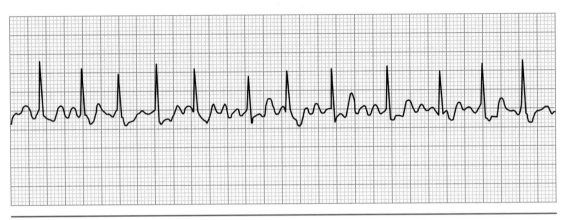

Figure 16.30

1. QRS duration _____
2. QT interval _____
3. Ventricular rate/rhythm _____
4. Atrial rate/rhythm _____
5. PR interval _____
6. Identification _____
7. Symptoms _____
8. Treatment _____

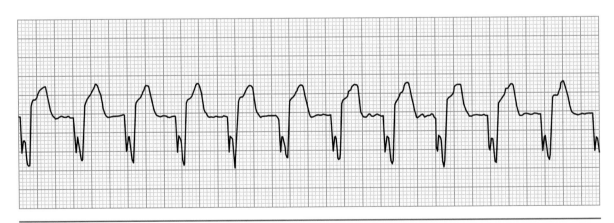

Figure 16.31

1. QRS duration _____
2. QT interval _____
3. Ventricular rate/rhythm _____
4. Atrial rate/rhythm _____
5. PR interval _____
6. Identification _____
7. Symptoms _____
8. Treatment _____

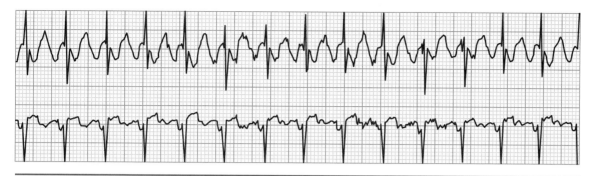

Figure 16.32

1. QRS duration _____
2. QT interval _____
3. Ventricular rate/rhythm _____
4. Atrial rate/rhythm _____
5. PR interval _____
6. Identification _____
7. Symptoms _____
8. Treatment _____

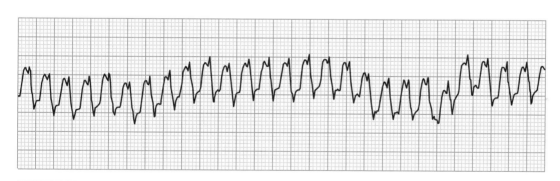

Figure 16.33

1. QRS duration _____
2. QT interval _____
3. Ventricular rate/rhythm _____
4. Atrial rate/rhythm _____
5. PR interval _____
6. Identification _____
7. Symptoms _____
8. Treatment _____

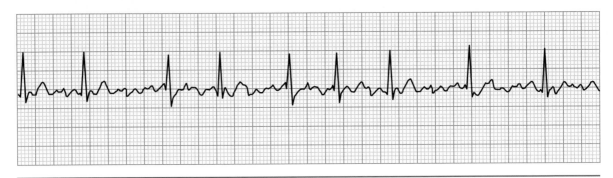

Figure 16.34

1. QRS duration _____
2. QT interval _____
3. Ventricular rate/rhythm _____
4. Atrial rate/rhythm _____
5. PR interval _____
6. Identification _____
7. Symptoms _____
8. Treatment _____

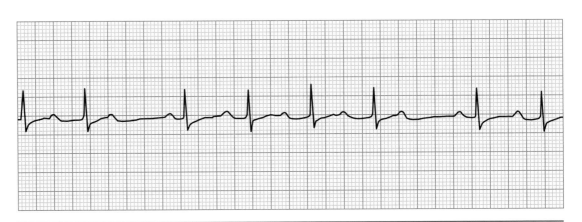

Figure 16.35

1. QRS duration _____
2. QT interval _____
3. Ventricular rate/rhythm _____
4. Atrial rate/rhythm _____
5. PR interval _____
6. Identification _____
7. Symptoms _____
8. Treatment _____

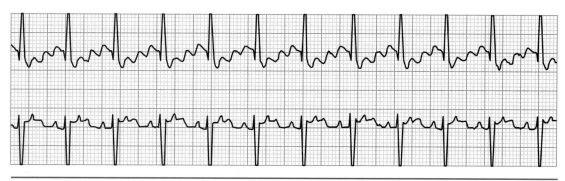

Figure 16.36

1. QRS duration _____
2. QT interval _____
3. Ventricular rate/rhythm _____
4. Atrial rate/rhythm _____
5. PR interval _____
6. Identification _____
7. Symptoms _____
8. Treatment _____

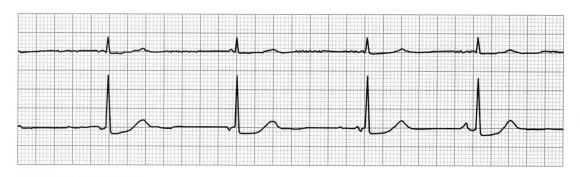

Figure 16.37

1. QRS duration _____
2. QT interval _____
3. Ventricular rate/rhythm _____
4. Atrial rate/rhythm _____
5. PR interval _____
6. Identification _____
7. Symptoms _____
8. Treatment _____

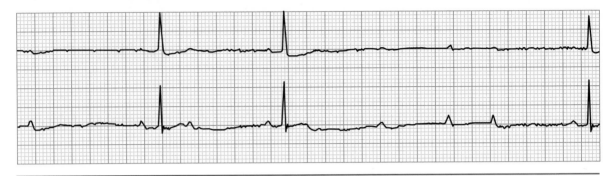

Figure 16.38

1. QRS duration _____
2. QT interval _____
3. Ventricular rate/rhythm _____
4. Atrial rate/rhythm _____
5. PR interval _____
6. Identification _____
7. Symptoms _____
8. Treatment _____

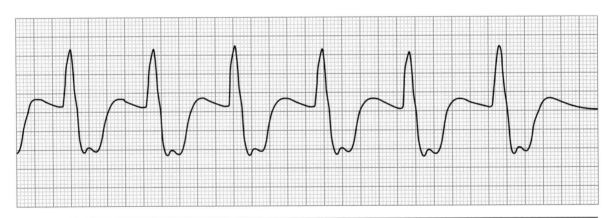

Figure 16.39

1. QRS duration _____
2. QT interval _____
3. Ventricular rate/rhythm _____
4. Atrial rate/rhythm _____
5. PR interval _____
6. Identification _____
7. Symptoms _____
8. Treatment _____

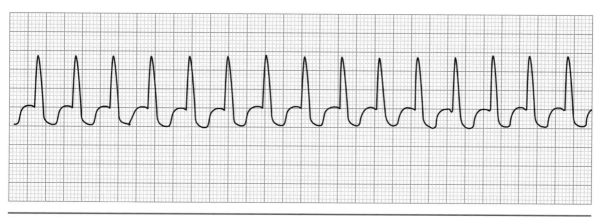

Figure 16.40

1. QRS duration _____
2. QT interval _____
3. Ventricular rate/rhythm _____
4. Atrial rate/rhythm _____
5. PR interval _____
6. Identification _____
7. Symptoms _____
8. Treatment _____

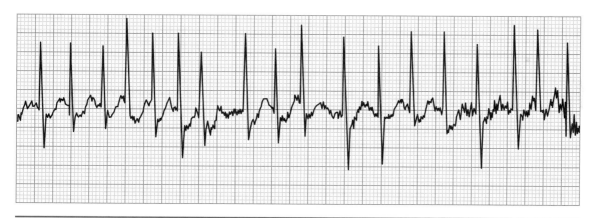

Figure 16.41

1. QRS duration _____
2. QT interval _____
3. Ventricular rate/rhythm _____
4. Atrial rate/rhythm _____
5. PR interval _____
6. Identification _____
7. Symptoms _____
8. Treatment _____

Answers to Self-Assessment Exercises

CHAPTER 1 REVIEW OF CARDIAC ANATOMY AND FUNCTION

Fill in the Blanks

1. function, musculature
2. systemic, lungs
3. oxygenated, lungs, body
4. thicker, systemic circulation
5. tricuspid, right
6. mitral, left
7. pulmonic, lungs, aortic, systemic circulation
8. rotated, anterior, posterior
9. aorta, downward, anterior, posterior, SA, AV
10. septal, bundle of His
11. left anterior descending, left circumflex
12. septum, right bundle branch, left bundle branch
13. circumflex, left posterior fascicle

CHAPTER 2 ELECTROPHYSIOLOGY OF THE HEART

Fill in the Blanks

1. electrical, mechanical
2. automaticity
3. excitability
4. conductivity
5. contractility
6. electrical activation, mechanical response (contraction).
7. SA node
8. atrial tissue
9. AV junction
10. AV node, bundle of His
11. right bundle branch
12. left main trunk, left anterior fascicle, left posterior fascicle
13. Purkinje system

CHAPTER 3 THE ECG AND THE MULTIPLE LEAD SYSTEM

Fill in the Blanks

1. left free wall
2. apical and inferior surfaces
3. right inferior surface
4. right bundle branch
5. right anterior surface
6. anterior septal surface
7. left anterior surface
8. left ventricle
9. left lateral surface
10. right ventricle

CHAPTER 4 RATE, RHYTHM, AND WAVE FORMS

ECG Rhythm Identification Practice

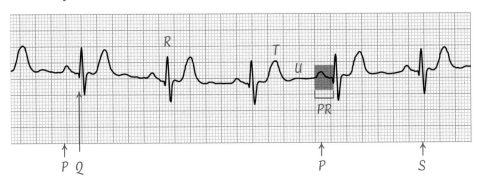

Figure 4-27

1. There are P, Q, R, S, T, and U waves. ST segment is on the line (isoelectric).
2. The P wave is positive (+).
3. QRS (ventricular) rate/rhythm = 56 bpm/regular.
4. P (atrial) rate/rhythm = 55 bpm/regular.
5. PR interval = 0.20 sec and consistent.

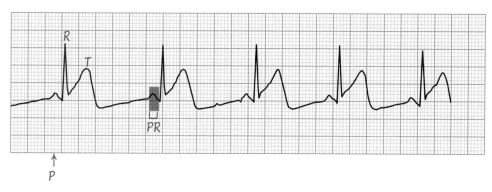

Figure 4-28

1.   There are P, R, and T waves.
2.   The P waves are positive (+).
3.   QRS (ventricular) rate/rhythm = 50–55 bpm/irregular.
4.   P (atrial) rate/rhythm = 50–55 bpm/irregular.
5.   PR interval = 0.12–0.16 sec.

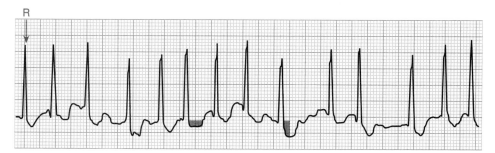

Figure 4-29

1.   The R waves are easily visible; other wave forms are not. ST segment is depressed and varies between 3 and 5 mm.
2.   There are no identifiable P waves.
3.   QRS (ventricular) rate/rhythm = 100–180 bpm/obviously irregular.
4.   P (atrial) rate/rhythm = no identifiable P waves.
5.   PR interval = none.

   COMMENT: The baseline is very erratic, referred to as a wandering baseline. Until a more even baseline is seen, simply note the variation in ST measurements, and give the rate, most shallow to the deepest.

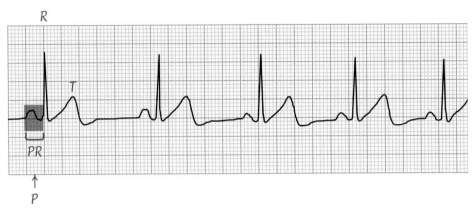

Figure 4-30

1. There are P, R, and T waves.
2. The P waves are (+).
3. QRS (ventricular) rate/rhythm = 53–60 bpm/irregular.
4. P (atrial) rate/rhythm = 53–60 bpm/irregular.
5. PR interval = 0.20 sec and consistent.

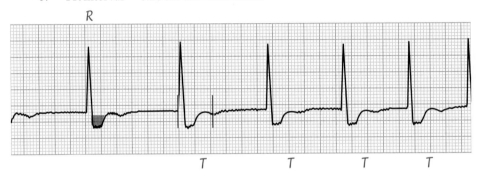

Figure 4-31

1. There are R and T waves; ST segment is ↓4 mm.
2. There are no visible P waves.
3. QRS (ventricular) rate/rhythm = 50–86 bpm/irregular.
4. P (atrial) rate/rhythm = no P waves;
5. There are no sinus P waves, therefore, no PR interval.

COMMENT: When it is difficult to identify the T wave, plot out 0.40 sec from a QRS that begins on a tall, dark line. The T wave should be more visible.

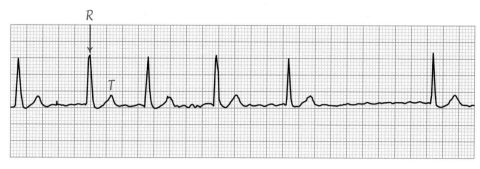

Figure 4-32

1. There are R and T waves.
2. There are no visible P waves.
3. QRS (ventricular) rate/rhythm = 30–85 bpm/irregular.
4. There are no visible P waves, therefore, no measurable atrial rate.
5. There are no P waves, therefore, no PR interval.

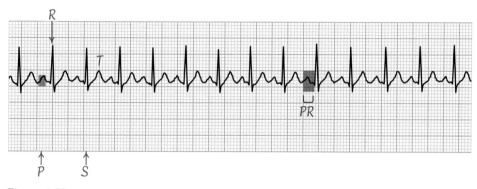

Figure 4-33

1. There are P, R, S, and T waves.
2. The P wave is (+).
3. QRS (ventricular) rate/rhythm = 150 bpm/regular.
4. P (atrial) rate/rhythm = 150 bpm/regular.
5. PR interval = 0.16 sec and consistent.

CHAPTER 5 AXIS DETERMINATION AND IMPLICATIONS

Matching

1. A   (E is not an option until voltage and axis are calculated.)

2. B   (B is not an option until voltage and axis are calculated.)

3. E

4. C

5. D

ECG Rhythm Identification Practice

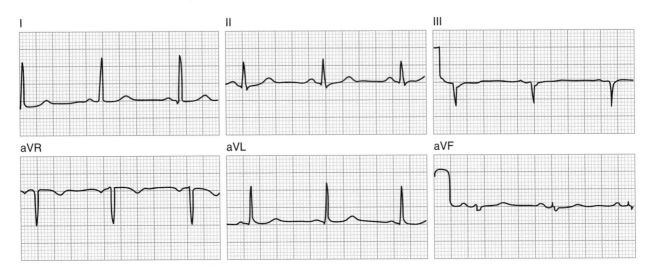

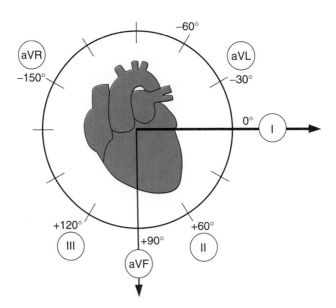

Figure 5-11

1. What is the underlying rhythm?
    Sinus at 67 bpm.

2. What is the axis?

    a. Look at leads I and II; are the QRS complexes positive?
        The QRS in leads I and II are positive. No other calculations are vital; axis is to the left at +0°, but we will continue to practice.

    b. Are there equiphasic deflections?
        Yes, in aVF. Draw an arrow pointing to aVF. Lead I is perpendicular to lead aVF and lead I is the greatest positive net area.

    c. Draw an arrow pointing to lead I. The area between your arrows shows the axis is within normal limits.

3. What is your interpretation? Sinus at about 67 bpm.

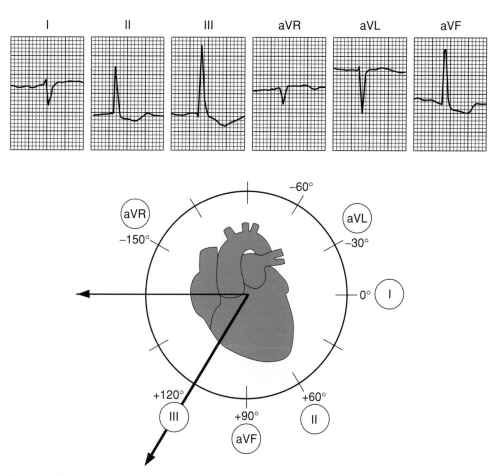

Figure 5-12

1. What is the underlying rhythm?
    Cannot tell. Unable to plot Ps with consistent PR intervals.

2. What is the axis?

    a. Look at leads I and II; are the QRS complexes positive?
        The QRS lead I is negative and II is positive; therefore calculation is in order.
        There are no equiphasic deflections. Using the circle, lead I is negative so the
        shift is away from lead I; lead III has the greatest positive net area; therefore
        axis is inferior and to the right at +120°.

    b. Are there equiphasic deflections? No, not really.

    c. Draw an arrow pointing away from lead I. Then draw an arrow pointing to
        lead III. The area between your arrows shows the axis is to the right.

3. What is your interpretation? Right axis deviation at +120°.

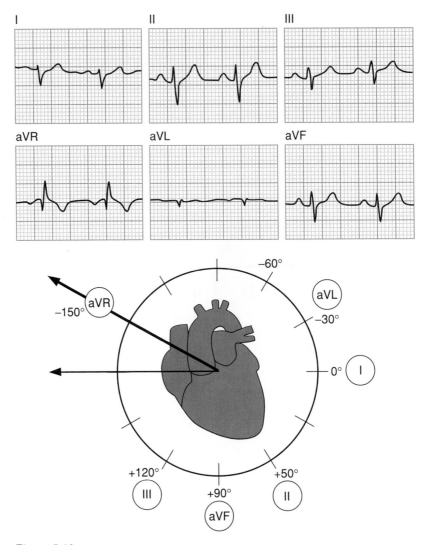

Figure 5-13

1. What is the underlying rhythm? Sinus at 86 bpm.
2. What is the axis?
   a. Look at leads I and II; are they positive?

      Lead I is negative and leads II and III are equiphasic; therefore calculation is in order. Leads II, III, and aVF are equiphasic. Lead I is negative, so the flow of current is away from lead I.
   b. Are there equiphasic deflections?

      Yes, that is what was confusing; II, III, and aVF are each equiphasic.
   c. Lead I has a direction, so draw an arrow away from lead I; lead aVR has a positive R wave, so draw an arrow pointing to aVR.
3. What is your interpretation?

   Sinus at 86 bpm with far right or northwest axis deviation at −150°. This is sometimes called no-man's-land.

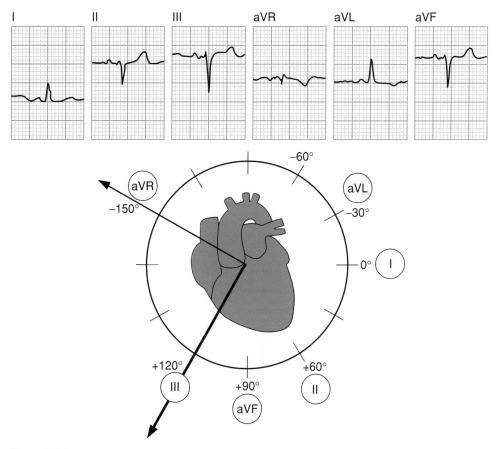

Figure 5-14

1. What is the underlying rhythm?
    Sinus.

2. What is the axis?

    a. Look at leads I and II; are they positive?
        Lead I is positive and II is negative, so calculation is in order.

    b. Are there equiphasic deflections?
        Yes, in aVR. The Q and R waves are very small, but on close inspection, the complex is pretty much equiphasic.

    c. Draw an arrow pointing to aVR since it is equiphasic. Since lead aVR is equiphasic and lead III is perpendicular to aVR, draw an arrow pointing to lead III. Lead III has the greatest net negative deflection, so the axis is inferior and to the right at +120°.

3. What is your interpretation?
    Sinus with right axis deviation at +120°.

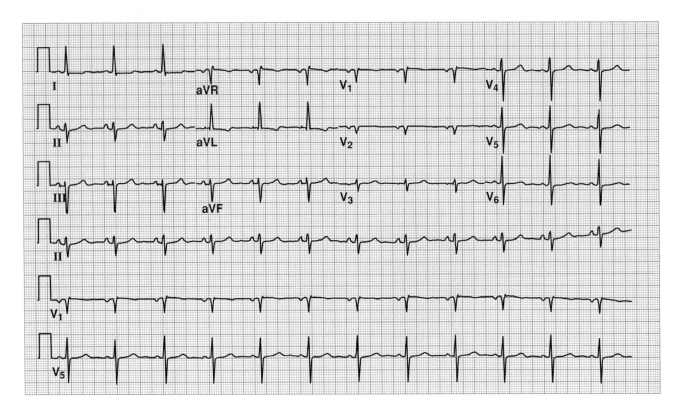

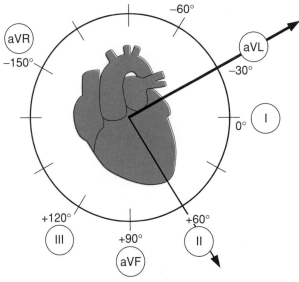

Figure 5-15

1. What is the underlying rhythm?
   Sinus at 75 bpm.
2. What is the axis?
   a. Look at leads I and II; are they positive?
      Lead I is positive and II is equiphasic; therefore calculation is in order.
   b. Are there equiphasic deflections?
      Yes, lead II.

c. Using the two-step method, lead II is equiphasic and lead aVL is perpendicular to lead II. So draw an arrow toward lead II and one to lead aVL. Lead III is negative, and the net area of leads I, III, and aVL are similar, so the average would be at aVL, or −30°.

3. What is your interpretation?

Sinus at 75 bpm with left axis deviation at −30°.

CHAPTER 6 THE SINUS MECHANISMS

Fill in the Blanks

	Sinus Rhythm	Sinus Bradycardia	Sinus Tachycardia
P wave	1(+) P wave/QRS	1(+) P wave/QRS	1(+) P wave/QRS
PR interval	0.12–0.20 sec	0.12–0.20 sec	0.12–0.20 sec
QRS complex	≤0.10 sec	≤0.10 sec	≤0.10 sec
QRS rate	60–100 bpm	<60 bpm	>100 bpm
QRS rhythm	Regular	Regular	Regular

	Sinus Rhythm	Sinus Arrhythmia	Sinus Block
P wave	1(+) P wave/QRS	1(+) P wave/QRS	Missing one P wave
PR interval	0.12–0.20 sec	0.12–0.20 sec	n/a
QRS complex	≤0.10 sec	≤0.10 sec	Missing a QRS
QRS rate	60–100 bpm	Usually 60–100 bpm	n/a
QRS rhythm	Regular	Irregular	Underlying rhythm usually regular

ECG Rhythm Identification Practice

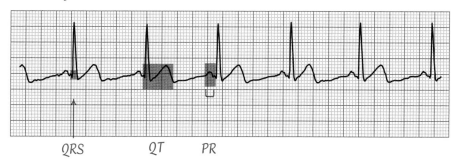

QRS   QT   PR

Figure 6-17

QRS duration	0.10 sec
QT interval	0.40 sec
Ventricular rate/rhythm	67 bpm/regular
Atrial rate/rhythm	67 bpm/regular
PR interval	0.12 sec
Identification	Sinus rhythm at 67 bpm
Symptoms	None anticipated
Treatment	Be supportive

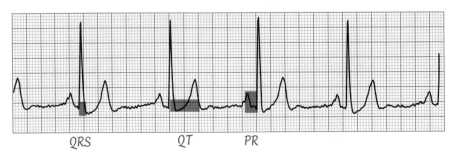

Figure 6-18

QRS duration	0.08 sec
QT interval	0.44 sec
Ventricular rate/rhythm	41–58 bpm/irregular
Atrial rate/rhythm	41–58 bpm/irregular
PR interval	0.20 sec
Identification	Sinus arrhythmia at 41–58 bpm, 2–3 mm ST seg ↓
Symptoms	None anticipated
Treatment	Be supportive

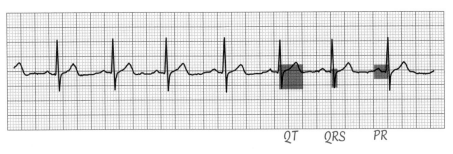

Figure 6-19

QRS duration	0.08 sec
QT interval	0.32 sec
Ventricular rate/rhythm	75 bpm/regular
Atrial rate/rhythm	75 bpm/regular
PR interval	0.16 sec
Identification	Sinus rhythm at 75 bpm
Symptoms	None anticipated
Treatment	Be supportive

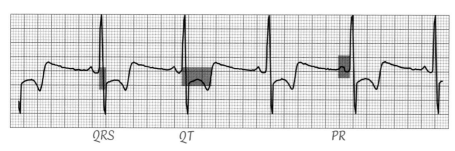

Figure 6-20

QRS duration	0.10 sec
QT interval	0.44 sec
Ventricular rate/rhythm	50 bpm/regular
Atrial rate/rhythm	50 bpm/regular
PR interval	0.16–0.20 sec
Identification	Sinus bradycardia at 50 bpm, 3 mm ST seg ↓ and T waves ↓
Symptoms	? ALOC, dizziness, s/s of hypoperfusion; syncopal and/or near-syncopal episodes
Treatment	If hypotensive and hypoperfusing, consider atropine, fluids, pace; pressor if necessary

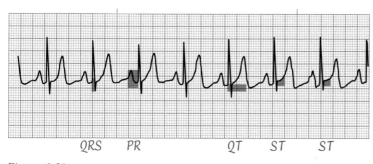

Figure 6-21

QRS duration	0.06–0.08 sec
QT interval	0.32 sec
Ventricular rate/rhythm	75 bpm/regular
Atrial rate/rhythm	75 bpm/regular
PR interval	0.16–0.20 sec
Identification	Sinus rhythm at 75 bpm; there is ST segment elevation noted in the last two complexes
Symptoms	None anticipated unless the ST ↑ persists and the patient presents with s/s of acute coronary syndrome (ACS)
Treatment	Be supportive; if there is no pain or discomfort, reassess, oxygen, fluids, Rx for pain, reassess

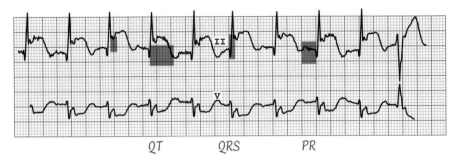

Figure 6-22

QRS duration	0.08 sec
QT interval	0.38 sec; need multiple leads to confirm a ↓ T wave and thus a longer QT
Ventricular rate/rhythm	125 bpm/regular
Atrial rate/rhythm	125 bpm/regular
PR interval	0.16–0.20 sec
Identification	Sinus tachycardia at 125 bpm with ST segment ↑, 3–4 mm Q waves; the last QRS is different than the rest; the QRS is predominantly negative and its T wave is positive; this is a PVC (Chapter 9)
Symptoms	? chest pain, SOB, diaphoresis
Treatment	Assess for s/s of ACS; assess vital signs to include multiple lead ECG; ASA, assess BP before considering nitroglycerin/morphine sulfate for pain; reassess

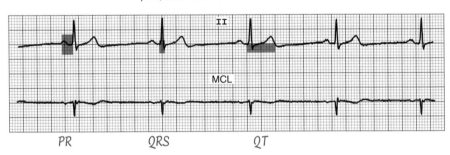

Figure 6-23

QRS duration	0.08 sec
QT interval	0.40 sec
Ventricular rate/rhythm	46 bpm/regular
Atrial rate/rhythm	46 bpm/regular
PR interval	0.16 sec
Identification	Sinus bradycardia at 46 bpm
Symptoms	? ALOC, dizziness, s/s of hypoperfusion; syncopal and/or near-syncopal episodes
Treatment	If hypotensive and hypoperfusing, consider atropine, fluids, pace, pressor if necessary

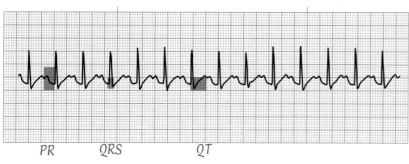

Figure 6-24

QRS duration	0.08 sec
QT interval	0.28 sec
Ventricular rate/rhythm	150 bpm/regular
Atrial rate/rhythm	150 bpm/regular
PR interval	0.16 sec
Identification	Sinus tachycardia at 150 bpm
Symptoms	? fever, anxiety, stress, anger, pain, medications—prescribed, borrowed, illegal, and/or recreational substances; s/s of CHF; s/s of ACS
Treatment	ID and Rx the cause; if s/s of ACS consider ASA, Rx the pain and reassess

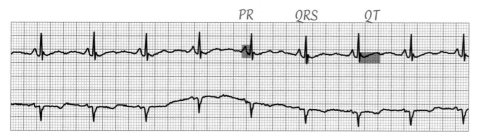

Figure 6-25

QRS duration	0.06–0.08 sec
QT interval	0.38 sec
Ventricular rate/rhythm	75 bpm/regular
Atrial rate/rhythm	75 bpm/regular
PR interval	0.12 sec
Identification	Sinus rhythm at 75 bpm
Symptoms	None anticipated
Treatment	Be supportive

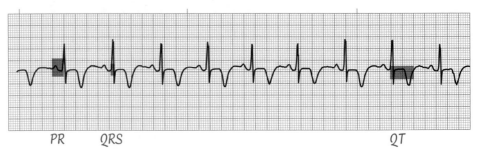

Figure 6-26

QRS duration	0.08 sec
QT interval	0.42 sec
Ventricular rate/rhythm	75 bpm/regular
Atrial rate/rhythm	75 bpm/regular
PR interval	0.16 sec
Identification	Sinus rhythm at 75 bpm; nadir ↓ T waves
Symptoms	None anticipated related to rate
Treatment	ID and Rx the cause; if s/s of ACS, consider ASA, Rx the pain, and reassess

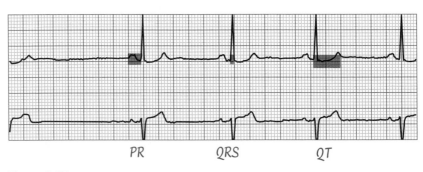

Figure 6-27

QRS duration	0.04–0.06 sec
QT interval	0.36 sec
Ventricular rate/rhythm	50 bpm/regular
Atrial rate/rhythm	50 bpm/regular
PR interval	0.16 sec
Identification	Sinus bradycardia at 50 bpm; possibly preceded by an episode of SA arrest or SA block
Symptoms	? ALOC, dizziness, s/s of hypoperfusion; syncopal and/or near-syncopal episodes
Treatment	If hypotensive and hypoperfusing, consider atropine, fluids, stand by for pacing, pressor as necessary

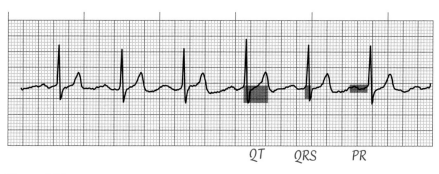

Figure 6-28

QRS duration	0.08–0.10 sec
QT interval	0.36 sec
Ventricular rate/rhythm	75 bpm/regular
Atrial rate/rhythm	75 bpm/regular
PR interval	0.20 sec
Identification	Sinus rhythm at 75 bpm
Symptoms	None anticipated
Treatment	Be supportive

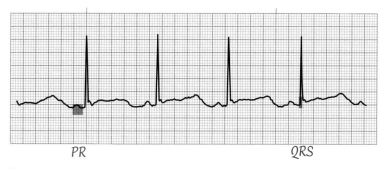

Figure 6-29

QRS duration	0.04–0.06 sec
QT interval	Unable to determine (UTD)
Ventricular rate/rhythm	54 bpm/regular
Atrial rate/rhythm	54 bpm/regular
PR interval	0.16 sec
Identification	Sinus bradycardia at 54 bpm
Symptoms	? ALOC, dizziness, s/s of hypoperfusion; syncopal near-syncopal episodes; ? meds/med Hx
Treatment	If hypotensive and hypoperfusing, consider atropine, fluids, pace, pressor

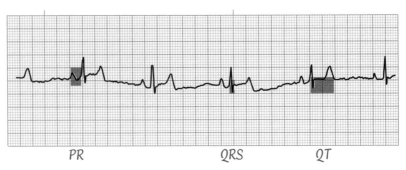

Figure 6-30

QRS duration	0.06 sec
QT interval	0.40 sec
Ventricular rate/rhythm	48–55 bpm
Atrial rate/rhythm	48–55 bpm
PR interval	0.16 sec
Identification	Sinus arrhythmia at 48–55 bpm, 1 mm ST seg ↑
Symptoms	? ALOC, s/s of hypoperfusion: rate may be "normal" for the patient, ? chest pain, ? med, assess for s/s of ACS
Treatment	ID and Rx the cause; if s/s of ACS consider ASA, Rx the pain and reassess

CHAPTER 7 THE JUNCTIONAL MECHANISMS

Matching

1. B
2. A
3. C
4. D

Fill in the Blanks

	Sinus Rhythm	Sinus Bradycardia	Junctional Rhythm
P wave	1(+) P wave/QRS	1(+) P wave/QRS	1(−) P′ wave or none
PR interval	0.12–0.20 sec	0.12–0.20 sec	0.12 sec
QRS complex	≤0.10 sec	≤0.10 sec	≤0.10 sec
QRS rate	60–100 bpm	<60 bpm	40–60 bpm
QRS rhythm	Regular	Regular	Regular

ECG Rhythm Identification Practice

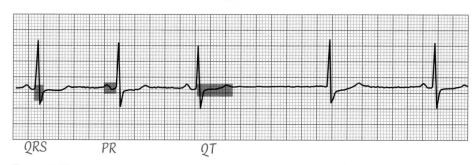

QRS   PR   QT

Figure 7-10

QRS duration	0.08 sec
QT interval	0.44 sec (may be related to rate)
Ventricular rate/rhythm	55 bpm prior to the event
Atrial rate/rhythm	55 bpm prior to the event
PR interval	0.16 sec
Identification	Sinus bradycardia at 55 bpm, ? SA arrest/block; junctional escape beat → sinus
Symptoms	? ALOC, dizziness, s/s of hypoperfusion; syncopal and/or near-syncopal episodes
Treatment	If s/s related to the slow rate, intervene as with narrow-complex bradycardia; ? meds; always wonder what happened to the sinus node; consider the causes of sinus node dysfunction

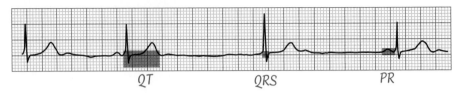

Figure 7-11

QRS duration	0.08 sec
QT interval	0.44 sec (there are U waves)
Ventricular rate/rhythm	47 bpm prior to event
Atrial rate/rhythm	47 bpm prior to event
PR interval	0.16 sec
Identification	Sinus bradycardia at 47 bpm, ? SA arrest/or SA block; junctional escape beat → sinus
Symptoms	? ALOC, s/s of hypoperfusion;? syncopal episodes
Treatment	If s/s related to the slow rate, intervene as with narrow-complex bradycardia; ? meds; always wonder what happened to the sinus node; consider the causes of sinus node dysfunction

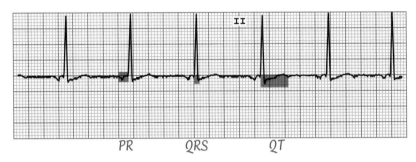

Figure 7-12

QRS duration	0.04–0.06 sec
QT interval	0.36 sec
Ventricular rate/rhythm	67 bpm/regular
Atrial rate/rhythm	67 bpm (note the P wave is inverted)
PR interval	0.10–0.12 sec
Identification	Accelerated junctional rhythm at 67 bpm
Symptoms	None anticipated related to rate
Treatment	? meds/med Hx; always wonder what happened to the sinus node

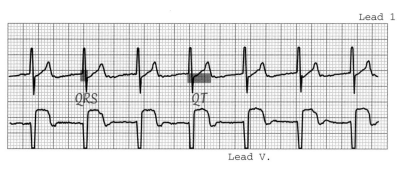

Figure 7-13

QRS duration	0.08 sec
QT interval	0.28 sec
Ventricular rate/rhythm	86 bpm/regular
Atrial rate/rhythm	UTD (no P wave)
PR interval	UTD
Identification	Accelerated junctional rhythm at 86 bpm; note the Q waves and 4 mm ST segment ↑ in V_1
Symptoms	Assess multiple lead ECG; assess for s/s of ACS
Treatment	If s/s of ACS consider ASA, Rx the pain, and reassess; consider why the sinus is not functioning

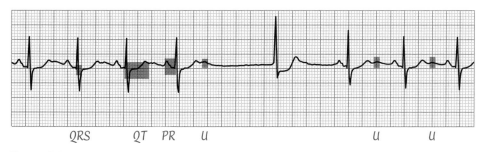

Figure 7-14

QRS duration	0.08 sec
QT interval	0.28 sec (there are U waves)
Ventricular rate/rhythm	75 bpm prior to event
Atrial rate/rhythm	75 bpm prior to event
PR interval	0.16 sec
Identification	Sinus at 75 bpm, U waves, ? SA arrest or SA block; junctional escape beat → sinus
Symptoms	? LOC, s/s of hypoperfusion; syncopal and/or near-syncopal episodes
Treatment	Consider what happened to the sinus node; the causes of sinus node dysfunction; underlying rhythm is within normal limits; be alert for recurrence of SA block or SA arrest

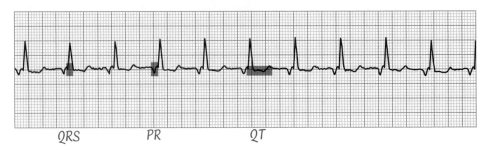

Figure 7-15

QRS duration	0.08 sec
QT interval	0.28 sec
Ventricular rate/rhythm	96 bpm/regular
Atrial rate/rhythm	96 bpm/regular (note that P waves are inverted)
PR interval	0.10 sec
Identification	Accelerated junctional rhythm at 96 bpm
Symptoms	May report syncopal episodes with a sudden onset
Treatment	Be supportive; consider why the sinus node is not functioning; what provoked the junction?

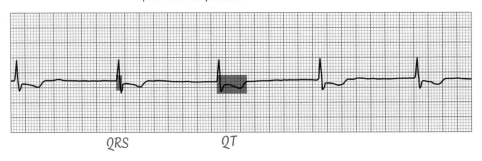

Figure 7-16

QRS duration	0.08 sec
QT interval	0.40 sec
Ventricular rate/rhythm	46 bpm/regular
Atrial rate/rhythm	UTD
PR interval	UTD
Identification	Junctional rhythm at 46 bpm
Symptoms	? ALOC, dizziness, s/s of hypoperfusion; syncopal and/or near-syncopal episodes
Treatment	If hypotensive and hypoperfusing, stand by for pacing, consider atropine, fluids, pressor; consider why the sinus is not functioning

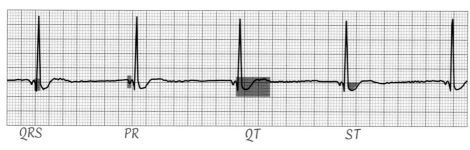

Figure 7-17

QRS duration	0.08 sec
QT interval	0.48 sec
Ventricular rate/rhythm	46 bpm/regular
Atrial rate/rhythm	46 bpm/regular
PR interval	0.06 sec (the segment is really short)
Identification	Junctional rhythm at 48 bpm, 2 mm ST ↓ and ↓ T
Symptoms	? ALOC, dizziness, s/s of hypoperfusion; syncopal and/or near-syncopal episodes
Treatment	If hypotensive and hypoperfusing, stand by for pacing, consider atropine, fluids, pressor; consider why the sinus is not functioning

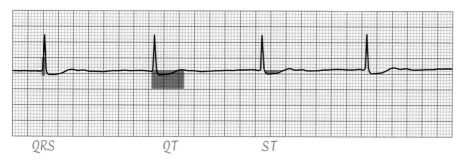

Figure 7-18

QRS duration	0.04 sec
QT interval	0.48 sec
Ventricular rate/rhythm	43 bpm/regular
Atrial rate/rhythm	UTD
PR interval	UTD
Identification	Junctional rhythm at 48 bpm, 1 mm ST ↓ and ↑ T
Symptoms	? ALOC, dizziness, s/s of hypoperfusion; syncopal and/or near-syncopal episodes
Treatment	If hypotensive and hypoperfusing, stand by for pacing, consider atropine, fluids, pressor; consider why the sinus is not functioning

CHAPTER 8 THE ATRIAL MECHANISMS

Matching

1. G
2. A
3. C
4. B
5. E

Fill in the Blanks

	Sinus Rhythm	Junctional Rhythm	PAC
P wave	1(+) P wave/QRS	1(−) P' wave before, during, or after the QRS	1 premature (+) P' wave
PR interval	0.12–0.20 sec	≤0.12 sec	Differs from sinus PRI
QRS complex	≤0.10 sec (usually)	≤0.10 sec	≤0.10 sec
QRS rate	60–100 bpm	40–60 bpm	Disturbs the sinus cadence
QRS rhythm	Regular	Regular	Disturbs the sinus rhythm

	Atrial Tach	Sinus Tach	Junctional Tach
P wave	Often UTD	1(+) P wave/QRS	1(−) P' wave or none
PR interval	UTD	0.12–0.20 sec	≤0.12 if P' is visible
QRS complex	≤0.10 sec	≤0.10 sec	≤0.10 sec
QRS rate	>160 bpm	100–160 bpm	100–130 bpm
QRS rhythm	Regular	Regular	Regular

ECG Rhythm Identification Practice

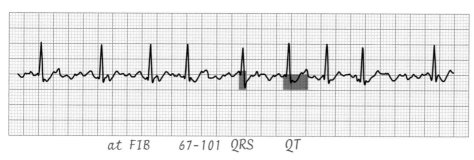

at FIB   67-101 QRS   QT

Figure 8-20

QRS duration	0.08 sec
QT interval	0.32 sec
Ventricular rate/rhythm	67–125 bpm
Atrial rate/rhythm	UTD
PR interval	UTD
Identification	A-fib vent rate at 67–125 bpm
Symptoms	None anticipated unless this is a new episode; ? chest pain ? SOB, SAo₂ dizziness, report of sudden onset; assess breath sounds; assess for ACS and s/s of pulmonary embolus (PE)
Treatment	? meds, particularly those associated with a-fib; if this is not new to the patient, Rx the pain, consider ASA unless the patient is on an anticoagulant

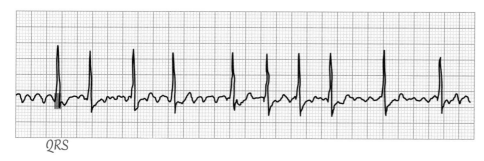

QRS

Figure 8-21

QRS duration	0.08 sec
QT interval	UTD
Ventricular rate/rhythm	80–125 bpm
Atrial rate/rhythm	UTD
PR interval	UTD
Identification	A-fib vent rate at 67–125 bpm
Symptoms	None anticipated unless this is a new episode; ? chest pain ? SOB, dizziness, report of sudden onset; assess breath sounds; SAo₂ assess for ACS and s/s of pulmonary embolus (PE)
Treatment	? meds, particularly those associated with a-fib; if this is not new to the patient, Rx the pain, consider ASA unless the patient is on an anticoagulant

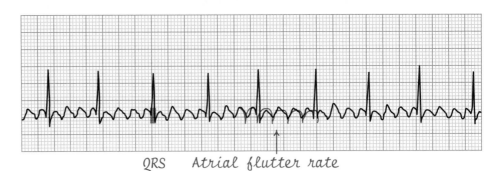

Figure 8-22

QRS duration	0.04–0.10 sec
QT interval	UTD
Ventricular rate/rhythm	86–100 bpm
Atrial rate/rhythm	300 bpm
PR interval	UTD
Identification	Atrial flutter vent rate at 86–100 bpm
Symptoms	None anticipated unless this is a new episode; ? chest pain ? SOB, SAo$_2$, dizziness, report of sudden onset; assess breath sounds; assess for ACS, CHF, and s/s of pulmonary embolus (PE)
Treatment	? meds, particularly those associated with a-fib; if this is not new to the patient, Rx the pain, consider ASA unless the patient is on an anticoagulant

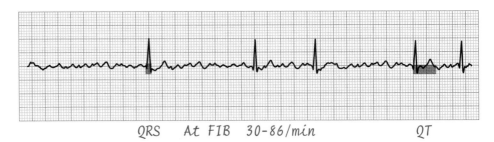

Figure 8-23

QRS duration	0.08–0.10 sec
QT interval	0.38 sec
Ventricular rate/rhythm	30–86 bpm
Atrial rate/rhythm	UTD
PR interval	UTD
Identification	A-fib vent rate at 30–86 bpm
Symptoms	May be related to the slow rate; ? digitalis; may have s/s related to digitalis toxicity
Treatment	? meds/med Hx; be supportive; consider fluids, if s/s of hypotension, hypoperfusion; stand by for pacing

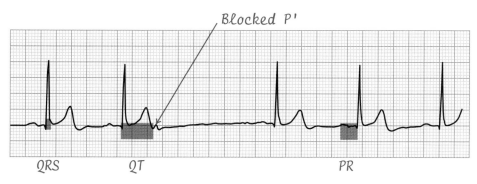

Figure 8-24

QRS duration	0.10 sec
QT interval	0.38 sec
Ventricular rate/rhythm	55–60 bpm
Atrial rate/rhythm	55–60 bpm
PR interval	0.20 sec
Identification	Sinus arrhythmia at 55–60 bpm with a nonconducted PAC (after second QRS)
Symptoms	May be related to the slow rate
Treatment	None anticipated unless this is new to the patient and there are s/s of hypotension, hypoperfusion, syncopal or near-syncopal episodes; then consider fluids, stand by for pacing; ? pressor if perfusion does not improve

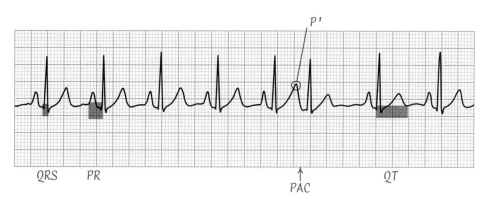

Figure 8-25

QRS duration	0.06 sec
QT interval	0.40 sec
Ventricular rate/rhythm	86 bpm
Atrial rate/rhythm	86 bpm
PR interval	0.16 sec
Identification	Sinus rhythm at 86 bpm with one PAC (6th complex) Note the P' on the T wave.
Symptoms	None anticipated
Treatment	Be supportive

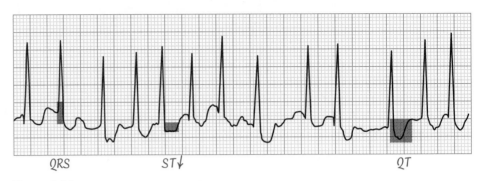

Figure 8-26

QRS duration	0.08–0.10 sec
QT interval	UTD
Ventricular rate/rhythm	107–187 bpm
Atrial rate/rhythm	UTD
PR interval	UTD
Identification	A-fib vent rate at 107–180 bpm, 3–4 mm ST seg ↓
Symptoms	May admit to "palpitations," light-headedness syncopal or near-syncopal episodes; ? chest pain, ? SOB, dizziness, report of sudden onset; assess breath sounds; SAo_2, assess for ACS and s/s of pulmonary embolus (PE)
Treatment	? meds, particularly those associated with Rx for a-fib; if this is not new to the patient, Rx the pain; consider ASA unless the patient is on an anticoagulant

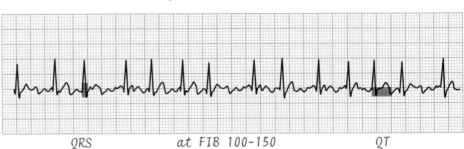

Figure 8-27

QRS duration	0.10 sec
QT interval	0.28 sec
Ventricular rate/rhythm	100–150 bpm
Atrial rate/rhythm	UTD
PR interval	UTD
Identification	A-fib vent rate at 100–150 bpm
Symptoms	May be asymptomatic if this is chronic to the patient; if new to the patient assess for light-headedness, syncopal or near-syncopal episodes; ? chest pain ? SOB, dizziness, report of sudden onset assess breath sounds; SAo_2, assess for ACS and s/s of pulmonary embolus (PE)
Treatment	? meds, particularly those associated with a-fib; if this is not new to the patient, Rx the pain, consider ASA unless the patient is on an anticoagulant

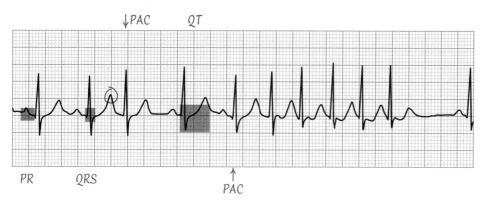

Figure 8-28

QRS duration	0.08 sec
QT interval	0.32 sec
Ventricular rate/rhythm	approx 100 bpm
Atrial rate/rhythm	approx 100 bpm for the sinus-conducted beats
PR interval	0.16 (sinus)
Identification	Sinus rhythm at about 100 bpm, frequent PACs (3rd and 6th complex), atrial tach at 150 bpm→sinus
Symptoms	None anticipated, except during bouts of PAT the patient may have episodes of syncopal or near-syncopal episodes
Treatment	? meds/med Hx; be supportive unless PAT recurs and patient response requires intervention

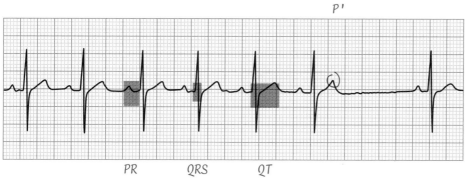

Figure 8-29

QRS duration	0.08–0.10 sec
QT interval	0.38–0.40 sec
Ventricular rate/rhythm	40–75 bpm
Atrial rate/rhythm	90 bpm/regular
PR interval	0.16 sec
Identification	Sinus at 90 bpm with one nonconducted PAC; note the sudden pause in the tracing; move to the left and look at the T wave—its amplitude is increased; this is the P′ on top of the T wave
Symptoms	Probably none
Treatment	Be supportive

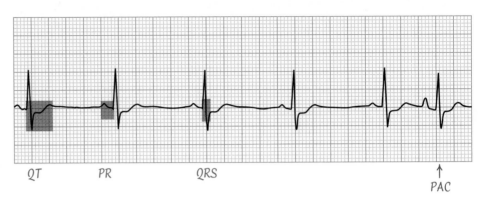

Figure 8-30

QRS duration	0.08 sec
QT interval	0.38 sec
Ventricular rate/rhythm	60 bpm
Atrial rate/rhythm	60 bpm
PR interval	0.16 sec
Identification	Sinus rate at 60 bpm, 1–2 mm ST ↓ with a PAC (last complex on the tracing)
Symptoms	May be related to slow rate; find out if this rate is new to the patient
Treatment	If the rate is new and considerably slower for the patient and there is hypotension and/or hypoperfusion, consider fluids; perhaps stand by for pacing 12-lead ECG to clarify the ST and other acute changes

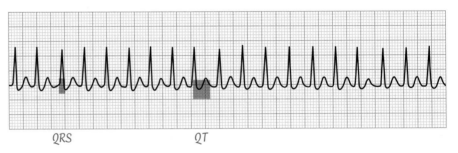

Figure 8-31

QRS duration	0.08–0.10 sec
QT interval	UTD
Ventricular rate/rhythm	188 bpm
Atrial rate/rhythm	UTD
PR interval	UTD
Identification	SVT vent rate at 188 bpm
Symptoms	? ALOC, ? SOB, anxiety, feelings of palpitations, syncopal or near-syncopal episodes
Treatment	If the patient is stable, attempt vagal maneuvers, pharmacologic intervention; if unstable, sedate and perform synchronized cardioversion

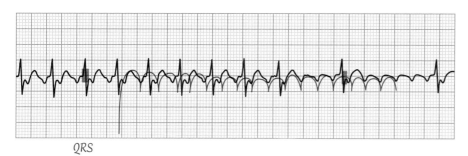

QRS

Figure 8-32

QRS duration	0.08 sec
QT interval	UTD
Ventricular rate/rhythm	150→75→50 bpm
Atrial rate/rhythm	Flutter waves at about 300 bpm
PR interval	UTD
Identification	Atrial flutter, vent rate 150→75→50 bpm
Symptoms	May admit to "palpitations"; some patients note the sudden change at the onset as "something happened," or "it just hit me"
Treatment	In this example, vagal maneuvers were performed causing the slowing of the ventricular rate; this was done to help differentiate between SVT and atrial flutter, and it did

PAC

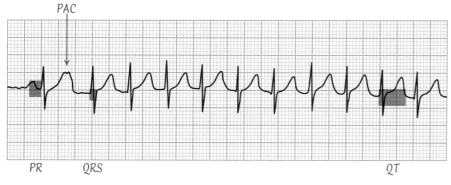

PR   QRS   QT

Figure 8-33

QRS duration	0.08 sec
QT interval	0.28 sec
Ventricular rate/rhythm	150 bpm/regular
Atrial rate/rhythm	UTD
PR interval	0.16 (sinus beat)
Identification	One sinus beat, a PAC→atrial tach at 150 bpm
Symptoms	? ALOC, ? SOB, anxiety, feelings of palpitations
Treatment	? meds/med Hx; if stable, consider vagal maneuvers, consider pharmacologic interventions; if the rhythm does persist and the patient becomes unstable, consider sedation and synchronized cardioversion

CHAPTER 9 THE VENTRICULAR MECHANISMS

Fill in the Blanks

	Sinus Rhythm	PJC	PAC	PVC
P wave	1(+) P wave/QRS	1 premature (−) P' wave/QRS; or none seen may be within the T wave	1 premature (+) P' wave; may be visible within the previous T wave	n/a
PR interval	0.12–0.20 sec	≤0.12 sec	Differs from sinus	n/a
QRS complex	≤0.10 sec	≤0.10 sec	≤0.10 sec	>0.10 sec*
QRS rate	60–100 bpm	n/a	n/a	n/a
QRS rhythm	Regular	Disturbs sinus cadence	Disturbs sinus cadence	Sinus cadence is not disturbed

*QRS opposite in polarity from its T wave.

	Atrial Tach	Sinus Tach	Ventricular Tach
P wave	May not see	1(+) P wave/QRS	As with underlying rhythm
PR interval	UTD	0.12–0.20 sec	As with underlying rhythm
QRS complex	0.10 sec	≤0.10 sec	>0.10 sec* (usually)
QRS rate	150+ bpm	101–150 bpm	>100 bpm
QRS rhythm	Regular	Regular	Regular

*QRS opposite in polarity from its T wave.
Atrial and ventricular tach are sudden onset; sinus tach is gradual onset.

ECG Rhythm Identification Practice

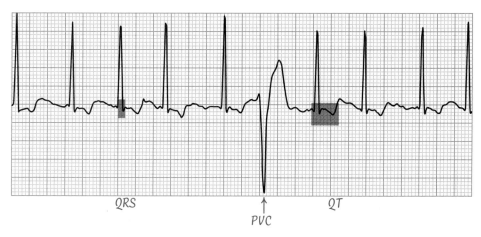

Figure 9-26

QRS duration	0.06–0.08 sec
QT interval	≤0.28 sec
Ventricular rate/rhythm	Irregular
Atrial rate/rhythm	UTD
PR interval	UTD
Identification	A-fib vent rate at 90–125 bpm with a PVC ? R on T; 1–2 mm ST ↓ ? ↓T wave.
Symptoms	Probably none
Treatment	? meds Hx, especially digitalis; PVCs frequently occur during digitalis therapy

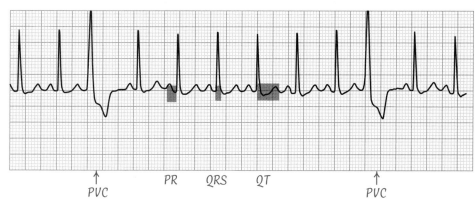

Figure 9-27

QRS duration	0.06 sec
QT interval	0.32 sec
Ventricular rate/rhythm	108 bpm/regular
Atrial rate/rhythm	108 bpm/regular
PR interval	0.16 sec
Identification	Sinus tach at 108 bpm/regular with freq uniform (u/f) PVCs; assess the underlying cause for the sinus tach
Symptoms	? pain, ? meds/med Hx
Treatment	Assess electrolytes; ? meds (i.e., diuretics, excessive use of caffeine); assess for s/s of ACS. ? nausea and/or vomiting; be supportive; if pain, Rx the pain and reassess; if PVCs persist or increase in frequency and duration, consider ventricular antiarrhythmics

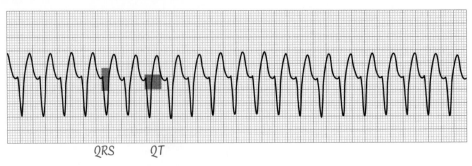

QRS   QT

Figure 9-28

QRS duration	0.12 sec
QT interval	0.32 sec
Ventricular rate/rhythm	168 bpm/regular
Atrial rate/rhythm	UTD
PR interval	UTD
Identification	Sustained ventricular tachycardia at 168 bpm
Symptoms	If conscious, the patient is probably unstable at this rate—confirm if the patient has a pulse
Treatment	If conscious with a pulse, consider sedation and synchronized cardioversion; if pulseless, begin immediate defibrillation

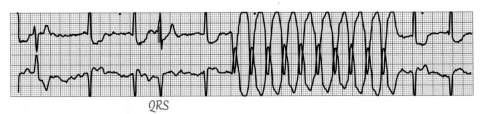

QRS

Figure 9-29

QRS duration	0.08 sec
QT interval	≤0.40 sec
Ventricular rate/rhythm	75–86 bpm (a-fib), 150 bpm (v-tach)
Atrial rate/rhythm	UTD
PR interval	UTD
Identification	A-fib vent rate at 75–86 bpm with m/f PVCs and a run of v-tach at about 150 bpm; there is ST ↓
Symptoms	Probably symptomatic with v-tach; light-headedness, dizziness, syncopal and/or near-syncopal episodes
Treatment	Antiarrhythmic meds; stand by for cardioversion if the v-tach persists and/or the patient becomes unstable; defibrillation if the patient is pulseless

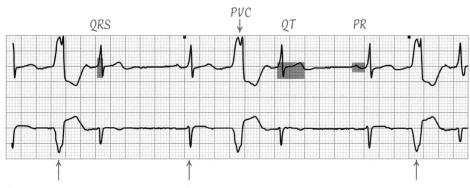

Figure 9-30

QRS duration	0.08–0.10 sec
QT interval	0.40 sec
Ventricular rate/rhythm	46 bpm/regular
Atrial rate/rhythm	46 bpm/regular
PR interval	0.16–0.20 sec
Identification	Sinus at 48 bpm with frequent u/f interpolated PVCs (note how the PVC is sandwiched between normal QRSs)
Symptoms	May be related to the brady; ? ALOC, dizziness, syncopal and/or near-syncopal episodes
Treatment	? meds, especially digitalis, and med Hx, vital signs; stand by for pacing

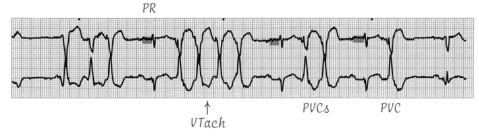

Figure 9-31

QRS duration	0.08–0.10 sec (sinus)
QT interval	0.38 sec (sinus)
Ventricular rate/rhythm	UTD
Atrial rate/rhythm	UTD
PR interval	0.16–0.20
Identification	Sinus→three- and -four-beat runs of v-tach; PVCs are uniform; there are fusion beats; symptoms probably with the v-tach, light-headedness, dizziness, syncopal and/or near-syncopal episodes
Treatment	If there is time, pay particular attention to med Hx and also excessive use of caffeine or other stimulants; multiple lead ECG and antiarrhythmic meds are indicated; stand by for cardioversion if the v-tach persists and the patient becomes unstable; defibrillation if the patient is pulseless

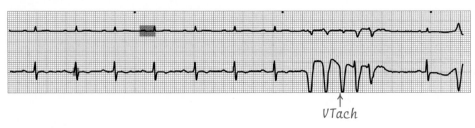

Figure 9-32

QRS duration	0.04 sec
QT interval	0.38 sec
Ventricular rate/rhythm	75 bpm/regular
Atrial rate/rhythm	75 bpm/regular
PR interval	0.24–028 sec
Identification	Sinus rhythm at 75 bpm→end-diastolic PVC→five-beat run of v-tach; PRI 0.28 sec (P wave is broad and notched and probably prolonged the PR interval)
Symptoms	Probably with the v-tach
Treatment	If the v-tach persists or increases in frequency or duration, consider antiarrhythmic meds; stand by for synchronized cardioversion if the v-tach persists and the patient becomes unstable; defibrillation if the patient is pulseless

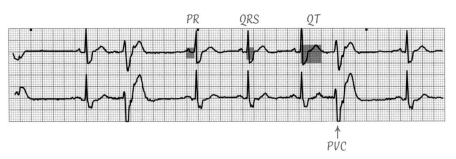

Figure 9-33

QRS duration	0.16 sec
QT interval	0.40 sec
Ventricular rate/rhythm	67 bpm/regular
Atrial rate/rhythm	67 bpm/regular
PR interval	0.16 sec
Identification	Sinus at 67 bpm with QRS 0.16 sec; frequent u/f PVCs (note the broad S wave and long QRS) ? RBBB; need to confirm on multiple lead ECG
Symptoms	May be none; assess for s/s of ACS; ? meds/med Hx
Treatment	Monitor and document frequency; be supportive

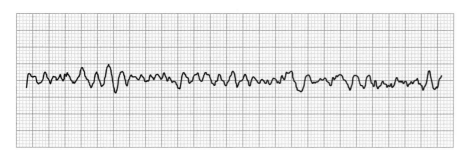

Figure 9-34

QRS duration	UTD
QT interval	UTD
Ventricular rate/rhythm	UTD
Atrial rate/rhythm	UTD
PR interval	UTD
Identification	Ventricular fibrillation; confirm no pulse
Symptoms	Pulseless
Treatment	Immediate defibrillation

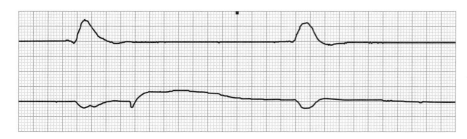

Figure 9-35

QRS duration	+0.40 sec
QT interval	UTD
Ventricular rate/rhythm	20 bpm
Atrial rate/rhythm	UTD
PR interval	UTD
Identification	Idioventricular rhythm at 20 bpm
Symptoms	? ALOC/pulseless
Treatment	Assess the scene; if appropriate, ask if there are advanced directives; CPR, oxygenate, ventilate, intubate IV, fluids; epinephrine, vasopressin, maybe atropine, perhaps TCP

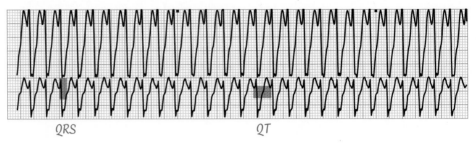

Figure 9-36

QRS duration	0.12 sec
QT interval	0.24 sec
Ventricular rate/rhythm	214 bpm/regular
Atrial rate/rhythm	UTD
PR interval	n/a
Identification	Ventricular tachycardia (or flutter) at 214 bpm
Symptoms	If conscious, the patient is probably unstable at this rate—confirm if the patient has a pulse
Treatment	If by chance the patient is conscious and with a pulse at this rate, consider sedation and synchronized cardioversion; if pulseless, immediate defibrillation

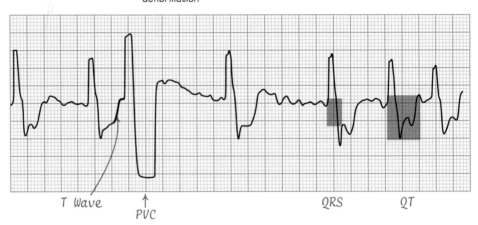

Figure 9-37

QRS duration	0.16–0.20 sec
QT interval	n/a
Ventricular rate/rhythm	50–100 bpm/irregular
Atrial rate/rhythm	n/a
PR interval	n/a
Identification	A-fib vent rate at 50–100 bpm, 4–6 mm ST ↓ and an R on T PVC
Symptoms	Assess for s/s of ACS
Treatment	? meds, medical history; concern for the PVC—may or may not be necessary for antiarrhythmics at this time

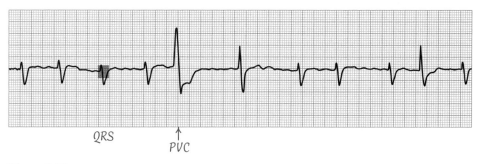

Figure 9-38

QRS duration	0.12–0.16 sec
QT interval	UTD
Ventricular rate/rhythm	67–86 bpm/irregular
Atrial rate/rhythm	UTD
PR interval	n/a
Identification	A-fib at 57–86 bpm, a PVC, QRS 0.12–0.16 sec
Symptoms	None noted
Treatment	? meds/med Hx; be supportive; assess multiple lead ECG for BBB

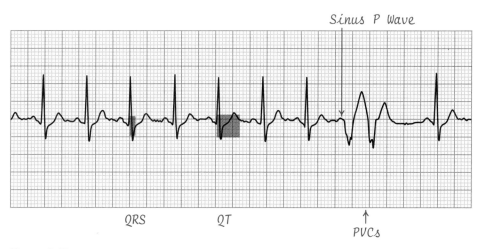

Figure 9-39

QRS duration	0.08 sec
QT interval	0.28 sec
Ventricular rate/rhythm	116 bpm/regular
Atrial rate/rhythm	116 bpm/regular
PR interval	0.16 sec
Identification	Sinus tach at 115 bpm with end-diastolic, paired PVCs
Symptoms	Assess for s/s of ACS
Treatment	Rx for pain if present; if PVCs persist or increase in frequency and/or duration, consider antiarrhythmics

CHAPTER 10 AV CONDUCTION DEFECTS

Fill in the Blanks

	Sinus Rhythm	First-Degree AV Block	Second-Degree AV Block Type I
P wave	1(+) P wave/QRS	1(+) P wave/QRS	1(+) P wave/QRS; sinus P plots through
PR interval	0.12–0.20 sec	>0.20 sec and consistent	Consistent after the dropped QRS; may progressively prolong as with Wenckebach phenomenon
QRS complex	≤0.10 sec	≤0.10 sec	≤0.10 sec
QRS rate	60–100 bpm	60–100 bpm	60–100 bpm
QRS rhythm	Regular	Regular	May be regular or irregular

	Sinus Rhythm	Complete AV Block	Second-Degree AV Block Type II
P wave	1(+)P wave/QRS	P waves independent of QRS	1(+) P wave/QRS; sinus P plots through
PR interval	0.12–0.20 sec	No consistent PRI	Sinus P plots through and is consistent after the dropped QRS
QRS complex	≤0.10 sec	≤0.10 sec junctional >0.10 sec ventricular	May be >0.10 sec or may be notched, or an rS, or have a broad, terminal S wave
QRS rate	60–100 bpm	40–60+ junctional 20–60+ ventricular	Usually slow
QRS rhythm	Regular	Regular	May be regular or irregular

ECG Rhythm Identification Practice

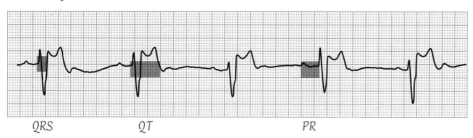

Figure 10-10

QRS duration	0.12–0.16 sec
QT interval	0.42 sec
Ventricular rate/rhythm	43 bpm/regular
Atrial rate/rhythm	46 bpm/regular
PR interval	0.28 sec and consistent
Identification	1° AV block, AR 86, VR 43 (QRS 0.12–0.16 sec), 2 mm ST ↑
Symptoms	Associated with bradycardia; dizziness, postural hypotension, syncopal and/or near-syncopal episodes; assess for s/s of ACS
Treatment	? meds/med Hx; stand by for pacing

COMMENT: At first glance you might think the U waves are in fact sinus P waves. However, they do not plot out. A 12-lead ECG confirmed the interpretation.

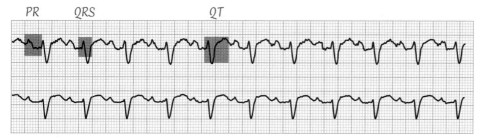

Figure 10-11

QRS duration	0.16 sec, ? broad S wave
QT interval	0.32–0.36 sec
Ventricular rate/rhythm	100 bpm/regular
Atrial rate/rhythm	100 bpm/regular
PR interval	0.24 sec and consistent
Identification	Sinus at 100 bpm with 1° AV block (QRS >0.12 sec), ? broad S wave, 1-2 mm ST ↑
Symptoms	Assess for s/s of ACS
Treatment	? meds/med Hx; multiple lead ECG to confirm BBB

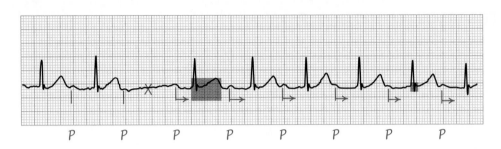

Figure 10-12

QRS duration	0.08–0.10 sec
QT interval	0.44 sec
Ventricular rate/rhythm	43–75 bpm
Atrial rate/rhythm	75 bpm/regular
PR interval	0.32, 0.38, 0.40, 0.42 sec (greatest increase between #1 and #2 PR in the group)
Identification	Sinus at 75 bpm with 2° AV block Type I Wenckebach (QRS 0.10 sec)
Symptoms	None noted
Treatment	? meds/med Hx; Rx for pain if present

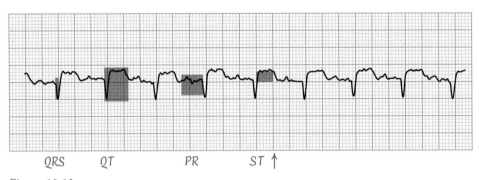

Figure 10-13

QRS duration	0.04–0.06 sec
QT interval	0.28 sec and consistent
Ventricular rate/rhythm	100 bpm
Atrial rate/rhythm	100 bpm
PR interval	0.24 sec and consistent
Identification	Sinus at 100 bpm with 1° AV block; Q waves 4-5 mm, 3 mm ST segment ↑
Symptoms	Assess for s/s of ACS
Treatment	Assess multiple lead ECG, especially V_{4R} for acute changes; perhaps when the rate slows down, the PR interval may improve

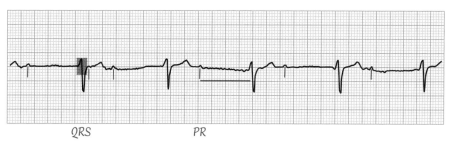

QRS   PR

Figure 10-14

QRS duration	0.10 sec
QT interval	0.38 sec
Ventricular rate/rhythm	50 bpm/regular
Atrial rate/rhythm	50 bpm/regular
PR interval	0.78 sec and consistent
Identification	Sinus brady at 50 bpm with 1° AV block
Symptoms	Associated with bradycardia (i.e., dizziness, postural hypotension)
Treatment	Multiple lead ECG to confirm sinus rate ? med/med Hx, especially digitalis; if symptomatic with bradycardia, may consider atropine, fluids, pressor; stand by for pacing

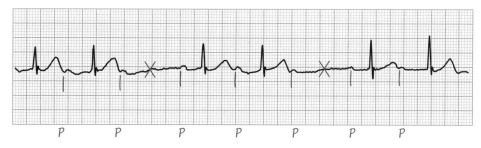

P   P   P   P   P   P   P

Figure 10-15

QRS duration	0.08 sec
QT interval	0.40 sec
Ventricular rate/rhythm	40–75 bpm/irregular
Atrial rate/rhythm	75 bpm/regular
PR interval	0.32, 0.38 sec; note the PRIs after the missed QRSs are consistent
Identification	Sinus at 75 bpm with vent rate at 40–75 bpm, 2° AV block, probably Type I Wenckebach (QRS 0.08 sec)
Symptoms	None unless the slower rate persists
Treatment	? meds/med Hx

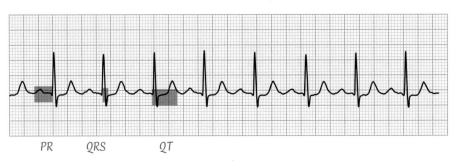

Figure 10-16

QRS duration	0.08 sec
QT interval	0.36 sec
Ventricular rate/rhythm	86 bpm/regular
Atrial rate/rhythm	86 bpm/regular
PR interval	0.24 sec and consistent
Identification	Sinus at 86 bpm with 1° AV block
Symptoms	None noted
Treatment	? meds/med Hx

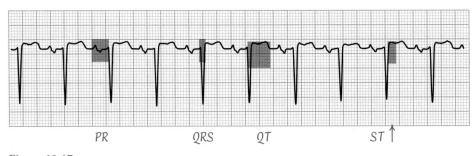

Figure 10-17

QRS duration	0.06–0.10 sec Q waves 17–20 mm
QT interval	0.32 sec
Ventricular rate/rhythm	100 bpm/regular
Atrial rate/rhythm	100 bpm/regular
PR interval	0.24–0.26 sec
Identification	Sinus at 100 bpm with 1° AV block, 2 mm ST segment ↑, and 17–20 mm Q waves
Symptoms	Assess for s/s of ACS
Treatment	12-lead ECG to confirm atrial rate, especially V_{4R} for acute changes

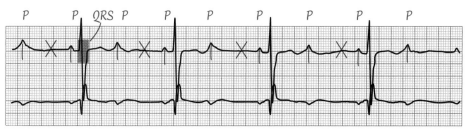

Figure 10-18

QRS duration	0.12 sec
QT interval	0.42–0.44 sec
Ventricular rate/rhythm	40 bpm/regular
Atrial rate/rhythm	75 bpm/regular
PR interval	0.20 sec and consistent
Identification	Sinus at 75 bpm with vent rate at 40 bpm, 2° AV block, 2:1; PR after missed beat is consistent; QRS 0.16 sec
Symptoms	Associated with bradycardia; assess for s/s of ACS
Treatment	Assess multiple lead ECG, especially V$_{4R}$ for acute changes; stand by for pacing

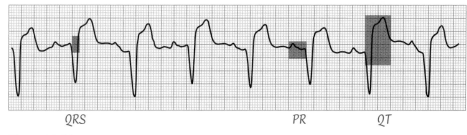

Figure 10-19

QRS duration	0.12 sec
QT interval	0.32–0.36 sec
Ventricular rate/rhythm	60 bpm
Atrial rate/rhythm	60 bpm
PR interval	0.24–0.26 sec
Identification	Sinus at 60 bpm with 1° AV block, 7 mm ST ↑, Q waves at 15–17 mm
Symptoms	Assess for s/s of ACS
Treatment	Assess multiple lead ECG, especially V$_{4R}$ for acute changes

CHAPTER 11 INTRAVENTRICULAR CONDUCTION DEFECTS

ECG Rhythm Identification Practice

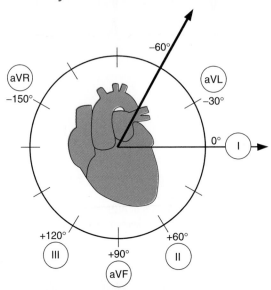

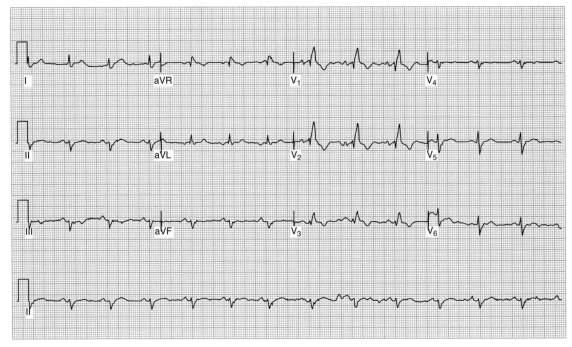

Figure 11-9

1. What is the underlying rhythm?

   Sinus at 77 bpm and regular.

2. What are the acute changes?

   rS in leads II, III, and F; rsR′ in V_1–V_3. There are broad S waves in leads I, II, aVF, V_5, and V_6. Axis is at −60°. There is RBBB.

3. What is your interpretation?

   Sinus at 77 bpm; left axis deviation at −60°; There is RBBB.

4. What can happen next?

   Observe for left anterior fascicular block.

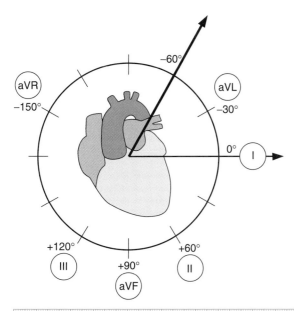

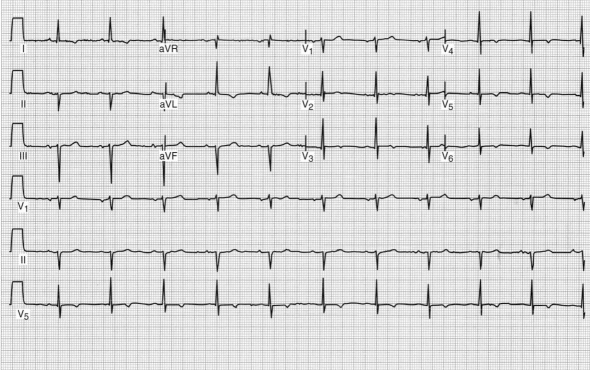

Figure 11-10

1. What is the underlying rhythm?
    Sinus at 63 bpm.

2. What are the acute changes?
    rS configuration in leads II, III, and aVF. Lead III is the greatest negative deflection. Axis is at −60°. There are inverted T waves in leads I, aVL, and V_3–V_6.

3. What is your interpretation?
    Sinus rhythm at 63 bpm; left anterior fascicular block (LAFB); assess for lateral ischemia.

4. What can happen next?
    Observe for V_1 RBBB. Observe for s/s of CHF.

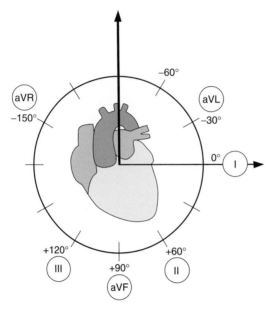

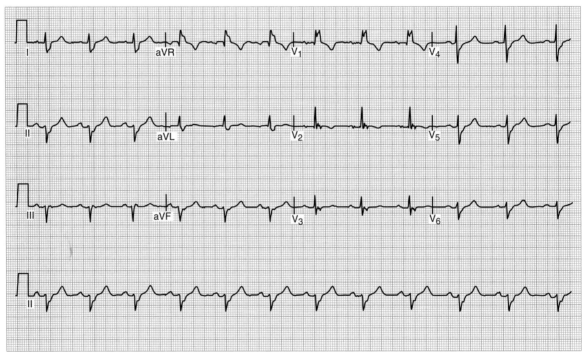

Figure 11-11

1. What is the underlying rhythm?
   Sinus at approximately 70 bpm.

2. What are the acute changes?
   QRS is 0.12–0.16 sec with broad S waves in leads I and aVL; terminal deflections in leads II, V_3–V_6. rS configuration in leads II, III, and aVF. Equiphasic deflection in lead I; lead aVF is negative, axis is abnormal at −90°. The R wave in V_1 is notched and the QRS measures 0.12 sec. The overall QT is 0.40–0.44 sec.

3. What is your interpretation?
   Sinus rhythm at 70 bpm with right bundle branch block (RBBB); consider left anterior fascicular block (LAFB).

4. What can happen next?
   Observe for AV conduction defects; s/s of CHF.

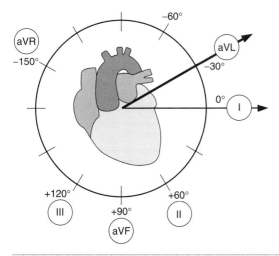

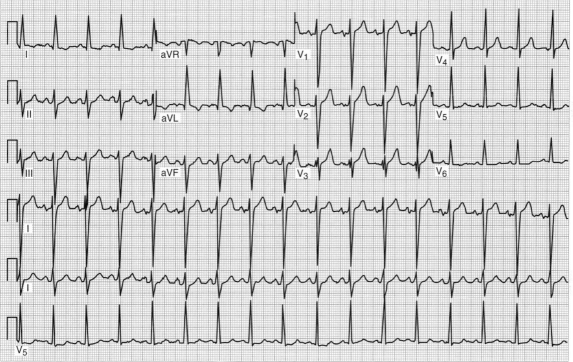

Figure 11-12

1. What is the underlying rhythm?

   Underlying rhythm is sinus at 100 bpm.

2. What are the acute changes?

   Acute changes are QRS is 0.10–0.12 sec with rS configuration in only leads III and aVF. Equiphasic deflection in lead II; in lead aVL the QRS is positive.

3. What is your interpretation?

   Interpretation is sinus rhythm at 100 bpm; abnormal QRS, consider rate-dependent LAFB. The equiphasic deflection is in lead II; lead aVL is positive, so the axis is at −30°. The overall QT is 0.36–0.40 sec. The R wave in lead I plus the S wave in lead III is greater than 21 mm and the height of the R wave in aVL is greater than 13 mm. Consider ventricular hypertrophy (see Chapter 12).

4. What can happen next?

   Observe for alterations in QRS if rate decreases. Observe for AV conduction defects; s/s of CHF.

CHAPTER 12 CHAMBER ENLARGEMENT AND HYPERTROPHY

ECG Rhythm Identification Practice

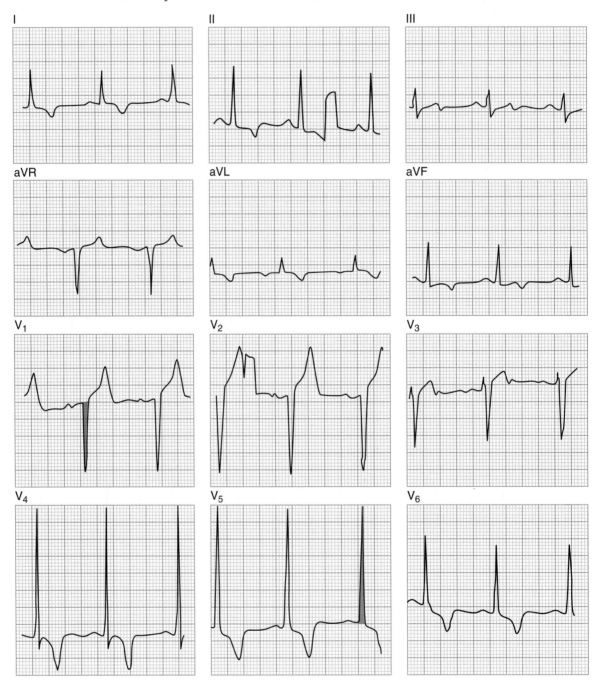

Figure 12-10

1. What is the underlying rhythm?

   Sinus at 68 bpm.

2. What are the acute changes?

   Inverted T waves in I, aVL and aVF, V_4–V_6. There are sagging (−) T waves in every lead with a tall R wave in V_4–V_6. There are rising ST segments and upright T waves in every lead with a deep S wave in V_1–V_3. Axis is +60°: (SV_1) 20 mm plus (RV_5) (35 mm) = 55 mm.

3. What is your interpretation?

    Sinus rhythm at 68 bpm; LVH by R/S voltage criteria and secondary ST-T changes.

4. What can happen next?

    Observe for s/s of ischemia, injury, any type of conduction defect.

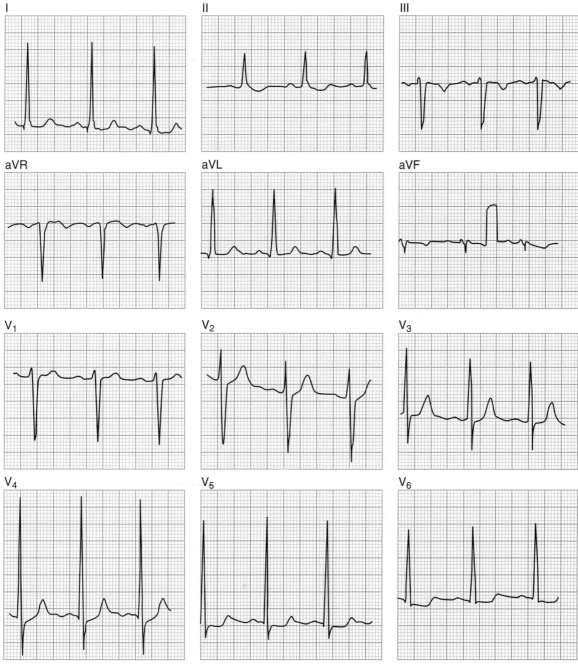

Figure 12-11

1. What is the underlying rhythm?

    Sinus at 78 bpm; 1 mm ST depression in II; T-wave inversion in III and aVF.

2. What are the acute changes?

    Axis is $+0°$: (SV_1) 29 mm plus (RV_5) (31 mm) = 60 mm.

3. What is your interpretation?

    Sinus rhythm at 78 bpm; LVH by R/S voltage criteria; also the S in V_1 plus RV_5 >35 mm.

4. What can happen next?

    Observe for s/s of ischemia, injury, any type of conduction defect.

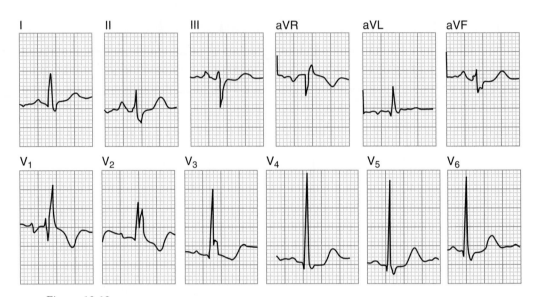

Figure 12-12

1. What is the underlying rhythm?

    Sinus at an undetermined rate.

2. What are the acute changes?

    rS configuration in leads II, III, and aVF. Lead III is the greatest negative deflection. Axis is at $-60°$. There are inverted T waves in leads V_1–V_3. There is a broad S wave in leads I, II, and aVF; R waves in V_4 are 23 mm; rSR' in V_1; tall, notched R waves in V_2 and V_3.

3. What is your interpretation?

    Sinus with RBBB; possible LVH.

4. What can happen next?

    Observe leads II, III, and aVF for LAFB. Observe for s/s of CHF.

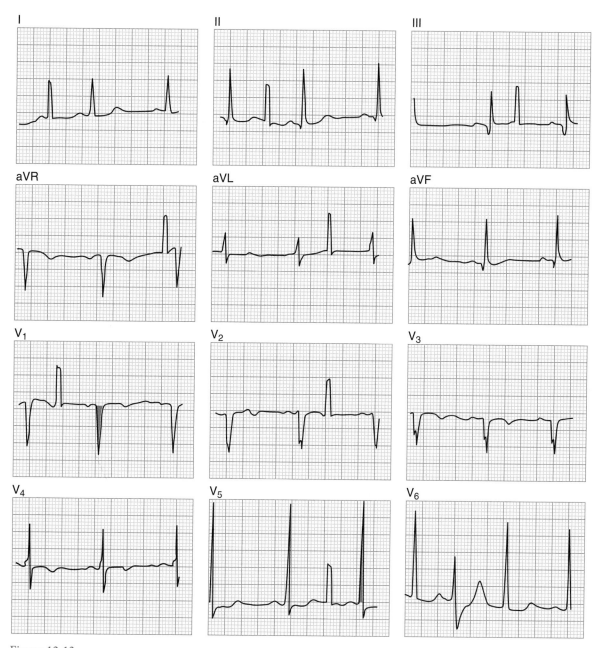

Figure 12-13

1. What is the underlying rhythm?

   Sinus at 67 bpm; 1 mm ST elevation in II and III; Q wave in leads II, III, and aVF. It appears the leads are not simultaneous; PACs appear in leads I, ? II, and V_6 (with aberration).

2. What are the acute changes?

   Axis is +60°: (SV_1) 14 mm plus (RV_5) 29 mm = 43 mm.

3. What is your interpretation?

   Sinus rhythm at 67 bpm with PACs; LVH by R/S voltage criteria; possible inferior MI; if so, age undetermined.

4. What can happen next?

   Observe for s/s of ischemia, injury, any type of conduction defect.

CHAPTER 13 ARRHYTHMIAS DUE TO ABNORMAL CONDUCTION PATHWAYS

ECG Rhythm Identification Practice

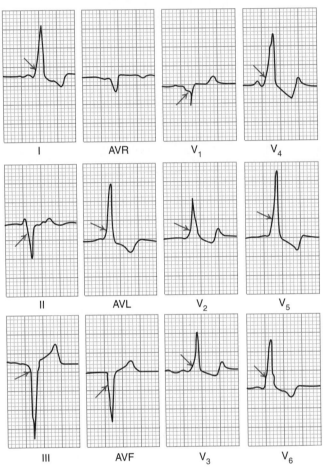

Figure 13-11

1. What is the underlying rhythm?

   Sinus.

2. What are the abnormalities?

   rS in lead II; QS in III and aVF; positive delta in I, aVL, and the precordial leads V_2–V_6. Negative delta in leads II, III, aVF, and V_1. PR interval <0.10 sec, with PR segment barely measureable at 0.04 sec; QRS 0.12 sec.

3. What is the interpretation?

   Sinus with pattern of preexcitation; shortened PR interval and delta waves in all leads.

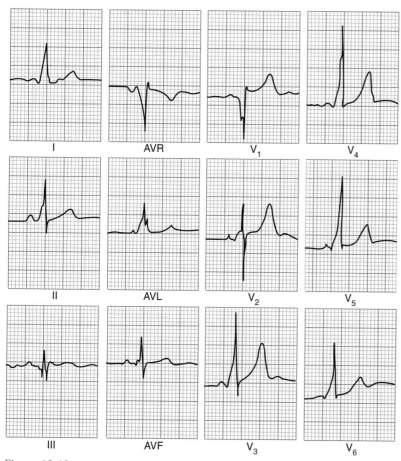

Figure 13-12

1. What is the underlying rhythm?

    Sinus

2. What are the abnormalities?

    Positive delta waves in I, II, aVR, aVL, and aVF. Negative delta waves in V_1, positive in V_2–V_6. PR interval 0.08–0.10 sec; QRS 0.12 sec.

3. What is the interpretation?

    Sinus with pattern of preexcitation; delta waves and shortened PR interval.

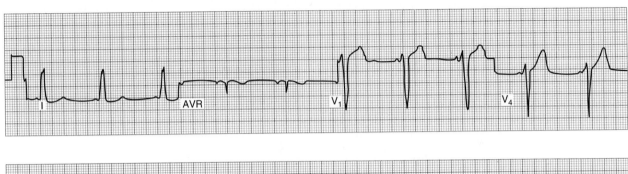
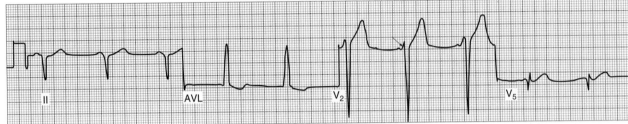
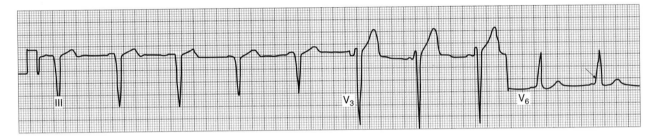

Figure 13-13

1. What is the underlying rhythm?

   Sinus at 60 bpm.

2. What are the abnormalities?

   QS in leads II, III, and aVF; positive delta waves in I, aVL, and V_6. PR interval 0.08 sec; QRS 0.14 sec.

3. What is the interpretation?

   Sinus with pattern of preexcitation. Delta waves and shortened PR interval. Remember that delta waves may not be readily visible in all the leads.

CHAPTER 14 MYOCARDIAL PERFUSION DEFICITS AND ECG CHANGES

Matching

1. D
2. B
3. C
4. E
5. A

ECG Rhythm Identification Practice

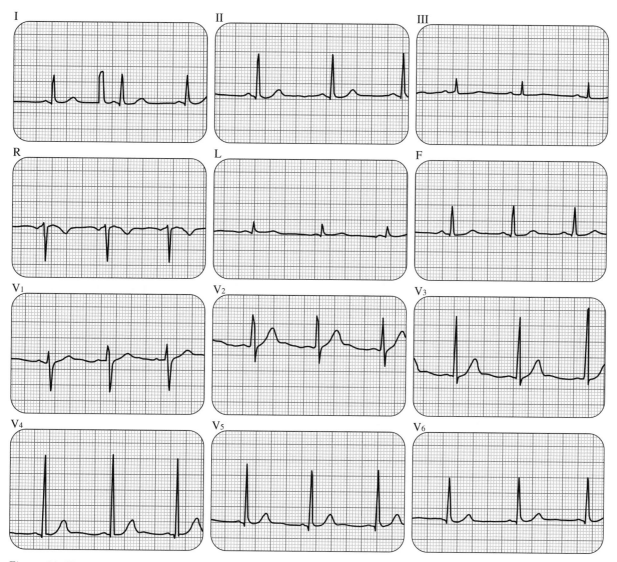

Figure 14-17

1. What is the underlying rhythm?
    Sinus at 60 bpm.
2. What are the acute changes?
    None noted.
3. What is your interpretation?
    Sinus rhythm at 50–55 bpm.
4. What can happen next?
    No acute changes; be vigilant with serial ECGs as necessary.

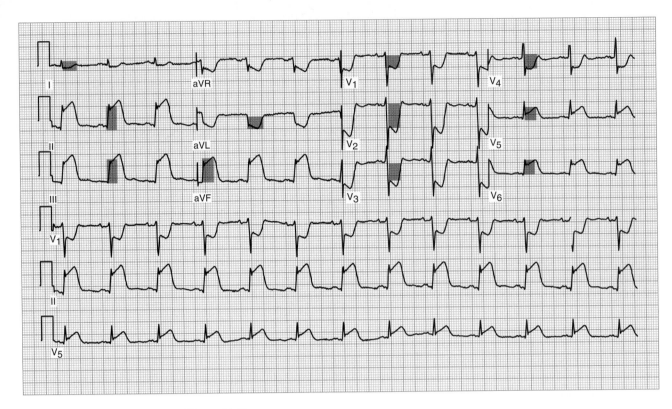

Figure 14-18

1. What is the underlying rhythm?

    Sinus at 75 bpm.

2. What are the acute changes?

    7 mm ST segment in leads II, III, and aVF, and with reciprocal changes (ST ↓) in I and aVL. ST elevation in III greater than in II (ST ↑ III > ST ↑ II [inferior]; ST ↓ in V_2–V_4 [reciprocal to the posterior surface]; ST ↑ in V_5 and V_6 [lateral]).

3. What is your interpretation?

    Acute right inferior MI; posterior MI (inferoposterior). There is extension to the left lateral surface. Probable occlusion of the RCA. Need full right precordial ECG analysis.

4. What can happen next?

    A high-risk patient; observe for SA and AV conduction defect, ventricular arrhythmias and CHF. Be alert for hypotension and hypoperfusion before administering medications causing vasodilation; assess right precordial leads; be vigilant with serial ECGs as necessary.

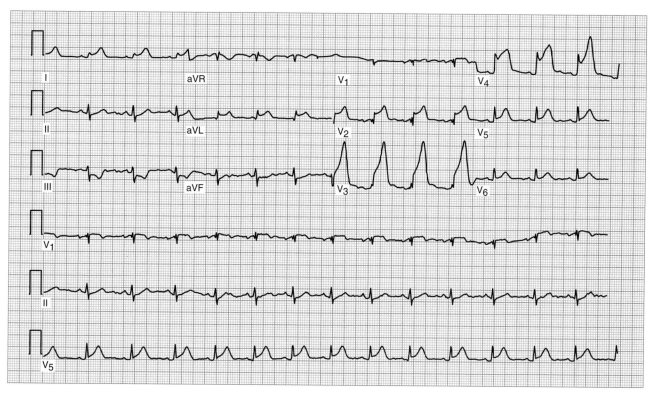

Figure 14-19

1. What is the underlying rhythm?

   Sinus at 75 bpm.

2. What are the acute changes?

   2 mm ST seg ↑ in I, aVL, and with reciprocal ST ↓ in II, III, and aVF. There are Q waves in V_1 and V_2. There is progressive ST ↑ in V_2–V_4, 2–3 mm ST ↑ in V_5 and V_6.

3. What is your interpretation?

   Sinus at 75 bpm with acute anteroseptal MI, extension of injury, and ischemia to the anterolateral surface.

4. What can happen next?

   Observe for AV and BB conduction problems, ventricular arrhythmias, and s/s of CHF.

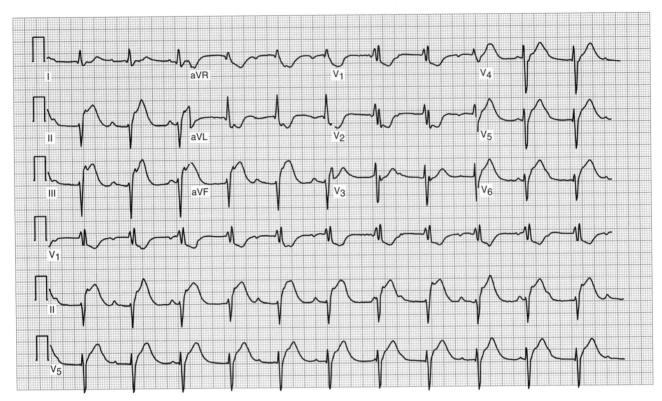

Figure 14-20

1.   What is the underlying rhythm?

Sinus at 86 bpm, complete AV block, and a junctional escape rhythm.

2.   What are the acute changes?

Broad, notched QRSs (rsr') (0.14 sec) in V_1–V_3 (? BBB pattern), ST ↓ in V_1 and V_2, ? V_3. There is ST ↑ leads II, III, elevation in III greater than in II (ST ↑ III > ST ↑ II) and aVF; reciprocal ST ↓ in I and aVL. There is ST ↓ in V_1, V_2, possibly V_3.

3.   What is your interpretation?

Sinus at 86 bpm with complete AV block and with a junctional rhythm at 50 bpm. This may be an acute inferoposterior MI. The BBB makes precise definition difficult. Need to assess previous ECGs. Need right precordial ECG analysis.

4.   What can happen next?

Observe for further conduction problems, extension of injury, ventricular arrhythmias, and s/s of CHF.

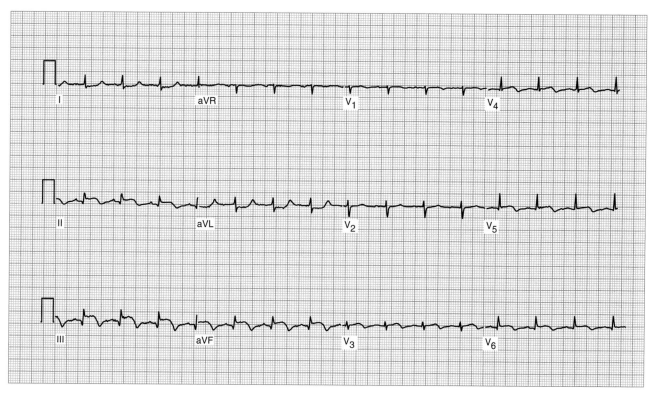

Figure 14-21

1. What is the underlying rhythm?

    Sinus at 86 bpm, QT interval 0.40 sec.

2. What are the acute changes?

    Small Qs and ST ↑ in leads II, III, and aVF reciprocal ST ↓ in I and aVL. ST in III is higher than in II (ST ↑ III > ST ↑ II) indicating possible RCA occlusion. There are T waves ↓ in V_4–V_6.

3. What is your interpretation?

    Sinus at 86 bpm with inferior wall MI. Need right precordial ECG analysis.

4. What can happen next?

    Observe for further conduction problems, extension of injury, ventricular arrhythmias, and s/s of CHF.

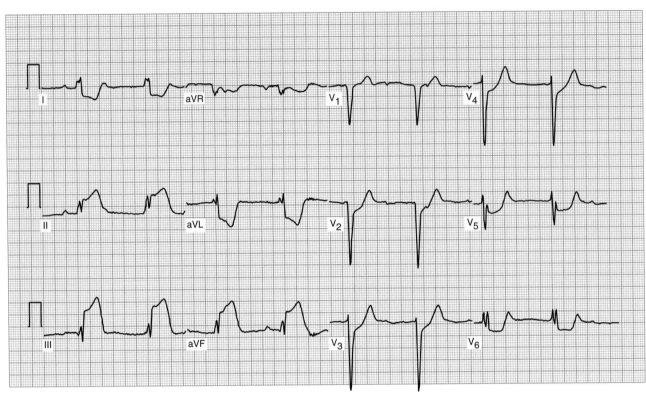

Figure 14-22

1. What is the underlying rhythm?

    Sinus at 86 bpm with complete AV block with ventricular rate at 50 bpm.

2. What are the acute changes?

    Broad QRS, notched, 0.14 sec in leads II, III and V_6. ST in III is higher than in II (ST ↑ III > ST ↑ II), with reciprocal ST ↓ in I and aVL. There are deep Qs with ST ↓ in V_1 and V_2. The is loss of R-wave progression. There is ST ↓ in V_2–V_6.

3. What is your interpretation?

    Sinus at 86 bpm with complete AV block and a junctional rhythm at 50 bpm. Current of injury pattern shows inferoposterior injury and ischemia; the broad, notched QRS in I and V_6 may indicate BBB. Need right precordial ECG analysis.

4. What can happen next?

    Observe for further conduction problems, extension of injury, ventricular arrhythmias, and s/s of CHF.

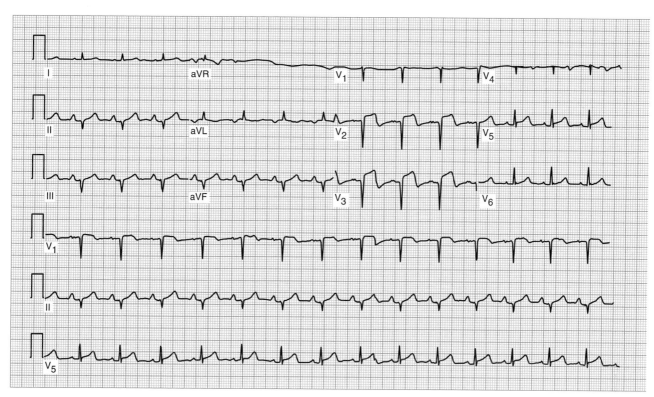

Figure 14-23

1. What is the underlying rhythm?

   Sinus at 86 bpm.

2. What are the acute changes?

   rS in leads II, III, and aVF. There are Qs with ST ↑ in V_2–V_4; ST ↑ V_5 and perhaps V_6.

3. What is your interpretation?

   Sinus at 86 bpm a current of injury pattern as with anteroseptal wall MI.

4. What can happen next?

   Observe for further conduction problems, extension of injury, ventricular arrhythmias, and s/s of CHF.

CHAPTER 15 ELECTRONIC PACEMAKERS

Matching

1.	H	8.	D	15.	L
2.	P	9.	B	16.	R
3.	J	10.	T	17.	O
4.	N	11.	V	18.	G
5.	K	12.	U	19.	A
6.	E	13.	Q	20.	M
7.	C	14.	F	21.	I

ECG Rhythm Identification Practice

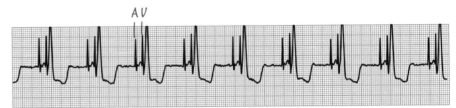

Figure 15-13

QRS duration	0.20 sec
QT interval	0.44 sec
Ventricular rate/rhythm	60 bpm/regular
Atrial rate/rhythm	60 bpm/regular
PR interval	None noted
Identification	Dual-chamber pacer at 60 bpm
Symptoms	None noted
Treatment	Be supportive

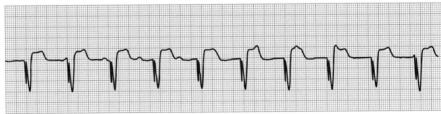

Figure 15-14

QRS duration	0.16 sec
QT interval	0.42 sec
Ventricular rate/rhythm	70 bpm/regular
Atrial rate/rhythm	UTD
PR interval	UTD
Identification	Ventricular pacer at 70 bpm; unable to determine if this is asynchronous (fixed-rate) or demand firing constantly since there are no intrinsic wave forms
Symptoms	Probably none
Treatment	Be supportive

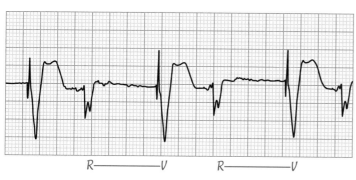

Figure 15-15

QRS duration	0.16 sec
QT interval	0.40 sec
Ventricular rate/rhythm	72 bpm/regular
Atrial rate/rhythm	UTD
PR interval	UTD
Identification	Vent demand pacer at 72 bpm; RV consistent
Symptoms	Probably none
Treatment	Be supportive

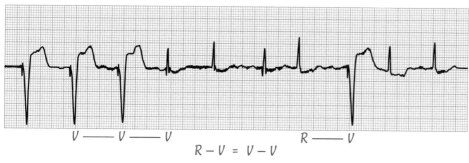

Figure 15-16

QRS duration	Intrinsic 0.04 sec; pacer 0.16 sec
QT interval	UTD QT interval pacer 0.44 sec
Ventricular rate/rhythm	Pacer at 75 bpm, a-fib at 75–110 bpm
Atrial rate/rhythm	None
PR interval	None
Identification	Vent demand pacer at 75 bpm with a-fib at 75–110 bpm; possible pacer artifacts fused with first and third QRS of a-fib-at that point the pacer is isorhythmic and there is no problem
Symptoms	None noted
Treatment	Be supportive

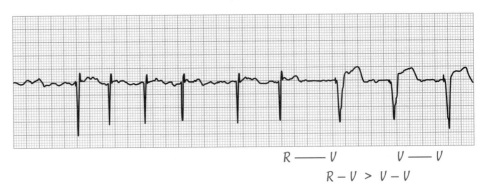

Figure 15-17

QRS duration	Intrinsic 0.08 sec; pacer 0.16 sec
QT interval	UTD pacer 0.44 sec
Ventricular rate/rhythm	75–125 bpm→75 bpm/regular
Atrial rate/rhythm	UTD
PR interval	UTD
Identification	A-fib at 75–125 bpm; vent demand pacer at 75 bpm; RV > VV (0.08 sec); ? hysteresis
Symptoms	Probably none
Treatment	Be supportive

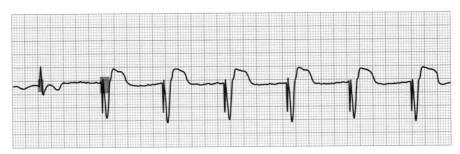

Figure 15-18

QRS duration	Intrinsic 0.08 sec; pacer 0.16 sec
QT interval	0.10 sec pacer; 0.44 sec
Ventricular rate/rhythm	Pacer at 61 bpm
Atrial rate/rhythm	UTD
PR interval	UTD
Identification	A-fib at 75–125 bpm; vent demand pacer at 61 bpm; RV = VV
Symptoms	Probably none
Treatment	Be supportive

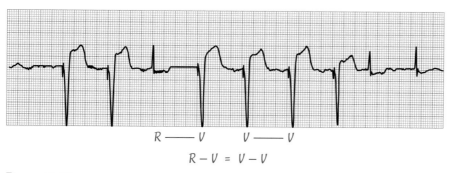

$$R \longrightarrow V \qquad V \longrightarrow V$$
$$R - V = V - V$$

Figure 15-19

QRS duration	Intrinsic 0.08 sec; pacer 0.16 sec
QT interval	UTD pacer; 0.44 sec
Identification	A-fib at 71 bpm; vent demand pacer at 75 bpm; RV = VV
Ventricular rate/rhythm	75–125 at bpm→75 bpm/regular
Atrial rate/rhythm	UTD
PR interval	UTD
Symptoms	Probably none
Treatment	Be supportive

PVC

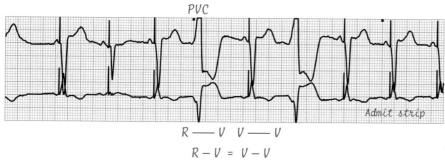

Admit strip

$$R \longrightarrow V \quad V \longrightarrow V$$
$$R - V = V - V$$

Figure 15-20

QRS duration	Pacer 0.16 sec
QT interval	Pacer 0.44 sec
Ventricular rate/rhythm	75 bpm/regular
Atrial rate/rhythm	75 bpm/regular
PR interval	UTD
Identification	Demand pacer 75 bpm with freq u/f PVCs; escape interval is OK
Symptoms	Probably none
Treatment	Be supportive

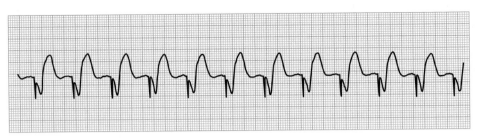

Figure 15-21

QRS duration	0.16 sec
QT interval	0.44 sec
Ventricular rate/rhythm	86 bpm/regular
Atrial rate/rhythm	UTD
PR interval	UTD
Identification	Vent pacer at 86 bpm; VV consistent
Symptoms	Probably none
Treatment	Be supportive

R ——— V

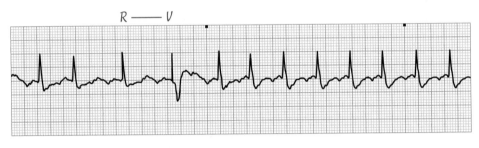

Figure 15-22

QRS duration	0.10 sec; pacer 0.16 sec
QT interval	Pacer 0.44 sec
Ventricular rate/rhythm	75–110 bpm
Atrial rate/rhythm	UTD (atrial flutter)
PR interval	UTD
Identification	Atrial flutter at 75–110 bpm; vent demand pacer
Symptoms	Probably none
Treatment	Be supportive

Paired PVC   V-Tach

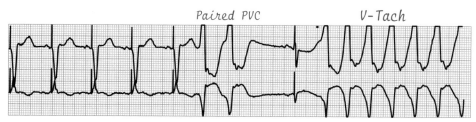

Figure 15-23

QRS duration	Pacer 0.16 sec
QT interval	Pacer 0.44 sec
Ventricular rate/rhythm	75 bpm/regular→150 bpm
Atrial rate/rhythm	75 bpm/regular
PR interval	n/a
Identification	Demand pacer at 75 bpm; paired PVCs (? R on T)→one paced beat→vent tach at 150 bpm
Symptoms	Associated with v-tach
Treatment	Rx the ventricular tachycardia; if by chance the patient is conscious and with a pulse at this rate, consider sedation and synchronized cardiover- sion; if pulseless, immediate defibrillation

CHAPTER 16 GENERAL REVIEW AND ASSESSMENT EXERCISES

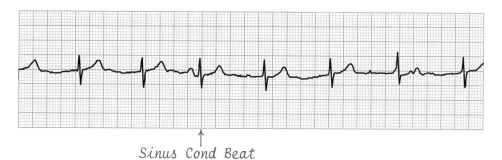

↑
Sinus Cond Beat

Figure 16-1

QRS duration	0.08 sec
QT interval	0.40 sec
Ventricular rate/rhythm	67 bpm/regular
Atrial rate/rhythm	100 bpm/regular
PR interval	None noted
Identification	Sinus rate at 100 bpm, complete AV block with accelerated junctional rhythm at 67 bpm; there is one sinus-conducted beat
Symptoms	? meds/med Hx, ? dizziness, s/s of hypoperfusion
Treatment	Stand by for TCP, fluids, and ? pressor for perfusion

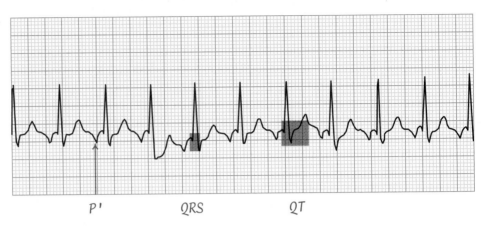

Figure 16-2

QRS duration	0.10 sec
QT interval	0.24 sec
Ventricular rate/rhythm	110 bpm/regular
Atrial rate/rhythm	110 bpm/regular
PR interval	0.12 sec
Identification	Junctional tachycardia vent rate at 110 bpm
Symptoms	? dizziness, postural hypotension
Treatment	Assess for s/s of ↓ perfusion; consider what happened to the sinus node

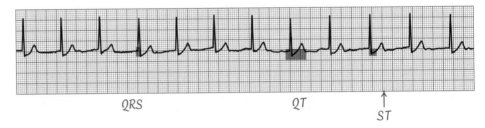

Figure 16-3

QRS duration	0.04 sec
QT interval	0.24 sec
Ventricular rate/rhythm	75 bpm/regular
Atrial rate/rhythm	UTD
PR interval	UTD
Identification	Accelerated junctional rhythm at 75 bpm
Symptoms	Probably none
Treatment	? meds/med Hx; consider what happened to the sinus node

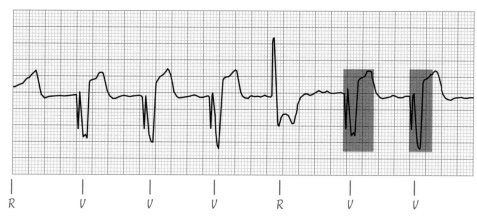

Figure 16-4

QRS duration	0.16 sec
QT interval	0.40 sec
Ventricular rate/rhythm	Pacer at 75 bpm (except for event)
Atrial rate/rhythm	UTD
PR interval	None noted
Identification	Vent demand pacer, a PVC, at 75 bpm with probably an underlying a-fib; RV is about 0.04–0.06 sec longer than the VV
Symptoms	Probably none
Treatment	Be supportive

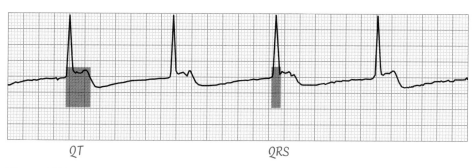

Figure 16-5

QRS duration	0.10 sec
QT interval	0.24–0.28 sec
Ventricular rate/rhythm	38 bpm/regular
Atrial rate/rhythm	UTD
PR interval	UTD
Identification	Junctional rhythm, vent rate at 46 bpm
Symptoms	? dizziness, postural hypotension, syncopal and/or near-syncopal episodes
Treatment	If hypotensive and hypoperfusing, may consider atropine, stand by for TCP, fluids, ? pressor for perfusion

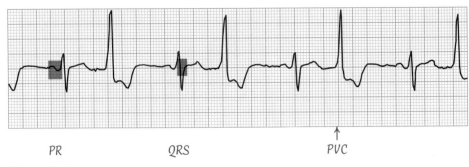

PR   QRS   PVC

Figure 16-6

QRS duration	0.12 sec
QT interval	0.36 sec
Ventricular rate/rhythm	Overall rate 70 bpm (bigeminy)
Atrial rate/rhythm	Visible sinus rate 35 bpm/regular
PR interval	0.16 sec
Identification	Sinus with ventricular bigeminy; overall rate at 70 bpm; sinus-induced QRS 0.12 sec; rS pattern
Symptoms	Probably none with an adequate overall vent rate; however, assess electrolytes, meds Hx, particularly digitalis
Treatment	? meds/med Hx; be supportive; multiple lead ECG to identify an intraventricular conduction defect

↓ PVC

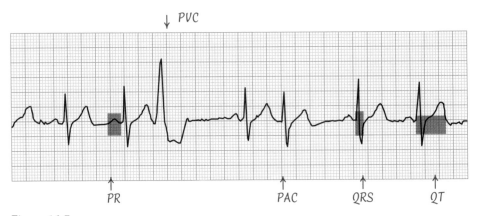

PR   PAC   QRS   QT

Figure 16-7

QRS duration	0.10 sec
QT interval	0.44 sec
Ventricular rate/rhythm	67 bpm/regular
Atrial rate/rhythm	67 bpm/regular
PR interval	0.16 sec
Identification	Sinus at 67 bpm with an R on T PVC and a PAC
Symptoms	Assess for s/s of ACS
Treatment	Rx for pain if present; if PVCs persist, or increase in frequency and/or duration, consider antiarrhythmics

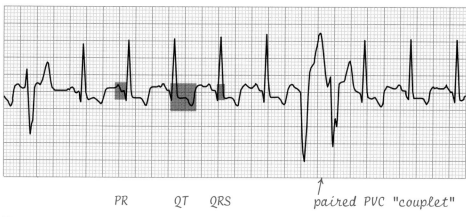

PR   QT   QRS   paired PVC "couplet"

Figure 16-8

QRS duration   0.10 sec
QT interval   0.44 sec
Ventricular rate/rhythm 100 bpm/regular
Atrial rate/rhythm   100 bpm/regular
PR interval   0.12–0.16 sec
Identification   Sinus at 100 bpm with frequent PVCs, R on T paired PVCs, Q waves, 2
                         mm ST ↓ and ↓ T waves
Symptoms   Assess for s/s of ACS
Treatment   Rx for pain if present; if PVCs persist, or increase in frequency and/or
                         duration, consider antiarrhythmics

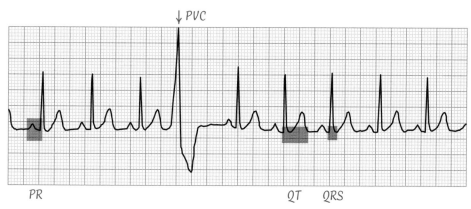

↓ PVC

PR   QT   QRS

Figure 16-9

QRS duration   0.08 sec
QT interval   0.32 sec
Ventricular rate/rhythm 100 bpm/regular
Atrial rate/rhythm   100 bpm/regular
PR interval   0.16 sec
Identification   Sinus at 100 bpm with a PVC
Symptoms   Assess for s/s of ACS
Treatment   Rx for pain if present; if PVCs persist, or increase in frequency and/or
                         duration, consider antiarrhythmics

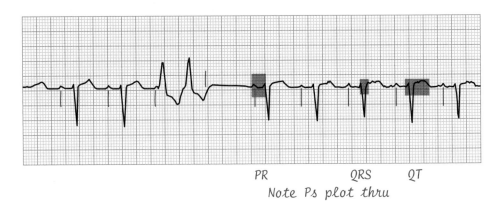

PR   QRS   QT

Note Ps plot thru

Figure 16-10

QRS duration	0.08 sec
QT interval	0.32 sec
Ventricular rate/rhythm	88 bpm/regular
Atrial rate/rhythm	88 bpm/regular
PR interval	0.16 sec
Identification	Sinus at 88 bpm with end-diastolic paired PVCs (note that the P waves plot through the event)
Symptoms	Assess for s/s of ACS
Treatment	Rx for pain if present; if PVCs persist, or increase in frequency and/or duration, consider antiarrhythmics

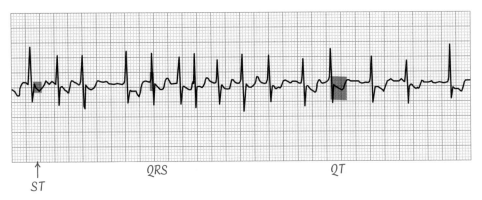

QRS   QT

↑
ST

Figure 16-11

QRS duration	0.06 sec
QT interval	0.32 sec
Ventricular rate/rhythm	100–296 bpm
Atrial rate/rhythm	UTD
PR interval	UTD
Identification	A-fib at 100–296 bpm with 2–3 mm ST ↓
Symptoms	Assess if this is new onset or recurrent; assess med Hx for antico-agulants, beta-blockers; assess breath sounds, s/s edema; assess for syncopal or near-syncopal episodes
Treatment	If tachycardia persists and patient is symptomatic, may consider beta-blockers if not already prescribed; if new onset and the patient is unstable consider sedation, synchronized cardioversion; if this is a long-term/recurrent problem the patient may be considered for ablation procedures

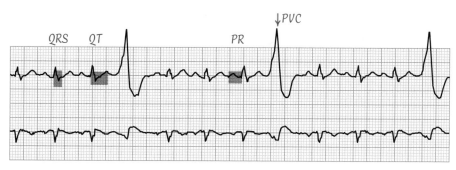

Figure 16-12

QRS duration	0.10 sec
QT interval	0.28 sec
Ventricular rate/rhythm	125 bpm/regular
Atrial rate/rhythm	125 bpm/regular
PR interval	0.16 sec
Identification	Sinus at 125 bpm with freq u/f PVCs (quadrageminy-every fourth beat is a PVC)
Symptoms	Assess for s/s of ACS; assess med Hx for digitalis or excessive use of caffeine
Treatment	Rx for pain if present; if PVCs persist, or increase in frequency and/or duration, consider antiarrhythmics

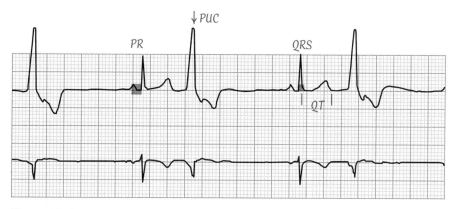

Figure 16-13

QRS duration	0.08 sec
QT interval	0.40 sec
Ventricular rate/rhythm	80 bpm/bigeminal
Atrial rate/rhythm	40 bpm/regular (P wave does not plot through)
PR interval	0.16 sec
Identification	Sinus at 40 bpm with bigeminal PVCs
Symptoms	Assess for s/s of ACS; assess med Hx for digitalis
Treatment	Rx for pain, reassess; if bradycardia persists, consider atropine, fluids, and pressor for perfusion; stand by for pacing

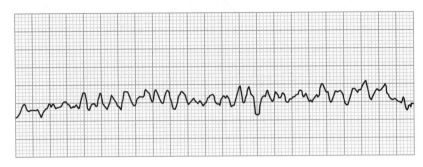

Figure 16-14

QRS duration	UTD
QT interval	UTD
Ventricular rate/rhythm	UTD
Atrial rate/rhythm	UTD
PR interval	UTD
Identification	Ventricular fibrillation confirm no pulse
Symptoms	Confirm no pulse
Treatment	Begin immediate defibrillation

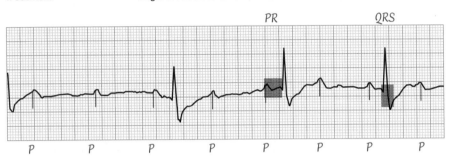

Figure 16-15

QRS duration	0.16 sec
QT interval	0.48 sec
Ventricular rate/rhythm	18–43 bpm
Atrial rate/rhythm	70 bpm/regular
PR interval	0.24 sec and consistent
Identification	Sinus at 70 bpm with 2° AV block, QRS 0.16 sec; PR after missed beat consistent
Symptoms	Associated with bradycardia; assess for s/s ACS
Treatment	Assess multiple lead ECG, especially V_{4R} for acute changes; stand by for pacing

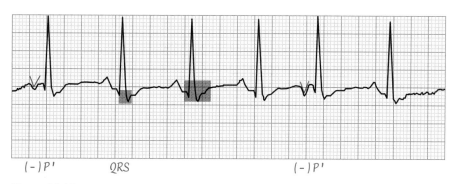

(-)P'   QRS   (-)P'

Figure 16-16

QRS duration	0.16 sec
QT interval	0.38 sec
Ventricular rate/rhythm	75 bpm/regular
Atrial rate/rhythm	75 bpm/regular
PR interval	0.20 sec
Identification	Sinus at 75 bpm with a premature junctional complex (PJC)
Symptoms	Probably none
Treatment	? meds/med Hx

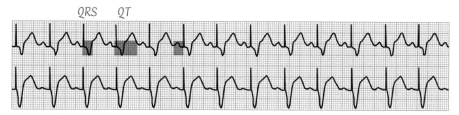

Figure 16-17

QRS duration	0.16 sec
QT interval	0.40 sec
Ventricular rate/rhythm	100 bpm/regular
Atrial rate/rhythm	100 bpm/regular
PR interval	0.24 sec and consistent
Identification	Ventricular paced rhythm ↓ 100 bpm; VV interval consistent; unable to determine if this is asynchronous (fixed-rate) or demand firing constantly since there are no intrinsic wave forms
Symptoms	Probably none
Treatment	Be supportive

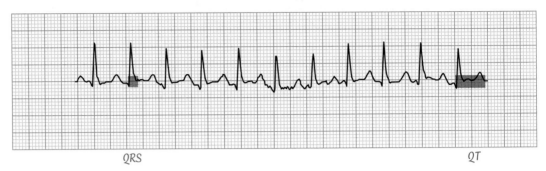

QRS   QT

Figure 16-18

QRS duration	0.10 sec
QT interval	0.38 sec
Ventricular rate/rhythm	136 bpm/regular
Atrial rate/rhythm	UTD
PR interval	UTD
Identification	Atrial tachycardia; don't mistake the T waves for P waves; there is the distortion between some of the QRS complexes that may be patient movement or artifact; there is a distortion in the descending arm of the R wave that may be flutter waves
Symptoms	? hypotension and/or hypoperfusion; assess for syncopal and/or near-syncopal episodes
Treatment	May try vagal maneuvers to slow ventricular response and try to "uncover" the atrial flutter

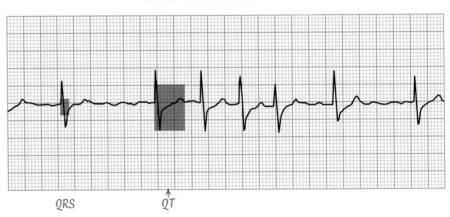

QRS   QT

Figure 16-19

QRS duration	0.10 sec
QT interval	0.40 sec
Ventricular rate/rhythm	50–150 bpm
Atrial rate/rhythm	UTD
PR interval	UTD
Identification	A-fib vent rate range ?50–150 bpm; 2 mm ST depression; don't call this "controlled"-one ECG does not tell you if this is appropriate for the patient who may be on several medications, or not
Symptoms	Probably none unless related to meds
Treatment	? meds/med Hx, especially for digitalis

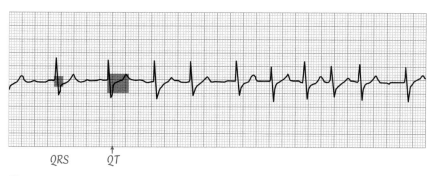

QRS   QT

Figure 16-20

QRS duration	0.10 sec
QT interval	0.40 sec
Ventricular rate/rhythm	75–150 bpm
Atrial rate/rhythm	UTD
PR interval	UTD
Identification	A-fib vent rate range at 75–150 bpm; 2 mm ST depression
Symptoms	? new onset or recurrence
Treatment	? meds/med Hx, especially for digitalis; unless the ventricular rate increases and persists as a tachycardia, observe and be supportive

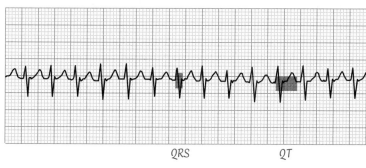

QRS   QT

Figure 16-21

QRS duration	0.06 sec
QT interval	0.24 sec
Ventricular rate/rhythm	188 bpm/regular
Atrial rate/rhythm	UTD
PR interval	UTD
Identification	SVT at 188 bpm—P' peeking out at the end of some of the QRS complexes
Symptoms	? ALOC, ? SOB, anxiety, feelings of palpitations, syncopal or near-syncopal episodes
Treatment	If the patient is stable, attempt vagal maneuvers, pharmacologic intervention; if unstable, sedate and perform synchronized cardioversion

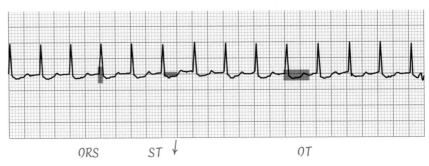

Figure 16-22

QRS duration	0.04 sec
QT interval	0.28 sec
Ventricular rate/rhythm	150 bpm/regular
Atrial rate/rhythm	UTD
PR interval	UTD
Identification	Atrial tachycardia, perhaps atrial flutter (note the distortion in the descending arm of the R wave—may be underlying atrial flutter wave; ventricular rhythm is regular)
Symptoms	? hypotension and/or hypoperfusion; assess for syncopal and/or near-syncopal episodes
Treatment	Multiple lead ECG to confirm the rhythm; may try vagal maneuvers to slow ventricular response and try to "uncover" the atrial flutter

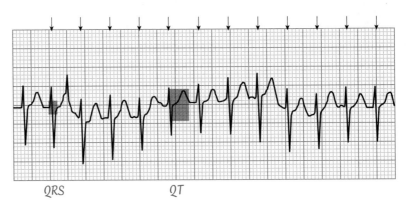

Figure 16-23

QRS duration	0.08 sec
QT interval	0.28 sec
Ventricular rate/rhythm	188 bpm/regular
Atrial rate/rhythm	UTD
PR interval	UTD
Identification	SVT at 188 bpm (note arrows in top margin; these are the "synch" markings as preparations were made for synchronized cardioversion)
Symptoms	This patient presented with ALOC, slow to respond
Treatment	Synchronized cardioversion was successful

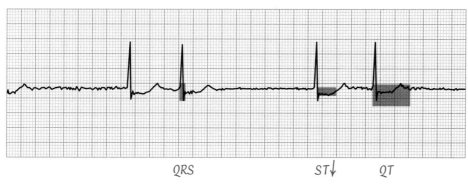

QRS   ST↓   QT

Figure 16-24

QRS duration	0.10 sec
QT interval	0.52 sec
Ventricular rate/rhythm	31–86 bpm
Atrial rate/rhythm	UTD
PR interval	UTD
Identification	A-fib at 31–86 bpm with 2 mm ST depression; a-fib perhaps with Wenckebach periodicity; needs a longer tracing
Symptoms	? dizziness, hypotension, ALOC
Treatment	? med Hx, digitalis; consider fluids, pacing, possibly a pressor for perfusion.

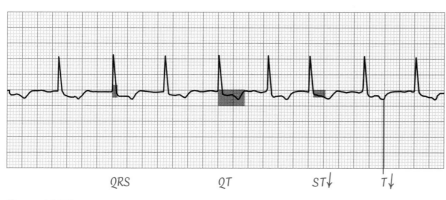

QRS   QT   ST↓   T↓

Figure 16-25

QRS duration	0.08 sec
QT interval	0.36 sec
Ventricular rate/rhythm	86–100 bpm
Atrial rate/rhythm	UTD
PR interval	UTD
Identification	A-fib at 86–100 bpm with 2 mm ST depression and inverted T waves
Symptoms	Probably none at this rate; ? med Hx, digitalis
Treatment	This a-fib is approaching regularity: if so, consider impending AV block because of dig ?; stand by for pacing; don't call this "controlled"-atrial fibrillation should not have a regular ventricular rhythm

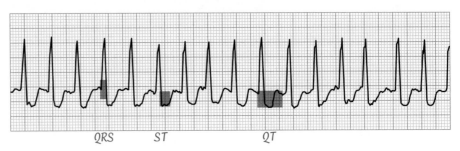

Figure 16-26

QRS duration	0.10 sec
QT interval	UTD
Ventricular rate/rhythm	136–166 bpm
Atrial rate/rhythm	UTD
PR interval	UTD
Identification	A-fib vent rate range at 136–166 bpm with 5 mm ST depression
Symptoms	? hypotension and/or hypoperfusion; assess for syncopal and/or near-syncopal episodes; ? if new onset or recurrence; assess electrolytes
Treatment	May try vagal maneuvers to slow ventricular response; consider adenosine, calcium channel blocker if new onset; if unstable, sedation, synchronized cardioversion

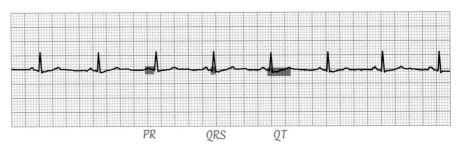

Figure 16-27

QRS duration	0.06 sec
QT interval	0.32 sec
Ventricular rate/rhythm	67 bpm/regular
Atrial rate/rhythm	67 bpm/regular
PR interval	0.16 sec
Identification	Sinus rhythm vent rate at 67 bpm
Symptoms	Probably none
Treatment	Be supportive

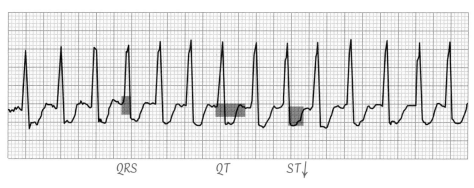

Figure 16-28

QRS duration	0.10 sec
QT interval	UTD
Ventricular rate/rhythm	150–188 bpm
Atrial rate/rhythm	UTD
PR interval	UTD
Identification	A-fib vent rate range at 150–188 bpm with 4 mm ST ↓
Symptoms	? hypotension and/or hypoperfusion; assess for syncopal and/or near-syncopal episodes; ? if new onset or recurrence
Treatment	May try vagal maneuvers to slow ventricular response; assess electrolytes; consider adenosine, calcium channel blockers; if unstable, consider sedation and synchronized cardioversion

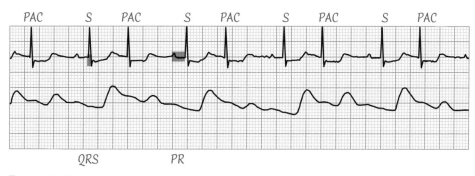

Figure 16-29

QRS duration	0.06 sec
QT interval	0.40 sec
Ventricular rate/rhythm	92 bpm/bigeminal
Atrial rate/rhythm	Visible sinus at 46 bpm
PR interval	Sinus PR 0.16 sec
Identification	Sinus with atrial bigeminy; overall rate at 92 bpm and bigeminal; there is 2 mm horizontal ST depression; below the ECG is a tracing from the arterial line-note the diminished systolic pressure with the ectopic
Symptoms	Perhaps none; assess breath sounds; assess for s/s of CHF; although you have to wonder why the patient has an artery line in, you don't know the underlying condition and/or diagnosis
Treatment	? meds/med Hx; be supportive; be alert for onset of SVT or a-fib or a-flutter

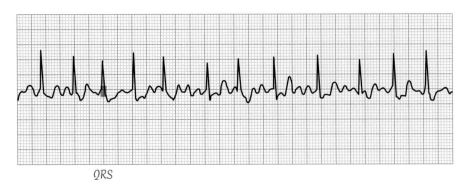

QRS

Figure 16-30

QRS duration	0.04 sec
QT interval	UTD
Ventricular rate/rhythm	100–150 bpm/irregular
Atrial rate/rhythm	UTD
PR interval	UTD
Identification	A-fib vent rate range at 100–150 bpm with 1–2 mm ST depression
Symptoms	? hypotension and/or hypoperfusion; assess for syncopal and/or near-syncopal episodes;? if new onset or recurrence
Treatment	May try vagal maneuvers to slow ventricular response; consider adenosine, calcium channel blocker if new onset; if unstable, consider synchronized cardioversion

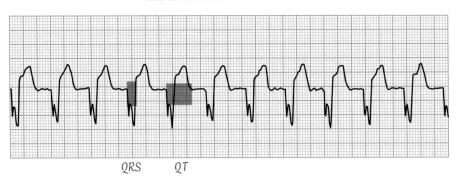

QRS   QT

Figure 16-31

QRS duration	0.12 sec
QT interval	0.40 sec
Ventricular rate/rhythm	100 bpm/regular; ? ventricular pacer
Atrial rate/rhythm	UTD
PR interval	UTD
Identification	Ventricular pacer at 100 bpm (confirmed on patient assessment); VV intervals are consistent
Symptoms	Probably none related to the pacer
Treatment	Be supportive

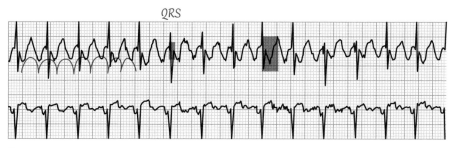

Figure 16-32

QRS duration	0.06 sec
QT interval	0.48 sec
Ventricular rate/rhythm	167 bpm/regular
Atrial rate/rhythm	Flutter waves at 300 bpm/regular
PR interval	UTD
Identification	Atrial flutter ventricular rate at 167 bpm/regular
Symptoms	? hypotension and/or hypoperfusion; assess for syncopal and/or near-syncopal episodes
Treatment	Vagal maneuvers to slow ventricular response; calcium channel blockers; if unstable, consider sedation and perform synchronized cardioversion

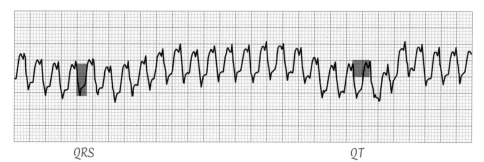

Figure 16-33

QRS duration	0.16 sec
QT interval	0.20 sec
Ventricular rate/rhythm	250 bpm/regular
Atrial rate/rhythm	UTD
PR interval	UTD
Identification	Sustained ventricular tachycardia at 250 bpm
Symptoms	Confirm if patient has a pulse; if conscious, patient is probably unstable at this rate
Treatment	If conscious with a pulse, consider sedation and synchronized cardioversion; if pulseless, begin immediate defibrillation

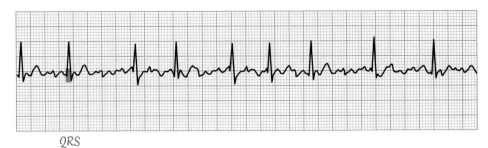

QRS

Figure 16-34

QRS duration	0.08 sec
QT interval	UTD
Ventricular rate/rhythm	67–125 bpm/irregular
Atrial rate/rhythm	UTD
PR interval	UTD
Identification	A-fib vent rate range at 67–125 bpm/irregular
Symptoms	Probably none with this rate; ? digitalis Hx
Treatment	? meds/med Hx; this a-fib may be controlled with meds for this patient; be alert for s/s of pulmonary embolism

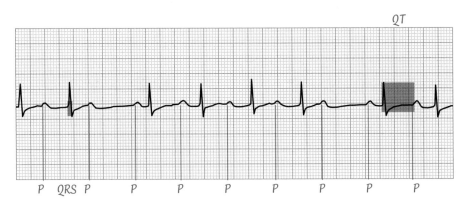

QT

P   QRS P   P   P   P   P   P   P   P

Figure 16-35

QRS duration	0.08 sec
QT interval	0.36 sec
Ventricular rate/rhythm	55–100 bpm/irregular
Atrial rate/rhythm	100 bpm/regular
PR interval	0.24, 0.32, 0.40 sec
Identification	Sinus at 100 bpm; 2° AV block, probably Type I Wenckebach (QRS 0.08 sec); PR interval progressively longer; PR after the missed QRS is consistent
Symptoms	Probably none
Treatment	? meds/med Hx

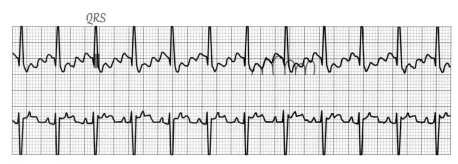

Figure 16-36

QRS duration	0.10 sec
QT interval	UTD
Ventricular rate/rhythm	125 bpm/regular
Atrial rate/rhythm	Flutter waves at 300 bpm
PR interval	UTD
Identification	Atrial flutter, vent rate at 125 bpm
Symptoms	? hypotension and/or hypoperfusion; assess for syncopal and/or near-syncopal episodes
Treatment	Vagal maneuvers to slow ventricular response; may not require pharmacologic intervention with this ventricular response

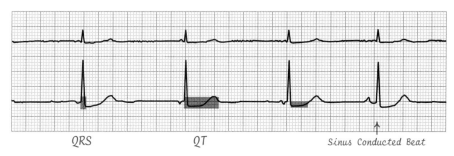

Figure 16-37

QRS duration	0.08 sec
QT interval	0.48 sec
Ventricular rate/rhythm	43–67 bpm/irregular
Atrial rate/rhythm	Sinus at 40 bpm, junction at 42 bpm
PR interval	One sinus beat PR 0.16 sec, junctional P'R 0.10 sec
Identification	The QRS complexes are narrow and consistent so the impulse originates above the ventricles; there is one clearly identified sinus beat at the far right; it is difficult with only these two leads to clearly identify other P waves, but the QRSs are regular and probably junctional in origin; although there is one sinus conducted beat, this is probably a junctional escape rhythm at 42 bpm; there is 2 mm ST segment depression
Symptoms	? dizziness, postural hypotension, syncopal and/or near-syncopal episodes
Treatment	If hypotensive and hypoperfusing, consider fluids, pacer, may consider pressor for perfusion consider what has happened to the sinus node

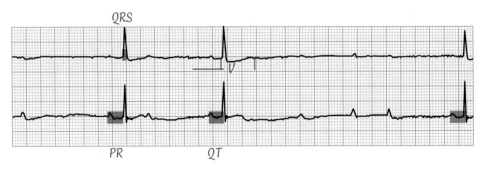

Figure 16-38

QRS duration	0.08 sec
QT interval	0.40 sec
Ventricular rate/rhythm	17–43 bpm/irregular
Atrial rate/rhythm	Sinus P at 50–125 bpm/irregular
PR interval	0.16 sec
Identification	Again, we only have two leads; sinus P-wave rate varies from 50 to 125 bpm; it looks like a nonconducted PAC in the bottom strip, after the first QRS complex; there are only two consistent PR intervals-then an RR interval of 3.2 sec
Symptoms	? dizziness, certainly postural hypotension, syncopal and/or near-syncopal episodes
Treatment	Patient needs to be paced; 12-lead ECG; consider fluids, consider pressor to support perfusion

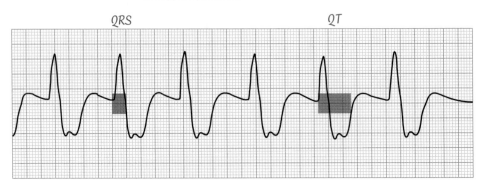

Figure 16-39

QRS duration	0.16–0.20 sec
QT interval	0.44 sec
Ventricular rate/rhythm	67 bpm/regular
Atrial rate/rhythm	UTD
PR interval	UTD
Identification	Accelerated vent rhythm rate at 55 bpm
Symptoms	? pulse; if pulse present, ALOC
Treatment	If pulseless, CPR; IV epinephrine/atropine, oxygenate, ventilate, intubate; if pulse is present, consider fluids; consider pacing

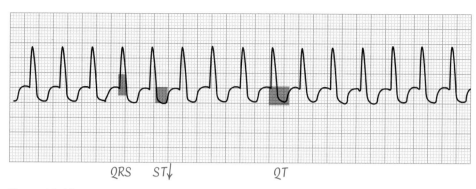

QRS   ST↓   QT

Figure 16-40

QRS duration	0.10 sec
QT interval	UTD
Ventricular rate/rhythm	150 bpm/regular
Atrial rate/rhythm	UTD
PR interval	UTD
Identification	Atrial tach at 150 bpm with 5 mm ST segment depression
Symptoms	? hypotension and/or hypoperfusion; assess for syncopal and/or near-syncopal episodes; ? new onset or recurrence
Treatment	Vagal maneuvers to slow ventricular response and perhaps unmask atrial flutter; may require pharmacologic intervention

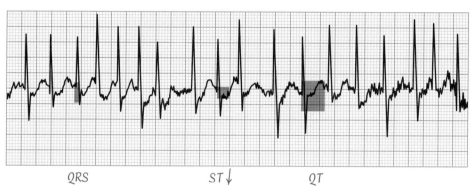

QRS   ST↓   QT

Figure 16-41

QRS duration	0.06 sec
QT interval	0.32 sec
Ventricular rate/rhythm	125–296 bpm/irregular
Atrial rate/rhythm	UTD
PR interval	UTD
Identification	A-fib with vent rate range at 125–296 bpm
Symptoms	? hypotension and/or hypoperfusion; assess for syncopal and/or near-syncopal episodes; ? if new onset or recurrence
Treatment	Assess electrolytes, med Hx, ? caffeine excess; may try vagal maneuvers to slow ventricular response; consider pharmacologic cardioversion if new onset; if unstable, consider synchronized cardioversion

Normal Ranges and Variations in the Adult 12-Lead Electrocardiogram

The following table can serve as a guide to the morphology of the wave forms and segments as reflected on the 12-lead ECG. It is one more tool to be used as a baseline as serial tracings are assessed in comparison. The ECG must be assessed and judged in the context of patient history and presentation.

Lead	P	Q	R	S	ST	T
I	Upright	< 0.04 sec < 25% of the R wave	Upright deflection of the QRS complex	< R or none	Isoelectric; may vary 1.0 mm (↑)	Upright
II	Upright	Small or none	Dominant with normal axis	< R or none with normal axis	Isoelectric; may vary 1.0 mm (↑) or (↓)	Upright
III	(+) or (−) flat or diphasic depending on frontal plane axis	Small or none 0.04–0.05 sec or >33% of the R wave is abnormal depending on frontal plane axis	None to dominant depending on frontal plane axis	None to dominant depending on frontal plane axis	Isoelectric; may vary 1.0 mm (↑) or (↓)	Upright, flat, diphasic, or inverted depending on frontal plane axis
aVR	Inverted	Small, none, or large	Small or none depending on frontal plane axis	Dominant; may appear as a QS configuration	Isoelectric	Inverted
aVL	Upright, flat, diphasic, or inverted depending on frontal plane axis	Small or none	Small or dominant depending on frontal plane axis	None to dominant, depending on frontal plane axis	Usually isoelectric; may vary from +1.0 to 0.5 mm	Upright, flat, diphasic, or inverted depending on frontal plane axis
aVF	Upright	Small or none	Small or none or dominant depending on frontal plane axis	None to dominant depending on frontal plane axis	Usually isoelectric; may vary from +1.0 to 0.5 mm	Upright, flat, diphasic or inverted depending on frontal plane axis
V₁	Flat or diphasic	None; may be a QS	Less than SV₁, or none (QS) Small R' may be present with incomplete RBBB	Dominant; may be a QS	0 to (+)1 mm	Upright, less commonly flat, diphasic, or inverted
V₂	Low amplitude or diphasic	None;	Less than SV₂₁ Small R' may be present with incomplete RBBB	Dominant	0 to (+)1 mm	Upright, less commonly flat, diphasic
V₃	Upright/low amplitude	none with R < S	R < S or R > S or R = S is the transitional complex	S > R or S < R or R = S	0 to (+)3 mm	Upright
V₄	Upright/low amplitude	Small or none	R > S	S < R	Usually isoelectric; (+)1.0 to 0.5 mm	Upright
V₅	Upright	Small or none	Dominant; < 26 mm	S < S₍V4₎	Usually isoelectric; (+)1.0 to 0.5 mm	Upright
V₆	Upright	Small or none	Dominant; < 26 mm	S < S₍V4₎	Usually isoelectric; (+)1.0 to 0.5 mm	Upright

Update courtesy Marshall Burns, MD, cardiologist and associate professor of medicine, University of Arizona Medical School, Phoenix Branch.

Emergency Cardiac Care Guidelines

The following information is derived primarily from the Emergency Cardiac Care Guidelines based on the American Heart Association's *2008 Handbook of Emergency Cardiovascular Care for Health Care Providers*. These are guidelines for possible interventions for the patient who presents with cardiac compromise. Regardless of the clinical setting, the provider must be aware of protocols, standards, and guidelines that affect and govern treatment modalities. Now, more than ever, changes in treatment, drugs, and drug dosages occur often, requiring frequent review of literature and communications among health care professionals.

At this printing, CPR has taken on several approaches. CPR refers to AHA standards and guidelines but is not limited to continuous chest compression CPR or minimally interrupted cardiac resuscitation (MICR), also referred to as cardiocerebral resuscitation, which is a new approach to out-of-hospital cardiac arrest for emergency medical services (EMS). The prudent practitioner will be ever vigilant to changing standards and guidelines in these procedures.

This appendix is not meant to be prescriptive, merely a baseline for assessment and a memory-jogger for the more common approaches to patient care. It is the responsibility of the provider to keep current with knowledge, care practices, and patient care standards and guidelines in a specific work environment.

Primary ABCD Survey

Survey Step	Assessment	Management
Airway	Patent?	If unresponsive, open the airway with head tilt–chin lift. In the case of suspected trauma, use jaw thrust maneuver and immobilize the C-spine.
Breathing	Chest rise and fall.	Provide oxygen.
	Breath sounds.	If conscious and responsive, assess for adventitious sounds.
		If unresponsive and no chest movement, assist ventilation with BVM and oxygen.
Circulation	Pulse present.	Assess rate and quality; determine what is normal for the patient. Is the rate appropriate for the circumstances?
		If no pulse, begin chest compressions, allowing chest recoil and minimizing interruptions.
		IV access, usually 500 cc normal saline (NS).
Defibrillation	V-fib; pulseless.	Defibrillate.
	V-tach; pulseless.	Defibrillate.

Secondary ABCD Survey

Survey Step	Assessment	Management
Airway	Adequate, protected.	If unresponsive, remove any obstruction; insert OPA, NPA.
		Suction as necessary on withdrawal of the catheter.
Breathing	Assess breath sounds.	Assess for adventitious sounds.
		During resuscitation, once airway is confirmed and patent, do not pause in chest compressions.
		Assess with pulse oximetry and $ETCO_2$ detector.
		Provide one breath every 6–8 seconds.
Circulation	Assess heart rate, and ECG rhythm Assess vital signs.	IV access, usually 500 cc NS. Consider antiarrhythmic medications to correct heart rate and rhythm, and reperfuse the patient. Assess pulse oximetry and blood glucose.
Differential Dx	Assess Hs and Ts.	Hs = hypovolemia, hypoxia, hydrogen ion (acidosis), hypokalemia, hyperkalemia, hypoglycemia, hypothermia.
		Ts = toxins, tamponade, tension pneumothorax, thrombosis (pulmonary or cardiac), trauma, medication or drug overdose; illegals and OTC.
		Assess for reversible causes.
		Assess blood glucose.
Disability	Assess mental status.	
	Pupillary response.	
	Glasgow Coma Scale.	
	Stroke screen.	
Expose/Examine	Assess for injuries.	Control bleeding; immobilize deformities.
	Inspect and palpate for soft tissue injuries, bleeding, and obvious deformities.	
	Assess for pregnancy.	
Foley catheter	In hospital: vaginal and rectal exams.	In hospital: insert Foley catheter; sample to lab for analysis, drug screen; monitor output.
Nasogastric tube	Assess for abdominal distention from ventilation techniques or prior conditions such as toxic ingestion.	Insert nasogastric tube; consider Rx for poisoning or overdose.
	Assess for blood.	
History	Communication and documentation.	Communicate with family, friends, bystanders.

SAMPLE

- **S:** Signs and symptoms
- **A:** Allergies
- **M:** Medications
- **P:** Pertinent past history and pregnancy
- **L:** Last oral intake (or last ins and outs)
- **E:** Events leading up to (the emergency)

Narrow QRS Complex Bradycardia

Heart rate <60 bpm or a slow rate unusual for the patient.

▼

Assess for altered mental status, chest pain, syncopal and/or near-syncopal episodes; treatable causes.

▼

If perfusion is adequate, be supportive and vigilant for s/s hypotension/hypoperfusion.

▼

Assess and maintain the airway; apply supplemental oxygen; monitor vital signs to include pulse oximetry and blood glucose monitoring.

▼

Assess for hypotension and hypoperfusion.

▼

Prepare for transcutaneous or transvenous pacing.

▼

While awaiting the pacer, consider atropine for narrow QRS complex bradycardia.

Be aware of the risk for worsening ischemia and/or infarction.

▼

Consider pressors such as dopamine or epinephrine infusions.

▼

Pacing may support adequate rate but additional fluids and pressors may be needed to support perfusion.

Narrow QRS Complex Tachycardia

Includes sinus, atrial tachycardias;
atrial, SVT, and junctional tachycardia.

Assess for altered mental status, chest pain, syncopal and/or
near-syncopal episodes; assess for treatable causes.

▼

If perfusion is adequate, be supportive and vigilant.

▼

Assess and maintain the airway; use supplemental oxygen; monitor vital signs to include pulse
oximetry and blood glucose monitoring.

▼

Sinus tachycardia—assess for treatable cause.

▼

Junctional tachycardia—assess for treatable cause; assess for digitalis toxicity.

▼

Atrial tachycardia—flutter or fibrillation with rapid ventricular response.

▼

Is this new to the patient or is there history of recurrence?

▼

Attempt vagal maneuvers.

▼

If unsuccessful and vital signs are stable, consider calcium channel blocker.

▼

Consider beta-blockers.

▼

If unstable, hypotensive, and hypoperfusing,

▼

Consider sedation and prepare for synchronized cardioversion.

VENTRICULAR FIBRILLATION AND PULSELESS VENTRICULAR TACHYCARDIA

Assess responsiveness; ABCs—avoid hyperventilation.

Perform CPR until defibrillator becomes available: if unwitnessed, 2 full minutes.

Push hard, push fast, ensure chest recoil, minimize interruptions of compressions.

▼

Defibrillate at 360 J or biphasic equivalent.*

▼

Perform CPR for 2 minutes five cycles of 30:2.

▼

Intubate, oxygenate, ventilate.

Endotracheal intubation; laryngeal mask airway (LMA), Combitube, or gum elastic bougie.

▼

IV access 500 cc NS.

▼

Epinephrine or vasopressin IV bolus.

▼

Consider treatable causes.

▼

Defibrillate at 360 J or biphasic equivalent.*

*Manual biphasic use device-specific dose, typically 120 J (rectilinear) or 150 J (truncated) to 200 J. If unknown use 200 J; subsequent shocks: same or higher energy.

▼

Resume CPR.

With advanced airway in place, compress 100 bpm and ventilate 8–10 bpm or 1 every 6–8 sec.

▼

Defibrillate at 360 J or biphasic equivalent.

▼

With advanced airway in place, compress 100 bpm and ventilate 8–10 bpm or 1 every 6–8 sec.

▼

Amiodarone IV bolus; may repeat in 3–5 minutes or lidocaine IVP; q5–10 minutes or magnesium sulfate.

▼

Defibrillate at 360 J or biphasic equivalent.

▼

Continue with CPR–drug–defibrillate–CPR–drug–defibrillate.

Asystole

▼

Confirmed on more than one ECG lead; check lead attachment; check the gain on the monitor.

Do not defibrillate!

Assess responsiveness.

ABCs—avoid hyperventilation.

Perform CPR for 2 full minutes.

Push hard, push fast, ensure chest recoil, minimize interruptions of compressions.

▼

CPR 2 minutes five cycles of 30:2.*

▼

Intubate, oxygenate, ventilate, bag-valve-mask (BVM).

Endotracheal intubation; laryngeal mask airway (LMA), or Combitube.

▼

IV access 500 cc NS.

▼

Epinephrine 1:10,000 1.0 mg IVP; may repeat every 3–5 minutes
or vasopressin 40 units IV bolus.

▼

Consider treatable causes.

▼

Resume CPR.

With advanced airway in place, compress 100 bpm and ventilate 8–10 bpm or 1 every 6–8 sec.

▼

Consider atropine 1 mg IV/IO; may repeat every 3–5 minutes to a total of 3 mg
or Consider termination of efforts.

*CPR refers to AHA standards and guidelines but is not limited to continuous chest compression CPR or minimally interrupted cardiac resuscitation (MICR), also referred to as cardiocerebral resuscitation, which is a new approach to out-of-hospital cardiac arrest for emergency medical services (EMS).

ACUTE CORONARY SYNDROME

Asssess, monitor, and support ABCs, vital signs to include pulse oximetry and blood glucose.

Monitoring.

▼

Oxygen.

▼

Monitor and obtain a multiple lead ECG.

▼

Aspirin 325 mg (nonenteric coated) or four 81 mg children's chewable.

▼

Establish an IV 500 cc NS.

▼

Assess vital signs; rule out ingestion of sexual enhancement medications prescribed, borrowed or over-the-counter, herbals; illegals and recreationals.

▼

Nitroglycerin 0.4 mg SL; may repeat every 5 minutes to a total of 1.2 mg (3 doses).

▼

If ineffective, consider morphine sulfate 2 mg increments IV.

▼

Perform targeted history and physical exam.

▼

Review fibrinolytic therapy checklist—assess for contraindications.

▼

Obtain initial cardiac biomarkers, serum electrolyte levels, and coagulation studies.

▼

Consider chest radiograph.

STE 8 or new LBB STEMI	ST 9 or T wave 9	Nondiagnostic Low-Risk UA UA/NSTEMI
Consider: Beta-blockers* Heparin	Beta-blockers Nitroglycerin IV	If unstable, UA/NSTEMI. If stable, assess cardiac bio-markers, multiple lead ECG. Consider echocardiography.

*If patient is not hypotensive and hypoperfusing.

Fibrinolytic Criteria for AMI

Patient symptomatic for less than 6 or even possibly 12 hours.

Chest pain suggesting an MI.

ST segment elevation >1 mm in two or more contiguous leads, with new or presumably new LBBB, strongly suspicious for injury (BBB obscuring ST segment analysis).

Age <75 years (age >75 years, Class IIa).

Absolute Contraindications

History of hemorrhagic stroke or intracranial hemorrhage.

Known structural cerebral vascular lesion (e.g., AVM).

Known malignant intracranial neoplasm (primary or metastatic).

Ischemic stroke or CVA within 3 months, EXCEPT acute ischemic stroke within 3 hours.

Active internal bleeding (menses excluded).

Suspected aortic dissection.

Significant closed head trauma or facial trauma within 3 months.

Relative Contraindications

Uncontrolled severe hypertension (BP sys >180 or dia >110).

Hx of chronic, severe, or poorly controlled hypertension.

Hx of prior ischemic CVA >3 months, dementia, or known intracranial pathology not covered in contraindications.

Current use of anticoagulants—the higher the INR, the higher the risk of bleeding.

Traumatic or prolonged (>10 minutes) CPR **or** major surgery (<3 weeks).

Noncompressible vascular punctures.

Pregnancy.

Recent (2–4 weeks) internal bleeding **or** active peptic ulcer disease.

For streptokinase/anistreplase—prior allergic reaction **or** prior exposure (more than 5 days ago).

Suspected Stroke: EMS Assessment and Actions

Support ABCs, begin oxygen.

Perform prehospital stroke assessment.

Establish time patient last known to be normal.

Transport and consider triage to stroke center.

Consider bringing a witness, family member, or caregiver.

Alert hospital.

Check glucose.

Immediate General Assessment and Stabilization

Assess ABCs, vital signs.

Provide oxygen if hypoxemic.

Obtain IV access, obtain blood samples (CBC, electrolytes, coagulation studies).

Check glucose; treat if indicated.

Perform general neurological screening assessment.

Activate stroke team, neurologist, radiologist, CT technician.

Order urgent noncontrast CT scan.

Obtain 12-lead ECG; check for arrhythmias.

Immediate Neurological Assessment by Stroke Team or Designee

Review patient history.

Establish onset (<3 hours required for fibrinolytics).*

Perform physical assessment.

Perform neurological examination.

Determine level of consciousness (Glasgow Coma Scale).

Determine level of stroke severity (NIH Stroke Scale or Canadian Neurologic Scale).

Does the CT scan show hemorrhage?

If No, Check for Probable Ischemic Stroke

Review for CT exclusions: are any observed?

Repeat neurological exam: are deficits variable or rapidly improving?

Review fibrinolytic exclusions: are any observed?

Review patient data: is symptom onset now >3 hours?

If No to All of the Above, Check the Following

Does the patient remain a candidate for fibrinolytic therapy?

Review the risks and benefits with patient and family: if acceptable.

Consider fibrinolytic treatment with tPA.

Monitor neurological status: emergent CT if deterioration.

Monitor BP; treat as indicated.

Admit to critical care unit.

No anticoagulants or antiplatelet treatment for 24 hours.

*Some clinicians will consider longer time limits on a case-by-case basis.

PREHOSPITAL STROKE CRITERIA: DETECTION DISPATCH DELIVERY

EMS assessment and actions to include the Cincinnati Prehospital Stroke Scale and Los Angeles Prehospital Stroke Screen. Alert hospital to possible stroke; arrange for rapid transport.

Cincinnati Prehospital Stroke Scale

Facial droop—have patients both smile and frown. Look for symmetry, and movement of all aspects of face, including forehead and eyebrows.

Arm drift—have patients close their eyes and hold their hands out in front. If one arm "drifts" away, this is considered abnormal.

Abnormal speech—completely aphasic, slurred, expressive or receptive aphasia, cannot grasp the correct word or finish a sentence or thought.

Expressive aphasic—know what you are asking, just can't express it appropriately and are frustrated with themselves.

Receptive aphasics—have no clue what you are asking; what they hear is not what was said. The patients are frustrated with you because you "do not seem to listen to their answers." The speech can be perfectly clear; it is their answers that are suspect.

Garbled or slurred speech—may never be clear; may start out clear and then drift off or into garbled, incomprehensible sounds.

Los Angeles Prehospital Stroke Screen—LAPSS

For evaluation of acute, noncomatose, nontraumatic neurologic complaint. If items 1–6 are all checked yes or unknown, provide prearrival notification to the hospital of a potential stroke patient. If any item is checked no, then return to the appropriate treatment protocol.

Criteria	Yes	Unkown	No
• Age > 45 years	—	—	—
• **Absent** history of seizures or epilepsy	—	—	—
• Duration of symptoms < 24 hours	—	—	—
• Patient is not wheelchair bound or bedridden, at baseline	—	—	—
• Blood glucose is between 60 and 400	—	—	—
• Obvious asymmetry (right vs. left) in any of the following 3 exam categories: *[must be lateral]:*	—	—	—

	Equal	R Weak	L Weak
Facial smile/grimace	—	—droop	—droop
Grip	—	—weak	—weak
Arm strength	—	—drifts down	—drifts down
	—	—falls rapidly	—falls rapidly

Airway Monitor	Vital Signs	Neuro Exam	GCS

Fibrinolytic Criteria for CVA

Inclusion Criteria (must have all yes boxes checked)

YES

Eighteen years or older.

Clinical diagnosis of ischemic stroke with a measurable neurologic deficit.

Time of onset was well established as <180 minutes or 3 hours before treatment would begin.

Exclusion Criteria (must have all no boxes checked under contraindications)

NO

Evidence of intracranial hemorrhage on pretreatment noncontrast head CT.

Clinical presentation suggestive of subarachnoid hemorrhage even with normal CT.

CT shows multilobar infarction.

History of hemorrhagic stroke or intracranial hemorrhage.

Uncontrolled severe hypertension (BP sys >185 or dia remains >110 despite repeated measurements).

Known structural cerebral vascular lesion (e.g., AVM).

Known malignant intracranial neoplasm (primary or metastatic).

Witnessed seizure at stroke onset.

Active internal bleeding or acute trauma (fracture).

Acute bleeding diathesis, including but not limited to:

Platelet count <100,000/mm

Heparin received within 48 hours, resulting in an activated PTT >upper norm limit for lab.

Current use of anticoagulants that has produced elevated INR >1.7 or PT >15 sec.

Within 3 months of intracranial or intraspinal surgery, serious head trauma or previous stroke.

Arterial puncture at a noncompressible site within the past 7 days.

Relative Contraindications

Recent experience suggests that under some circumstances—with careful consideration and weighing of risk-to-benefit ratio—patients may receive fibrinolytic therapy despite one or more relative contraindications.

Consider the pros and cons of tPA administration carefully if any of the relative contraindications is present:

Only minor or rapidly improving stroke symptoms (clearing spontaneously).

Trauma **or** major surgery within 14 days.

Recent GI or urinary tract hemorrhage within previous 27 days.

Recent AMI within previous 3 months.

Postmyocardial infarction pericarditis.

Abnormal blood glucose level (<50 or >400 mg/dL).

APPROACH TO ELEVATED BLOOD PRESSURE IN ACUTE ISCHEMIC STROKE

NOT ELIGIBLE FOR FIBRINOLYNIC THERAPY:

Systolic 220 mmHg or diastolic 120 mm Hg	Observe unless other end-organ involvement.
	Treat other s/s of stroke.
	Treat other complications of stroke.
Systolic >220 mmHg or diastolic 121–140 mm Hg	Labetalol 10–20 mg IV for 1–2 minutes.
	Nicardipine 5 mg/h IV initial.
Diastolic >140 mm Hg	Nitroprusside 0.5 mcg/kg/min IV initial.

ELIGIBLE FOR FIBRINOLYTIC THERAPY:	
Pretreatment systolic >185 mm Hg or diastolic >110 mm Hg	Labetalol 10–20 mg IV for 1–2 minutes (MR x 1).
During and after treatment, monitor BP:	
Diastolic >140 mm Hg	Nitroprusside 0.5 mcg/kg/min IV initial.
Systolic >230 mm Hg or diastolic 121–140 mm Hg	Labetalol or nicardipine
Systolic 180–230 mm Hg or diastolic 105–120 mm Hg	Labetalol 10 mg

Quick Review of Assessment and Interventions for Patients with Arrhythmias

APPROACH TO PATIENTS

Once attention to ABCs and oxygen therapy has begun, securing an IV for possible administration of fluids and medications is usually the next step. Assessing and documenting vital signs and initial ECG analysis should follow. Remember, dialogue with the patient, friends, and significant others is important.

In cases where more than one advanced life support (ALS) provider is present, there is almost simultaneous assessment, history taking, noting of the physical environment, and detailed physical examination. Questions should be appropriate to assess the chief complaint, history of present illness, medical history, any medication history, and allergies that may contribute to patient care decisions.

The patient's statements describing signs and symptoms are documented in the patient's own words. Clinical assessment, vital signs, and reassessment are done after each intervention. For example, if the patient received pain medication, the reassessment would include the patient presentation, vital signs, effect on the ECG rhythm, and the effect on the ectopics if applicable.

What follows are guidelines for possible interventions for the patient who presents with cardiac compromise, such as arrhythmias, CHF, and/or pulmonary edema. Regardless of the clinical setting, the provider must be aware of protocols and guidelines that direct, affect, and govern treatment modalities. Changes in treatment often occur as a result of aggressive world wide investigations in the area of cardiovascular disease.

This section is not meant to be prescriptive, merely a baseline for assessment and a memory-jogger for the more common approaches to patient care. The content is based on the *2008 Handbook of Emergency Cardiovascular Care for Health Care Providers* by the American Heart Association as well as other references. It is the responsibility of the provider to keep current with knowledge, care practices, and patient care standards and guidelines in a specific work environment.

For Slow Rates in Hypotensive and Hypoperfusing Patients

Narrow QRS

Atropine sulfate for rate.

Pacemaker: Although the pacemaker may capture and provide a pulse, the patient may still need support for perfusion.

Inotropic drugs for perfusion.

Wide QRS

Pacemaker.

Inotropic drugs for perfusion.

AV Block with Narrow QRS Bradycardia and Rapid Sinus Rate

Inotropic drugs for perfusion.

Pacemaker.

For Ventricular Fibrillation

Confirm "No Pulse"

Goal is to depolarize the fibrillating myocardium.

Defibrillation.

Epinephrine or vasopressin.

Lidocaine.

Amiodarone.

Magnesium sulfate.

For the Narrow QRS Tachycardia

Stable

Goal is to slow down AV conduction and provide a better perfusing ventricular rate.

Vagal maneuvers.

Adenosine.

Calcium channel blockers.

Unstable

Patient is hypotensive and hypoperfusing.

Goal is to terminate the ectopic or reentrant tachycardia.

Synchronized cardioversion (also known as synch CV)

For Asystole

Confirmed in Other Leads

Goal is to maintain the patient and try to support an underlying escape rhythm.

CPR, oxygenate, intubate, ventilate.

Epinephrine.

May consider atropine.

May consider pacemaker.

Assess patient circumstance, environment, and presentation to attempt to discover the cause. Ask if there is a DNR document.

Do not defibrillate!

For the Wide QRS Tachycardia

VT Stable

Goal is to terminate the ectopic or reentrant tachycardia.

Assess 12-lead ECG to confirm ventricular tachycardia.

Lidocaine.

Amiodarone.

VT Unstable

Patient is hypotensive and hypoperfusing.

Sync CV.

VT Torsades de Pointes

Defibrillation.

Magnesium sulfate.

Consider overdrive suppression if arrhythmia recurs.

VT Pulseless

Defibrillation.

For Pulseless Electrical Activity

Identify the Rhythm

Goal is to identify any mechanical impairment to pulse and cardiac output.

CPR (assess for pulses; ? MI tamponade/rupture).

Intubate (assess breath sounds; ? pneumothorax).

IVs (fluid challenge; ? hypovolemia).

Epinephrine.

May consider atropine if there is a bradycardia.
As you treat, continually reassess as this may help determine the cause.

Grid for Assessing the Narrow QRS

Look at the P waves:

S → 1(+) P wave/QRS

J → (−) P wave/QRS or none

A → $\begin{cases} \text{Tachy} = \text{regular} \\ \text{Flutter} = \text{flutter waves you can count} \\ \text{Fib} = \text{junk—no identifiable Ps; QRS rhythm is irregular} \end{cases}$

Analyzing the Narrow QRS Complex

Sinus Rhythm (+) P Wave per QRS

60–100 bpm = sinus rhythm

<60 bpm = sinus bradycardia

>100 bpm = sinus tachycardia

Irregular = sinus arrhythmia

SA block missed one PQRST

SA arrest misses more than one PQRST

Junctional (−) P Wave or None

40–60 bpm = junctional rhythm

61–100 bpm = accelerated junction rhythm

>100 bpm = junctional tachycardia

Atrial

Flutter waves between QRS complex = atrial flutter

Irregular, chaotic baseline = atrial fibrillation

Persistent, regular rate >100 bpm = atrial tachycardia

Premature P waves

(−) or absent = junctional

(+) premature P′ wave/QRS = PAC

(+) premature P wave, no QRS = blocked PAC

Analyzing the Wide Complex QRS

Ventricular

QRS different than underlying rhythm
> QRS (+) and T wave (−)
> QRS (−) and T wave (+)

Sinus P wave plot through the event

20–40 bpm = idioventricular rhythm

41–100 bpm = accelerated ventricular rhythm

>100 bpm = ventricular tachycardia

>3 in a row = ventricular tachycardia
> AV dissociation supports ventricular tachycardia
> Fusion/capture QRS complexes support ventricular tachycardia
> Precordial negative concordance supports ventricular tachycardia
> Right axis deviation—QRS (+) in lead aVR supports ventricular tachycardia

Chaotic baseline = ventricular fibrillation

Confirm no pulse and that all leads are attached

Assess for somatic tremors and seizure activity that may mar the baseline

Aberrant Ventricular Conduction

QRS premature

QRS different than underlying rhythm

QRS and T wave (+)

QRS (+) and T wave (−) (rare)

QRS preceded by PAC

PACs seen with the underlying rhythm

Torsades de Pointes

Spindlelike effect

QRS is (+) and rapid; a twist in polarity occurs and is followed by (−) QRS

PVCs

Uniform	=	similar in appearance
Multiform	=	vary in appearance
Bigeminy	=	every other beat is a PVC
Paired	=	two PVCs in succession (also known as couplet)
Interpolated	=	the PVC is sandwiched between two normal QRS complexes
End-diastolic	=	immediately after a regularly anticipated P wave
R-on-T	=	appears on any part of the preceding T wave

How to Assess a Monitor Pattern

- Is the rhythm supraventricular or ventricular in origin?
  - If the QRS is ≤0.10 sec: it is likely supraventricular in origin.
  - If the QRS is >0.12 sec: may be ventricular in origin.
- If the QRS is 0.10 sec: look to the left of the QRS:
  If there is a P for every QRS and the P wave is
  - (+) regular and consistent: it is probably sinus in origin.
  - (−) or absent and the QRS rhythm is regular: it is probably junctional.
- Is the PR interval ≤0.20 sec and consistent?
  - If the PR interval is >0.20 sec: consider AV conduction defect.
  - Progressive prolongation of the PR interval (segment): consider an AV conduction defect.
  - No consistent PR interval and P-wave rate different than ventricular rate: consider complete AV block.
  - P waves and QRS are independent of each other: consider complete AV block.
- Analyze if *different* QRS complexes are premature (early) or escape (late). Plot out the P waves:
  - If P waves plot out regularly: the ectopic is probably ventricular in origin, regardless of how it looks.
  - If P waves do not plot out regularly: the ectopic is probably supraventricular in origin, most commonly, atrial.

- Calculate the rate:
  - Plot P to P and QRS to QRS at the baseline, *not* peak to peak.
  - If Ps and/or QRSs are regular: count the number of large (0.20 sec) between two regularly occurring wave forms and divide into 300.
  - In rapid rates: divide the number of small (0.04 sec) boxes between two regularly occurring wave forms and divide into 1,500.
  - For irregular rhythms, calculate using the widest and narrowest RR for the accurate rate range.
- Describe any other deviation including:
  - ST segment elevation or depression.
  - T wave changes such as inversion or in appearance (deep, symmetrical).
  - QRS notching.
  - Any change in the rhythm.

How to Look at a Monitor Pattern Using the Multiple Lead ECG

- What is the standard? This is the measurement against which we compare the amplitude of the wave forms.
- What is the underlying rhythm?
- Look for the acute changes, according to the surfaces of the heart: Q waves, ST segment changes, T-wave inversion:
  - Initially look at all the limb leads:
    - ST ↑ in lead II, look at lead III.
    - ST ↑ in lead III, look for reciprocal changes in lead I.
    - ST ↑ in lead III > lead II, immediately assess the right sided precordial leads.
    - ST OK in lead II, look at lead I.
    - ST ↑ in lead I, look for reciprocal changes in lead III: assess the precordial leads.
  - Leads II, III, aVF: the inferior.
  - Leads I, aVL, V_6: left lateral.
  - Leads $V_1 \rightarrow V_4$: anterior.
  - Lead $V_{3R} \rightarrow$ right anterior.
- Look for ventricular conduction disturbances:
  - Leads II, III, aVF: left anterior fascicle.
  - Leads I, aVL, V_6: left posterior fascicle.
  - Lead V_1 for RBBB.
  - For wide QRS complex tachycardia, look for positive or negative concordance in precordial leads.
  - If the QRS is positive in aVR, go to the precordial leads and determine concordance. Concordant negativity in precordial leads supports ventricular tachycardia.
- Calculate the axis. Northwest axis deviation (aVR) with wide QRS complex supports ventricular tachycardia.
- What can happen next?
- Which lead should be monitored and observed?

Medication Profiles

Premise

To know a drug, when to use it, what to expect, and, most important, when NOT to use it, is a key to the intervention and care of the patient in cardiac compromise.

Introduction

The purpose of this appendix is to review common medications used in the care of patients with cardiovascular disease. This is a quick reference only, and is not all-inclusive; knowledge of the pharmacokinetics should be maintained with intense study and review of pharmacological references. Also, practitioners must be aware of current standards, guidelines, and oversight that guide patient care in their specific environment.

ACETYLSALICYLIC ACID (ASA)

Generic Name: acetylsalicylic acid (ASA).

Trade Names: Aspirin®, Bayer®, Excedrin®, Bufferin®, Goldline Children's Chewable Aspirin®, others.

Classes: platelet aggregator inhibitor, analgesic, antipyretic, anti-inflammatory.

Mechanism of Action:
- Blocks formation of thromboxane A_2, which prevents platelet clumping and blood clot formation (specifically in the coronary arteries).

Indications:
- Chest pain consistent with an AMI.
- Prevention and treatment of unstable angina (USA).

Contraindications:
- Bleeding disorders.
- Known hypersensitivity to the medication.
- Has been known to cause bronchospasm in asthma patients.

Adverse Reactions:
- Gastrointestinal irritation.
- Gastrointestinal bleeding.

Notes on Administration

Route of Administration:

- Oral (chewed or swallowed).

Onset of Action:

- 20–30 minutes.

Drug Interactions:

- None in an emergency setting.

Adult Dosage:

- 325 mg tablet

  or

- Up to four 81 mg children's flavored chewable tablets

  or

- Administer this medication according to current standards and guidelines.

ABCIXIMAB

Generic Name: Abciximab.

Trade Name: Reopro.

Classes: Antiplatelet agent, glycoprotein (GP) IIb/IIIa inhibitor.

Standard Supply: 2.0 mg/1.0 ml in 5.0 ml vial (must be refrigerated).

Mechanism of Action:

- Reversibly binds with GP IIb/IIIa receptors on the surface of platelets by inhibiting the binding of fibrinogen, von Willebr and factor, and other adhesive molecules. Binding with GP IIb/IIIa receptors effectively prevents formation of intravascular thrombus and may contribute to the resolution of preexisting thrombus. This is termed stenic hindrance.

Indications:

- Adjunctive to, or in preparation for, percutaneous transluminal coronary angioplasty (PTCA) for the prevention and management of acute coronary syndrome and associated acute cardiac ischemic complications in patients at risk for abrupt closure of the treated coronary vessel. Includes intravenous infusion monitoring during prehospital interfacility transportation.
- Thrombotic arterial disease.

Contraindications:

- Active internal bleeding or recent history (within 30 days) of clinically significant gastrointestinal or genitourinary bleeding.
- History of stroke with current residual neurological deficit, or within the past 2 years.
- Bleeding disorder, condition, or predisposition
- Concomitant use of Coumadin (warfarin), or use within the past 7 days unless prothrombin time is <1.2 times control.
- Thrombocytopenia (<100,000 cells/µl).

- Trauma or major surgery within the past 6 weeks.
- Intracranial neoplasm.
- Arteriovenous malformation, aneurysm, or evidence of aortic dissection.
- Severe uncontrolled hypertension (systolic blood pressure >180 mmHg/diastolic blood pressure >110 mmHg).
- History of vasculitis.
- Concomitant use of another GP IIb/IIIa inhibitor.
- Acute pericarditis.
- Concomitant use of IV Dextran (results in a high incidence of bleeding).
- Known hypersensitivity to abciximab or murine proteins.

Adverse Reactions:
- Bleeding.
- Hemorrhagic stroke and intracranial bleeding.
- Thrombocytopenia.

The most common sites of spontaneous bleeding include venous and arterial access sites. Major bleeding has been demonstrated to occur more often in patients who are >65 years old, who are <75 kg, who have a history of gastrointestinal disease, and who are receiving thrombolytics or heparin.

Notes on Administration

- Heparin should be concomitantly administered and monitored with abciximab.
- Due to the risk of spontaneous bleeding during administration of abciximab, the following procedures should be avoided whenever possible: arterial and venous punctures, intramuscular injection, placement of a urinary catheter, placement of a nasogastric tube, and nasotracheal intubation.

Routes of Administration:
- IVP.
- Continuous intravenous infusion.

Onset of Action:
- Several minutes.

Drug Interactions:
- Other medications that affect hemostasis: thrombolytics, oral anticoagulants, aspirin and other nonsteroidal anti-inflammatory drugs (NSAIDs), dipyridamole, ticlopidine, and clopidogrel.
- Herbal products containing ginkgo, biloba, ginger, and garlic. Ginkgo may potentiate the risk of bleeding associated with anticoagulants, platelet inhibitors, and thrombolytic agents. Ginkgolide B, a component of ginkgo, inhibits platelet-activating factor by displacing it from its receptor-binding site, resulting in reduced platelet aggregation.

Adult Dosage:
- 0.25 mg/kg slow IVP over 5 minutes.

If the patient weighs <80 kg:
- 0.125 µg/kg/minute (0.09 mg/kg) intravenous infusion.

If the patient weighs >80 kg:

- 10 µg/minute (7.2 mg) in 250 ml of D_5W or normal saline 21 ml/hour for 12 hours.

Caveats

Weight-based dosing of abciximab and concomitant heparin are essential to decrease the incidence of bleeding. An infusion pump is required for intravenous infusion administration of abciximab. Abciximab infusions must be administered through a low-protein binding 0.2- or 0.22-micron in-line filter.

ADENOSINE

Generic Name: Adenosine.

Trade Name: Adenocard.

Classes: Antiarrhythmic, endogenous nucleoside.

Standard Supply: 6.0 mg/2.0 ml.

Mechanism of Action:

- Slows conduction of electrical impulses through the AV node.
- Interrupts reentry pathways and can terminate paroxysmal SVT (PSVT).

Indications:

- PSVT, including that caused by WPW syndrome refractory to common vagal maneuvers.
- Wide complex tachycardia of uncertain origin after administering lidocaine.

NOTE: Whenever possible, first assess multiple lead ECG for differentiation of the source of the tachycardia.

Contraindications:

- Second-degree block.
- Complete (third-degree) block.
- Sick-sinus syndrome.
- Known hypersensitivity to the drug.

Adverse Reactions:

- Transient flushing of the skin.
- Chest pain.
- Dyspnea.
- Brief period of asystole or bradycardia.
- Hemodynamic instability.

Notes on Administration

Onset of Action:

- Seconds (adenosine has a 5–10 second half-life).

Drug Interactions:

- Concomitant use of methylxanthines may inhibit desired effects.
- Concomitant use of carbamazepine (Tegretol) can create high degree of AV block.
- Higher doses may be necessary when theophylline has been taken.

Adult Dosage:

- 6.0 mg rapid IVP followed by rapid infusion of normal saline.
- If the rhythm does not convert within 2 minutes, administer 12 mg rapid IVP followed by rapid infusion of normal saline.
- If the rhythm does not convert within 2 minutes after the second dose, administer 12 mg rapid IVP followed by a rapid fluid infusion of normal saline.

AMIODARONE HCl

Generic Name: Amiodarone HCl.

Trade Names: Cordarone, Pacerone.

Class: Antiarrhythmic Class III.

Standard Supply: 150 mg/3.0 ml.

Mechanism of Action:

- Antiarrhythmic, potent vasodilator.
- Prolongs action potential.
- Prolongs effective refractory period in all cardiac tissue including accessory pathways.
- Noncompetitive block of alpha- and beta-adrenergic receptors.
- Reduces heart rate through beta-blocking effects.
- Blocks sodium, potassium, and calcium channels.

NOTE: Grapefruit juice increases by 50 percent the bioavailabiity of amiodarone when taken orally. St. John's Wort will decrease amiodarone levels.

Indications:

- Atrial fibrillation with rapid ventricular response.
- Recurring ventricular fibrillation.
- Recurring unstable ventricular tachycardia.
- Paroxysmal atrial fibrillation with rapid ventricular response.
- Prophylaxis of recurring ventricular fibrillation and unstable ventricular tachycardia.

Contraindications:

- Known hypersensitivity to the medication.
- SA node dysfunction.
- Marked sinus bradycardia.
- Second-degree heart block.
- Complete (third-degree) heart block.
- Cardiogenic shock.
- Electrolyte imbalance (hypocalcemia, hypomagnesemia).
- Thyroid disease.

Adverse Reactions:

- Hypotension.
- Pulmonary toxicity and fibrosis.
- Asystole/cardiac arrest/PEA.
- Bradycardia.

- Atrioventricular block.
- Torsades de Pointes.
- Congestive heart failure.
- GI disturbances with oral dosage.

Notes on Administration

Route of Administration:
- Intravenous infusion.
- By mouth (not in the emergency setting).

Onset of Action:
- Various response.

Drug Interactions:
- None in the emergency setting.
- Concomitant use of beta-blockers or calcium channel blockers.
- Concomitant use of digoxin and procainamide causes an additive effect.

Adult Dosage:

Patient with Pulse and Blood Pressure
- 150 mg IV infusion over 10–30 minutes, then add 3.0 ml of the medication (150 mg) to 100 ml of D_5W and infuse 10–30 minutes monitoring blood pressure.
- 360 mg slow IV infusion controlled over the next 6 hours (= 1.0 mg/minute).
- 540 mg IV infusion (with controller) over the next 18 hours (= 0.5 mg/minute) (not to exceed 2.2 g in 24 hours).

Patient in Ventricular Fibrillation, Pulseless Ventricular Tachycardia
- 300 mg IVP.
- May repeat 150 mg IVP.
- Follow with IV infusion.

ATROPINE SULFATE

Generic Name: Atropine sulfate.

Trade Name   Atropine.

Class: Anticholinergic.

Standard Supply:
- 1.0 mg/10 ml.
- 8.0 mg/20 ml.

Mechanism of Action:
- Blocks or antagonizes the effects of acetylcholine, thus inhibiting parasympathetic stimulation.

Systemic Effects:
- Decreases salivary and gastrointestinal secretions/motility.
- Causes bronchodilation.
- Decreases mucus production.

- Decreases urinary bladder tone.
- Causes mydriasis (pupillary dilation).
- Decreases sweat production.

Cardiac Effects:
- Increases the rate of SA node discharge.
- Enhances conduction through the node.

Indications:
- Hemodynamically significant bradycardia.
- Asystole.
- PEA with ventricular rate less than 60 bpm.
- Narrow-complex second-degree block.
- Narrow-complex complete (third-degree) block.
- Antidote for cholinergic poisonings (e.g., organophosphate and carbamates).

Contraindications:
- Wide complex second-degree (Type II) block.
- Wide complex complete (third-degree) block.

Adverse Reactions:
- Anxiety.
- Blurred vision.
- Delirium.
- Dilated pupils.
- Dry mouth.
- Headache.
- Palpitations.
- Tachycardia.

Notes on Administration

Routes of Administration
- IVP.
- IO.
- ETT.

Onset of Action:
- 1 minute.

Drug Interaction:
- Sodium bicarbonate inactivates.

Adult Dosage:
- For hemodynamically significant bradycardia: 0.5–1.0 mg IVP or 1.0–2.5 mg ET every 3–5 minutes to a total dose of 3.0 mg or 0.03–0.04 mg/kg.
- For asystole and slow PEA: 1.0 mg IVP (or IO) or 2.0–2.5 mg ET every 3–5 minutes to a total dose of 3.0 mg or 0.03–0.04 mg/kg.
- For cholinergic poisonings: 2.0–5.0 mg IVP every 5–10 minutes, or administer this medication according to local protocol.

CALCIUM CHLORIDE

Generic Name: Calcium chloride.

Trade Name: Calcium chloride.

Class: Electrolyte.

Standard Supply: 1.0 g/10 ml.

Mechanism of Action:

Action Potential Threshold Regulation

- Increases myocardial contractility.
- Increases ventricular automaticity.

Indications:

- Calcium channel blocker toxicity (e.g., verapamil, nifedipine).
- Acute hyperkalemia (e.g., renal failure with cardiovascular compromise).
- Magnesium sulfate toxicity.
- Acute hypocalcemia.
- Black widow spider envenomation.

Contraindications:

- None in the emergency setting.

Adverse Reactions:

- Arrhythmias.
- Hypotension.
- Syncope.
- Bradycardia.
- Nausea and vomiting.
- Cardiac arrest.
- Large doses increase the effects of digoxin.

Notes on Administration

NOTE: May precipitate with many medications.

Route of Administration:

- IVP.

Onset of Action:

- Immediate.

Drug Interactions:

- Sodium bicarbonate inactivates.
- Thoroughly flush IV tubing with normal saline before and after administration of this medication.

Adult Dosage:

- 2.0–4.0 mg/kg IVP.
- Repeat 2.0–4.0 mg/kg IVP every 10 minutes

  or
- Administer this medication according to current standards and guidelines.
- For calcium channel blocker overdose: 100 mg q2–3 minutes.

DIAZEPAM

Generic Name: Diazepam.

Trade Name: Valium, Diastat.

Classes: Anticonvulsant, sedative.

Standard Supply:

Parenteral

- 10 mg/2.0 ml.
- 2 ml ampules and syringes.

Oral

- *Tablets:* 2 mg, 5 mg, 10 mg.
- *Liquid:* 5 mg and 10 mg unit dose.

Rectal

- *Suppositories:* 5 mg and 10 mg.
- *Prefilled Syringe (Diastat):* 2 mg, 5 mg, 10 mg, and 15 mg.

Mechanism of Action:

- Inhibits neuronal transmission in the central nervous system.
- Causes muscle relaxation.
- Binds to stereo specific benzodiazepine receptors on postsynaptic GABA neuron.
- Causes increase in neuronal membrane permeability to chloride ions.

Indications:

- Major motor seizures.
- Status epilepticus.
- Sedation before cardioversion or external transthoracic pacing.
- Skeletal muscle relaxation.
- Acute anxiety state.
- Alcohol and opiate withdrawal syndrome.
- Diazepam is a benzodyazepine that is used clinically as a hypnotic.

Contraindication:

- Known hypersensitivity to the medication.

Adverse Reactions:

- Hypotension.
- Respiratory depression or arrest.
- Blurred vision.
- Nausea and vomiting.
- Drowsiness.

NOTE: Tolerance to the anticonvulsant effects of diazepam may develop within 6 to 12 months of treatment, effectively rendering it useless for this purpose and also because of side effects—in particular, sedation.

Notes on Administration

Routes of Administration:

- IVP.
- IM.
- Rectal: Suppository or liquid solution.

Onset of Action:

- IVP 1–5 minutes.
- IM 15–20 minutes.
- Rectal: 1–5 minutes.

NOTE: Duration of diazepam's peak pharmacological effects is 15 minutes to 1 hour for IVP and IM routes of administration.

Drug Interactions:

- Incompatible with many medications.

Adult Dosage:

Sedation

- *IV/IM:* 2 mg to 10 mg, repeated at intervals of at least 5 to 10 minutes, until adequate sedation and/or anxiolysis is achieved.

Status Epilepticus

- *Oral:* 2 mg to 10 mg, 2 to 4 times daily.
- *IV/IM:* 5 mg to 10 mg. May be repeated every 5 to 10 minutes until termination of seizures. Maximum dose of 40 mg to 60 mg can be used; if this dose is ineffective, other anticonvulsant drug therapy should be instituted.
- *Rectal Solution:* 10 mg as a single dose. May be repeated after 5 minutes, if necessary. The oral solution can also be administered rectally.

DILTIAZEM HCl

Generic Name: Diltiazem HCl.

Trade Names: Cardizem, Dilacor, Tiazac.

Classes: Calcium channel blocker, slow channel blocker, calcium antagonist (nondihydropyridine, benzodiazepine calcium channel blocker).

Standard Supply: 5.0 mg/1.0 ml in 5.0 ml and 10 ml vials (requires refrigeration).

Mechanism of Action:

- Depresses contractility, impulse conduction, and automaticity in myocardial and vascular smooth muscle (reduced peripheral vascular resistance). (This is due to inhibiting the movement of calcium ions across the cell membranes of specialized contractile cells, specifically through slow calcium channels.)
- Decreases sinoatrial (SA) and atrioventricular (AV) conduction (this prolongs the atrial-His-Purkinje refractory period, which prolongs PR interval and decreases heart rate).
- Increases cardiac output in the presence of supraventricular tachyarrhythmias.
- Calcium channel antagonism may dilate coronary vasculature (results in increased blood flow and oxygen delivery, of particular value in vasospastic conditions).
- Reduces blood pressure (due to dilation of peripheral arterioles and negative inotropy or depressed contractility).
- Reduces afterload (due to dilation of peripheral arterioles and negative inotropy or depressed contractility).

Indications:

- Rate reduction and control of atrial fibrillation, atrial flutter, and PSVT.
- Unstable angina.
- Severe hypertension.

Contraindications:

- Sick-sinus syndrome.
- Second-degree AV block.
- Hypotension (systolic blood pressure <100 mmHg).
- AMI.
- Concomitant use of a beta-blocker medication (relative contraindication).
- Pulmonary congestion.

Adverse Reactions:

- Hypotension.
- Congestive heart failure.
- Angina.
- Bradycardia.
- Headache.
- Bausea and vomiting.
- Dizziness.

Notes on Administration

Routes of Administration:

- IVP.
- Intravenous infusion.
- Oral.

Onset of Action:

- IVP: immediate.
- Oral: 30–60 minutes.

Drug Interactions:

- Concomitant use of amiodarone, digoxin, and beta-blockers may produce additive cardiac depression.
- Concomitant use of cimetidine may increase the bioavailability of diltiazem.
- Diltiazem may increase the bioavailability of carbamazepine, digoxin, and theophylline.

Adult Dosage:

Initial Dose

- 0.25 mg/kg IVP over 2 Minutes.
    - 40 kg = 10 mg (2.0 ml).
    - 60 kg = 15 mg (3.0 ml).
    - 80 kg = 20 mg (4.0 ml).

Second Dose (If Necessary) after 15 Minutes

- 0.35 mg/kg IVP over 2 minutes.
    - 40 kg = 14 mg (2.8 ml).
    - 60 kg = 21 mg (4.2 ml).
    - 80 kg = 28 mg (5.6 ml).

Initial Intravenous Infusion

- 5.0–10 mg/hour; dilute 125 mg (25 ml) in 100 ml of normal saline (1.0 mg/1.0 ml).

Adjusted Intravenous Infusion

- 15 mg/hour; dilute 150 mg (30 ml) in 150 ml of normal saline (1.0 mg/1.0 ml).

Oral Maintenance Therapy

- 120–360 mg per day (diltiazem is packaged in 30 mg tablets or 120 mg, 180 mg, or 240 mg CD capsules).

DOPAMINE

Generic Name: Dopamine.

Trade Name: Intropin.

Class: Sympathomimetic.

Standard Supply:

- 400 mg/5.0 ml.
- 400 mg in a 250 ml bag of D_5W (1,600 μg/ml premixed solution).

Mechanism of Action:

- Increases cardiac rate and contractility.
- Causes peripheral vasoconstriction.

Dose-Dependent Effects:

- *1.0–2.0 μg/kg/minute:* May dilate vessels in the kidneys and mesentery; may increase urine output; may decrease blood pressure.
- *2.0–10.0 μg/kg/minute:* Increases heart rate and myocardial contractility.
- *10–20 μg/kg/minute:* Causes peripheral vasoconstriction and hypertension.

Indications:

- Cardiogenic shock.
- Hemodynamically significant hypotension associated with CHF.
- Hemodynamically significant hypotension that is unresponsive to IV fluid resuscitation.
- Hemodynamically significant hypotension commensurate with the return of spontaneous pulses.

Contraindications:

- Hypovolemic shock.
- Pheochromocytoma (a tumor of the adrenal gland).

Adverse Reactions:

- Arrhythmias.
- Chest pain.
- Dyspnea.
- Extravasation may cause tissue necrosis.
- Headache.
- Hypertension.
- Nausea and vomiting.
- Palpitations.
- Tachycardia.

Notes on Administration

Route of Administration:

- Intravenous infusion.

Onset of Action:

- Immediate.

Drug Interaction:

- This medication may be deactivated by sodium bicarbonate.

Adult Dosage:

- *2.5–20.0 µg/kg/minute:* Initiate the infusion at 2.5 µg/kg/minute and titrate to effect.
- *5.0 µg/kg/minute:* If the patient's blood pressure is less than 70 mm Hg systolic, initiate the infusion at this rate.
- *2.5 µg/kg/minute:* If the patient's blood pressure is greater than 70 mm Hg systolic, initiate the infusion at this rate.

EPINEPHRINE

Generic Name: Epinephrine.

Trade Name: Adrenalin.

Class: Catecholamine.

Standard Supply:

- 1.0 mg/10 ml (1:10,000).
- 1.0 mg/1.0 ml (1:1,000).
- 30 mg/30 ml (1:1,000).

Mechanism of Action:

- Stimulates α-adrenergic receptors.
- Stimulates β-adrenergic (β_1 and β_2) receptors; β-adrenergic effects of epinephrine are more profound.
- Epinephrine also activates *ß-adrenergic receptors* of the liver and muscle cells, thereby activating the <u>adenylate cyclase</u> signaling pathway, which will in turn increase <u>glycogenolysis</u>.
- β_2 receptors are found primarily in <u>skeletal muscle</u> blood vessels where they trigger <u>vasodilation</u>. However, α-adrenergic receptors are found in most <u>smooth muscles</u> and <u>splanchnic</u> vessels, and epinephrine triggers <u>vasoconstriction</u> in those vessels.
    - Arterial vasoconstriction.
    - Increased systemic vascular resistance.
- β_1-adrenergic effects.
    - Increased heart rate.
    - Increased cardiac automaticity.
    - Increased cardiac contractility.
    - Lowers the threshold for defibrillation.
    - May restore electrical activity in asystole.
- β_2-adrenergic effects.
    - Relaxes bronchial smooth muscle, resulting in bronchodilation.

Indications:

- Asthma.
- Reversible bronchospasm associated with COPD.

- Severe allergic reaction (anaphylaxis).
- Hemodynamically significant bradycardia.
- Cardiac arrest.
    - Ventricular fibrillation.
    - Pulseless ventricular tachycardia.
    - Asystole.
    - PEA.

Contraindications:
- None in the emergency setting.

Adverse Reactions:
- Angina.
- Anxiety.
- Arrhythmias.
- Headache.
- Hypertension.
- Nausea.
- Palpitations.
- Sweating.
- Tachycardia.
- Tremors.
- Vomiting.

Notes on Administration

Routes of Administration:
- IVP.
- ET.
- IM.
- IO.
- Subcutaneous (SC).
- Intravenous infusion.

Onset of Action:
- Immediate.

Drug Interactions:
- Potentiates effects of other sympathomimetic drugs.
- May be deactivated by sodium bicarbonate.
- May not achieve desired effects in the presence of acidosis.

Adult Dosage:
In Cardiac Arrest
- 1.0 mg (1:10,000) IVP every 3–5 minutes
  or
- 2.0–2.5 mg (1:1,000) ET every 3–5 minutes.

For Anaphylaxis, Asthma, and Reversible Bronchospasm Associated with COPD
- 0.1–0.3 mg (1:1,000) SC or IM.
- 0.2–0.75 mg (1:10,000) ET or IVP if cardiovascular collapse occurs.

As a Vasopressor Agent

- Add 1.0 mg into a 250 mL bag of normal saline (4.0 µg/1.0 ml concentration) and infuse at 2.0–10 µg/minute (30–150 gtts/minute).

Eptifibatide

Generic Name: Eptifibatide.

Trade Name: Integrlin.

Classes: Antiplatelet agent, glycoprotein (GP) IIb/IIIa inhibitor.

Standard Supply:

- 20 mg/10 ml vial.
- 75 mg/100 ml bottle (requires refrigeration).

Mechanism of Action:

- Reversibly binds with GP IIb/IIIa receptors on the surface of platelets, inhibiting platelet aggregation. (GP IIb/IIIa receptor blockade interferes with the binding of fibrinogen and other platelet aggregation modulators to the surface of platelets, thus preventing aggregation.)

Indications:

- Acute coronary syndrome.
- Unstable angina.
- PTCA or atherectomy.
- Reduce complications associated with PTC.
- Non–Q-wave MI.

Contraindications:

- Active internal bleeding or recent history (within 30 days) of clinically significant gastrointestinal or genitourinary bleeding.
- History of stroke with current residual neurological deficit, or within the past 2 years.
- Bleeding disorder, condition, or predisposition.
- Concomitant use of Coumadin (warfarin), or use within the past 7 days unless prothrombin time is <1.2 times control.
- Thrombocytopenia (<100,000 cells/µl).
- Trauma or major surgery within the past 6 weeks.
- Intracranial neoplasm.
- Arteriovenous malformation, aneurysm, or evidence of aortic dissection.
- Severe uncontrolled hypertension (systolic blood pressure >180 mm Hg/diastolic blood pressure >110 mm Hg).
- History of vasculitis.
- Concomitant use of another GP IIb/IIIa inhibitor.
- Acute pericarditis.
- Known hypersensitivity to eptifibatide.

Adverse Reactions:

- Bleeding. The most common sites of spontaneous bleeding include venous and arterial access sites. Major bleeding has been demonstrated to occur more often in patients who are >65 years old, who are who are <75 kg, who have a history of gastrointestinal disease, and who are receiving thrombolytics or heparin.

- Hemorrhagic stroke and intracranial bleeding.
- Thrombocytopenia.

Notes on Administration

- Heparin should be concomitantly administered and monitored with eptifibatide.
- Due to the risk of spontaneous bleeding during administration of eptifibatide, the following procedures should be avoided whenever possible: arterial and venous punctures, intramuscular injection, placement of a urinary catheter, placement of a nasogastric tube, and nasotracheal intubation.

Routes of Administration:

- IVP.
- Intravenous infusion.

Onset of Action:

- Several minutes.

Drug Interactions:

- Other medications that affect hemostasis: thrombolytics, oral anticoagulants, aspirin and other nonsteroidal anti-inflammatory agents, dipyridamole, ticlopidine, and clopidogrel.
- Eptifibatide is not compatible in the same IV line with Lasix (furosemide).
- Herbal products containing ginkgo, biloba, ginger, and garlic.

Adult Dosage:

For acute coronary syndrome, there are several recommendations. The presiding physician will make the final decision.

- 180 μg/kg IVP

  then

- 2.0 μg/kg/minute intravenous infusion for 72 hours, until discharge or if angioplasty or coronary artery bypass graft (CABG) procedure, then 20–24 hours post this procedure (IV pump required for intravenous infusion of eptibibatide).

For percutaneous coronary intervention (PCI) in patients not presenting with an acute coronary syndrome, the following is recommended.

- 135 μg/kg IVP immediately before PTCA.
- 0.5 μg/kg/minute, continued for 20–24 hours

  or

- 180 μg/kg bolus; 180 μg/kg 10 minutes later. Then 1 μg/kg/minute.

Caveats: Weight-based dosing of eptifibatide and concomitant heparin essential to decrease the incidence of bleeding; infusion pump required for intravenous infusion administration of eptifibatide.

FUROSEMIDE

Generic Name: Furosemide.

Trade Name: Lasix.

Class: Diuretic.

Standard Supply:

- 40 mg/4.0 ml.
- 20 mg/2.0 ml.

Mechanism of Action:

- Causes excretion of large volumes of urine within 5–30 minutes of administration.
- Inhibits sodium and chloride reabsorption in the kidney in the ascending loop of Henle and the distal renal tubule.
- Causes venous vasodilation.

Indications:

- Fluid overload in CHF.
- Pulmonary edema.

Contraindications:

- Hypovolemia.
- Hypotension.
- Pregnancy (furosemide has been known to cause fetal abnormalities).

Adverse Reactions:

- Dehydration.
- Electrolyte disturbances.
- Hypotension.
- Arrhythmias.
- Nausea and vomiting.

Notes on Administration

Route of Administration:

- IVP.

Onset of Action:

- 5 minutes.

Drug Interactions:

- Incompatible with diazepam, diphenhydramine, and thiamine.
- Lithium (may cause toxic levels of this medication).

Adult Dosage:

- 0.5–1.0 mg/kg (usually 20–40 mg) slow IVP.
- A patient already taking prescribed furosemide may require a larger dose to achieve desired effects.

ISOPROTERENOL

Generic Name: Isoproterenol.

Trade Name: Isuprel.

Class: Sympathomimetic.

Mechanism of Action:

- Isoproterenol is a synthetic catecholamine that stimulates both beta-1 and beta-2 adrenergic receptors (no alpha receptor capabilities).

- Isoproterenol affects the heart by increasing inotropic and chronotropic activity. In addition, isoproterenol causes arterial and bronchial dilation, and is sometimes administered via aerosolization as a bronchodilator to treat bronchial asthma and bronchospasm.

Indications:

- Temporary control of bradycardia in heart transplant patients with denervation unresponsive to atropine.
- Hemodynamically significant bradycardias unresponsive to atropine, dopamine, and epinephrine or when external pacing is not available.
- Management of Torsades de Pointes refractory to magnesium sulfate.
- Poisoning from beta-blockers.

Contraindications:

- Hypotension (non–rate related).
- Cardiac arrest.
- Ischemic heart disease.
- Do not give with epinephrine.
- Do not give with poison-induced shock except in cases of beta-blocker poisoning.

Adverse Reactions:

- Arrhythmias.
- Hypotension.
- Precipitation of angina.
- Facial flushing.

Onset of Action:

- 1–5 minutes.

Duration:

- 15–30 minutes.

Drug Interactions:

- MAO inhibitors potentiate the effects of catecholamines.
- Beta-adrenergic antagonists may blunt inotropic response.
- Sympathomimetic and phosphodiesterase inhibitors may exacerbate arrhythmia response.

Supplied:

- 5 ml (0.2 mg/ml) vial.

Dose/Administration:

Adult

- *Infusion:* 2–10 µg/minute titrated to increase HR and perfusion. Typical preparation: dilute 1 mg in 250 ml for a concentration of 4 µg/ml. Titrate to response.

Pediatric

- *Infusion:* 0.5 µg/kg/minute titrated to increased HR and perfusion. Typical preparation: dilute 0.6 mg/kg to create 100 ml solution.

Special Considerations:

- For pregnancy safety, Category C.

- Isoproterenol increases myocardial oxygen demand, and can induce serious arrhythmias (including VT and VF).
- Administer via infusion pump to ensure precise flow rates.
- May exacerbate arrhythmias due to digitalis toxicity or hypokalemia.
- Newer inotropic agents have replaced isoproterenol in most clinical settings.

NOTE: If electronic pacing is available, it should be used instead of isoporterenol, or as soon as possible after the drug has been initiated.

LIDOCAINE HCl 2%

Generic Name: Lidocaine HCl (2%).

Trade Name: Xylocaine.

Class: Antiarrhythmic.

Standard Supply:
- 100 mg/5 ml.
- 1 g/25 ml.
- 1 g/250 ml (4 mg/ml) or 2 g/250 ml (8 mg/ml premixed solution).
- 2 g in a 500 ml bag of D_5W (4.0 mg/ml premixed solution).

Mechanism of Action:
- Suppresses ventricular ectopy.
- Increases ventricular fibrillation threshold.

Indications:
- Alternative to amiodarone in cardiac arrest from ventricular tachycardia and/or ventricular fibrillation.
- Pulseless ventricular tachycardia.
- Stable monomorphic ventricular tachycardia with preserved ventricular function.
- Stable polymorphic ventricular tachycardia with normal baseline QT interval; ischemia is treated and electrolyte balance ensured.
- Wide complex tachycardia of uncertain origin.
- Premature ventricular complexes (PVCs):
    - More than six PVCs per minute.
    - Two or more PVCs in a row.
    - Frequent multiformed PVCs.
    - R-on-T phenomenon.
- Post successful defibrillation from ventricular tachycardia or ventricular fibrillation.

Contraindications:
- Known hypersensitivity to the medication.
- Ventricular escape rhythm.
- Idioventricular rhythm.
- Usually in second-degree Mobitz II and complete (third-degree) heart block.
- Do not administer lidocaine to treat ventricular ectopy if the heart rate is less than 60 bpm.
- Do not administer lidocaine in patients with impaired liver function.

Adverse Reactions:

- Cardiac arrest.
- Central nervous system depression, including coma.
- Drowsiness.
- Heart blocks.
- Hypotension.
- Nausea and vomiting.
- Paraesthesia.
- Seizures.
- Tremors.

Notes on Administration

Routes of Administration:

- IVP.
- Intravenous infusion.
- ET.

Onset of Action:

- 1–5 minutes.

Drug Interactions:

- None in the emergency setting.

Adult Dosage:

Rhythms with a Pulse

- 1.0–1.5 mg/kg IVP.
- Additional IVP boluses: 0.5–0.75 mg/kg every 10 minutes to a total of 3.0 mg/kg.

Rhythms without a Pulse (Ventricular Fibrillation and Pulseless Ventricular Tachycardia)

- 1.5 mg/kg IVP may repeat in 3–5 minutes to a total of 3.0 mg/kg.

Following the Return of Pulses

- 2.0–4.0 mg/minute intravenous infusion.

NOTE: The dosage may need to be decreased for older patients as well as patients with liver disease.

MAGNESIUM SULFATE

Generic Name: Magnesium sulfate.

Trade Name: Magnesium Sulfate.

Classes: Electrolyte, anticonvulsant, antiarrhythmic.

Standard Supply: 1.0 g/2.0 ml.

Mechanism of Action:

- DecreasesACh in motor nerve terminals.
- Slows SA node impulse formation and conduction time.
- Stabilizes muscle cell membranes by interacting with the sodium/potassium exchange system.
- Alters calcium's effect on myocardial conduction.

- Depresses the central nervous system.
- Causes smooth muscle relaxation.

Indications:

Obstetrical

- Pregnancy-induced hypertension.
- Seizures associated with preeclampsia.
- Preterm labor.

Cardiac Arrhythmias

- Torsades de pointes.
- Ventricular fibrillation/pulseless ventricular tachycardia.

There is growing support in advanced cardiac life support for use of magnesium sulfate as a first-line agent in the treatment of myocardial ischemia, MI, and cardiac arrhythmias.

Contraindications:

- Heart blocks.
- Respiratory depression.
- Kidney failure.

Adverse Reactions:

- Hypotension.
- Respiratory depression or arrest.
- Cardiac arrest.
- Hypotension.
- Drowsiness.
- Arrhythmias.

NOTE: Calcium chloride should be administered as an antidote to magnesium sulfate if respiratory depression occurs.

Notes on Administration

Routes of Administration:

- IVP.
- IM.
- Intravenous infusion.

Onset of Action:

- Immediate.

Drug Interactions:

- None in the emergency setting.

Adult Dosage:

For Seizures Associated with Preeclampsia

- 3.0–6.0 g IVP or infusion delivered over 15–20 minutes.
- Repeat bolus 2–4 g IVP or infusion over 10–15 minutes.
- If intravenous access cannot be established: 2–4 g IM.

Because of the volume of this medication, the IM dose should be divided in half and administered IM at separate sites (usually each gluteus). An infusion may be prepared by adding the medication to a 50 ml or 100 ml bag of normal saline.

For Preterm Labor

- 4–6 g IVP or infusion delivered over 10–15 minutes.
- Follow initial bolus with 2.0 g/hour infusion, which may be continued until uterine contractions are reduced to one or less every 10 minutes.

For Cardiac Arrhythmias

- 1–2 g IVP or infusion delivered over 1–2 minutes.

For Torsades de Pointes

- 1–2 g IVP or infusion delivered over 1–2 minutes.
- Follow initial bolus with 1–2 g infusion delivered over 1 hour.

MIDAZOLAM

Generic Name: Midazolam.

Trade Names: Dormicum, Hypnovel, Midacum, and Versed.

Classes: An ultra-short-acting benzodiazepine derivative. It has potent anxiolytic, amnesic, hypnotic, anticonvulsant, skeletal muscle relaxant, and sedative properties.

Mechanism of Action:

- Like other benzodiazepines, midazolam acts on the benzodiazepine binding site of $GABA_A$ receptors. When bound it enhances the binding of GABA to the $GABA_A$ receptor, which results in inhibitory effects on the central nervous system. Capable of producing all levels of CNS depression, from mild sedation to coma.

Indications:

- Premedication before procedures.
- Anticonvulsant.
- Sedation.
- Management of acute agitation; treat the cause first.
- Induction for intubation.

Contraindications:

- Acute narrow angle glaucoma.
- Known hypersensitivity to the medication.
- Relative contraindication in myasthenia gravis or other neuromuscular disorders; acute alcohol intoxication; severe, chronic obstructive pulmonary disease (COPD); and acute pulmonary insufficiency.

Adverse Reactions:

- *Impaired psychomotor and cognitive functions:* May persist with patients taking the drug at night for insomnia.
- *CV:* Hypotension (especially in patients premedicated with narcotic); cardiac arrest; irregular or fast heartbeat.
- *Respiratory:* Apnea; respiratory depression, respiratory arrest; hyperventilation; wheezing or difficulty in breathing; hiccups; coughing.
- *CNS:* Emergence delirium; muscle tremor; uncontrolled or jerky movements of body; unusual excitement, irritability, or restlessness; dizziness, light-headedness, or feeling faint; prolonged drowsiness; headache.
- *GI:* Nausea and/or vomiting.

Notes on Administration

Midazolam administered intravenously has been associated with respiratory depression and respiratory arrest, especially when used concomitantly with opioid analgesics for conscious sedation or when rapidly administered. Midazolam may cause phlebitis. May need to adjust midazolam dose down for patients on erythromycin.

Route of Administration:

- For IM administration, inject deep into large muscle mass.
- For IV bolus and infusion, administer slowly in small increments over at least 2 minutes and allow 2 more minutes between doses to evaluate effect.

Onset of Action:

- IM for 15 minutes.
- IV immediately.

Peak Effects

- IM for 15 to 60 minutes.
- IV for 3 to 5 minutes.

Duration of Action

- 2 to 6 hours.

Drug Interactions:

- Midazolam may potentiate the action of other CNS depressants, including opiate agonists or other analgesics, barbiturates or other sedatives, anesthetics, or alcohol.
- Erythromycin may double the half-life of midazolam.

Adult Dosage:

Patients 14 to 60 Years of Age

- 2 to 5 mg IM.
- 1 to 5 mg IV, titrate to effect, administer slowly in small increments of no more than 2.5 mg over at least 2 minutes.

Patients over 60 Years of Age

- 1 to 3 mg IM.
- 1 to 3.5 mg IV, titrate to effect, administer slowly in small increments of no more than 1.5 mg over at least 2 minutes.

Total Dose

- Should not exceed 20 mg.

For Emergency Intubation

- 0.1 mg/kg up to 0.3 mg/kg with dosage limit of 20 mg.

Seizures

- 0.2 mg/kg IM for status seizures if no IV access.

Pediatric Dosage

- 0.05 to 0.1 mg/kg slow IV push.
- 0.2 mg/kg IM for status seizures if no IV access.

MORPHINE SULFATE

Generic Name: Morphine sulfate.

Trade Name: Morphine sulfate.

Class: Narcotic analgesic.

Standard Supply:

- 10 mg/1.0 ml.
- 2 mg/ml.
- 4 mg/ml.

Mechanism of Action:

- Provides relief of pain.
- Causes central nervous system depression.
- Causes peripheral venous dilation ($\downarrow$ preload).
- Decreases systemic vascular resistance ($\downarrow$ afterload).

Indications:

- Chest pain in MI.
- Pain associated with burns.
- Pain associated with musculoskeletal injuries.
- Pain associated with kidney stones.
- Pulmonary edema.

Contraindications:

- Known hypersensitivity to the medication.
- Acute bronchospasm or asthma.
- Respiratory depression.
- Head injury.
- Abdominal pain of unknown etiology.
- Hypotension.

Adverse Reactions:

- Central nervous system depression.
- Constricted pupils.
- Hypotension.
- Nausea and vomiting.
- Respiratory arrest.
- Respiratory depression.

Notes on Administration

Routes of Administration:

- IVP.
- IM.
- SQ (SC).

Onset of Action:

- Immediate.

Drug Interactions:

- Central nervous system and respiratory depression can occur when administered with antihistamines, sedatives, hypnotics, barbiturates, antidepressants, and alcohol.
- Effects of this medication can be reversed by administration of naloxone (Narcan).

Adult Dosage:

- *For Relief of Pain:* 2.0–10.0 mg slow IVP or IM.
- *For Cardiogenic Chest Pain:* 1.0–3.0 mg slow IVP.
- Additional doses of 2.0 mg every 2–10 minutes may be administered to titrate for relief of pain.
- *For Pulmonary Edema:* 1.0–3.0 mg IVP or according to protocol.

NITROGLYCERIN

Generic Name: Nitroglycerin.

Trade Names: Nitrostat, Nitro-Bid sustained release.

Classes: Vasodilator, antianginal.

Standard Supply:

- 0.4 mg tablet.
- Nitrolingual pump spray (nitroglycerin lingual spray) 400 μg per spray, 60 or 200 metered sprays.

Mechanism of Action:

- Mitochondrial aldehyde dehydrogenase transforms nitroglycerin to nitric acid, which promotes relaxation of vascular smooth muscle resulting in vasodilator effect on peripheral veins and arteries:
  - Coronary artery vasodilation.
  - Relief of chest pain by dilating coronary arteries.
  - Decreased return of blood to the heart (preload).
  - Decreased myocardial oxygen demand.
  - Decreased workload on the heart.
  - Decreased systemic vascular resistance (afterload).

Indications:

- Signs and symptoms associated with angina pectoris.
- Signs and symptoms associated with MI.
- Congestive heart failure with pulmonary edema.

Contraindications:

- The patient already has taken the maximum prescribed dose of the medication.
- Hypotension.
- Shock.
- Head injury.

Adverse Reactions:

- Bitter taste.
- Bradycardia.
- Burning or tingling sensations in the mouth.
- Dizziness.
- Fainting.
- Flushing and feelings of warmth.
- Headache.

- Hypotension.
- Nausea and vomiting.
- Tachycardia.
- Weakness.

Notes on Administration

Route of Administration:
- Sublingual (SL).
- Nitrolingual Pumpspray.

Onset of Action:
- Immediate.

Drug Interactions:
- Increased effects with other vasodilators.
- Alcohol (may cause severe hypotension).
- Beta-adrenergic blockers (may cause orthostatic hypotension).
- Sexual enhancement drugs (concomitant use may cause severe hypotension).

Adult Dosage:
- 0.4 mg SL.
- 0.4 mg SL may be repeated after 5 minutes, and then again after 5 more minutes, for a total of 3 doses (1.2 mg).
- One to two sprays of Nitrolingual Pumpspray for 0.5–1.0 second at 5-minute intervals provides 0.4 mg per dose. Maximum is three sprays within 15 minutes.

Caveat: Nitroglycerin must be protected from light and expires quickly once the bottle has been opened.

OXYGEN

Generic Name: Oxygen.

Trade Name: Oxygen.

Class: Natural gas.

There is 21 percent oxygen present in atmospheric air. Arterial partial pressure is represented by the abbreviation *Pa*. The normal arterial partial pressure for oxygen (Pao_2) = 100 torr (range = 80–100 torr).

Standard Supply:
- Oxygen is stored in steel-green or aluminum gray cylinders under pressure of 2,000–2,200 pounds per square inch (psi).
- Oxygen cylinders are designated by letters to identify their size. D, E, and M cylinders are the most common in emergency care.
- Oxygen flow from a cylinder is controlled by a regulator that reduces high pressure and controls liter flow.

Mechanism of Action:
- Rapidly diffuses across the alveolar walls and binds to hemoglobin in the red blood cells.

- Reverses deleterious effects of hypoxemia on the brain, heart, and other tissues in the body.
- Increases arterial oxygen tension (Pao_2).
- Increases hemoglobin saturation.
- Is necessary for the efficient breakdown of glucose into a usable energy: adenosine triphosphate (ATP). This process is known as *aerobic metabolism*, metabolism that occurs in the presence of oxygen.

Indications:
- Any condition in which systemic or local hypoxemia may be present, including:
  - Dyspnea or respiratory arrest from any cause.
  - Chest pain.
  - Shock.
  - Cardiopulmonary arrest.
  - Unconsciousness.
  - Any submersion accident.
  - Toxic inhalations.
  - Stroke.
  - Head injury.
  - Seizures.
  - Any critical patient, including all forms of trauma and medical emergencies.

Contraindications:
- None in the emergency setting.
- There is concern that patients with COPD may experience respiratory depression with the administration of high-flow oxygen. COPD patients' respiration tends to be regulated by a hypoxic drive in which respiration is stimulated by the brain's perception of a low oxygen level, rather than by a high carbon dioxide level, as in normal patients. High flow oxygen administration to the COPD patient does not have a clinically significant effect on respiration if used for a brief time in an emergency setting.

Adverse Reactions:
- None in the emergency setting.

Notes on Administration

Routes of Administration:
- Inhalation.
  - Nasal cannula.
  - Simple face mask.
  - Nonrebreather mask.
- Ventilation.
  - Any ventilatory device; for example, bag-valve-mask (BVM), automatic transport ventilator (ATV), or pocket mask with oxygen inlet.

Onset of Action:
- Variable.

Drug Interaction:
- None in the emergency setting.

Oxygen Delivery Devices:

Device	Flow Rate	Percentage of O_2 Delivered
Nasal cannula	1–6 L/minute	24–44%
Simple face mask	8–10 L/minute	35–60%
Nonrebreather mask	15 L/minute	95%

Caveat:

NOTE: Other oxygen delivery systems include the pocket mask, BVM, flow-restricted oxygen-powered ventilation device, and ATV.

PROCAINAMIDE HCl

Generic Name: Procainamide HCl.

Trade Names: Pronestyl, Procan.

Class: Antiarrhythmic.

Standard Supply:
- 1.0 g/10 ml.
- 1.0 g/2.0 ml (for infusion).

Mechanism of Action:
- Suppresses ventricular ectopy.
- Slows intraventricular conduction.
- Increases ventricular fibrillation threshold.
- Shortens effective refractory period of the AV node.
- Prolongs the refractory period in the ventricles.

Indications:
- Wide complex tachycardias which cannot be distinguished from ventricular tachycardia.
- Stable monomorphic ventricular tachycardia with normal QR interval and preserved left ventricular function.
- Atrial fibrillation with a rapid ventricular response in Wolff-Parkinson-White.
- Reentry SVT uncontrolled by vagal maneuvers, adenosine if blood pressure is stable.

Contraindications:
- Second-degree heart block.
- Complete AV block.
- PVCs in conjunction with bradycardia.

Adverse Reactions:
- Hypotension, especially in patients with impaired left ventricular function.
- Lengthening of the baseline PR interval or QT interval.
- AV block.
- Cardiac arrest.
- Torsades de pointes.
- Preexisting QT prolongation.

Route of Administration:

- IVP.
- IV infusion.

Adult Dosage:

- Recurrent ventricular fibrillation/ventricular tachycardia 20 mg/minute IV infusion (maximum dose: 17 mg/kg).
- In urgent situations up to 50 mg/minute may be administered to a total dose of 17 mg/kg.
- 20 mg/minute IV infusion.

Adverse Reactions:

- Decrease the maintenance infusion in patients with renal failure, CHF, or liver dysfunction.
- Proarrhythmic in the setting of AMI, hypokalemia or hypomagnesemia if renal dysfunction is present reduce total maximum dose to 12 µg/kg and infusion to 1–2 mg/minute.
- Discontinue administration of this drug if any of the following occur:
  - The arrhythmia is suppressed.
  - Hypotension.
  - The QRS complex is widened by >50 percent of its original width.
  - 17 mg/kg has been administered.

SODIUM BICARBONATE

Generic Name: Sodium bicarbonate.

Trade Name: Sodium Bicarbonate.

Class: Alkalinizing agent.

Standard Supply: 50 mEq/50 ml.

Mechanism of Action:

- Increases pH (alkalinization) in the blood and urine
- Acts as buffering (neutralizing) agent for acids in the blood and interstitial fluid.
- Increases tricyclic antidepressant excretion from the body in an overdose setting (by making the urine more alkaline).

Indications:

- Severe acidosis refractory to ventilation.
- Tricyclic antidepressant overdose.
- Documented metabolic acidosis.
- Considered after 10 minutes in resuscitation of cardiac arrest.

NOTE: Prompt defibrillation, ventilatory management, the administration of epinephrine and ventricular antiarrhythmics, assessment of blood gas analysis at the onset, and serial studies should precede use of sodium bicarbonate.

Contraindications:

- None in the emergency setting.

Adverse Reactions:

- Paradoxical intracellular acidosis.
- Metabolic alkalosis.

NOTE: Sodium bicarbonate transiently raises arterial P_{CO_2}. Administration of this medication must be accompanied by efficient ventilation to blow off excess carbon dioxide.

Notes on Administration

Route of Administration:

- IVP.

Onset of Action:

- Immediate.

Interactions:

- Inactivates sympathomimetic medications (e.g., epinephrine, dopamine, and isoproterenol) when they come in contact (i.e., when given together).
- May produce a chalky precipitate of calcium carbonate when administered together with calcium chloride, calcium gluconate, atropine, morphine sulfate, aminophylline, and magnesium.

Adult Dosage:

- 1.0 mEq/kg IVP.
- Repeat every 10 minutes: 0.5 mEq/kg.

TIROFIBAN

Generic Name: Tirofiban.

Trade Name: Aggrastat.

Classes: Antiplatelet agent, GP IIb/IIIa inhibitor.

Standard Supply:

- 250 µg/ml in 50 ml vial premixed.
- 50 µg/ml in 500 ml D_5W or normal saline.

Mechanism of Action:

- Reversibly binds with GP IIb/IIIa receptors on the surface of platelets, inhibiting platelet aggregation. (GP IIb/IIIa receptor blockade interferes with the binding of fibrinogen and other platelet aggregation modulators to the surface of platelets, thus preventing aggregation.)

Indications:

- Acute coronary syndrome.
- PTCA; intravenous infusion monitoring during prehospital interfacility transportation.
- Unstable angina.
- AMI.

Contraindications:

- Known hypersensitivity.
- Active internal bleeding or recent history (within 30 days) of clinically significant gastrointestinal or genitourinary bleeding.

- History of stroke with current residual neurological deficit, or within the past 2 years.
- Bleeding disorder, condition, or predisposition.
- Concomitant use of Coumadin (warfarin), or use within the past 7 days unless prothrombin time is <1.2 times control.
- Thrombocytopenia (<100,000 cells/μl).
- Trauma or major surgery within the past 6 weeks.
- Intracranial neoplasm.
- Arteriovenous malformation, aneurysm, or evidence of aortic dissection.
- Severe uncontrolled hypertension (systolic blood pressure >180 mm Hg/diastolic blood pressure >110 mm Hg).
- History of vasculitis.
- Concomitant use of another GP IIb/IIIa inhibitor.
- Acute pericarditis.
- Known hypersensitivity to tirofiban.

Adverse Reactions:

- Bleeding. The most common sites of spontaneous bleeding include venous and arterial access sites. Major bleeding has been demonstrated to occur more often in patients who are >65 years old, who are <75 kg, who have a history of gastrointestinal disease, and who are receiving thrombolytics or heparin.
- Fever, chills, diaphoresis, and dizziness.
- Hemorrhagic stroke and intracranial bleeding.
- Sinus bradycardia.
- Thrombocytopenia.

Notes on Administration

- Heparin should be concomitantly administered and monitored with tirofiban.
- Due to the risk of spontaneous bleeding during administration of tirofiban, the following procedures should be avoided whenever possible: arterial and venous punctures, intramuscular injection, placement of a urinary catheter, placement of a nasogastric tube, and nasotracheal intubation.

Route of Administration:

- IVP.
- Intravenous infusion.

Onset of Action:

- Several minutes.

Drug Interactions:

- Medications that affect hemostasis: thrombolytics, oral anticoagulants, aspirin and other NSAIDs dipyridamole, ticlopidine, and copidogrel
- Herbal products containing ginkgo biloba, ginger, and garlic.

Adult Dosage:

- 0.4 μg/kg/minute IVP for 30 minutes

then

- 0.1 μg/kg/minute intravenous infusion, for a minimum of 48 hours and 12–24 hours postangioplasty.

Caveat: Weight-based dosing of tirofiban and concomitant heparin is essential to decrease the incidence of bleeding. An infusion pump is required for intravenous infusion administration of tirofiban.

VASOPRESSIN

Generic Name: Vasopressin.

Brand Name: Pitressin.

Class: Pituitary (antidiuretic) hormone.

Standard Supply: 20 units/1.0 cc vial.

Mechanism of Action:
- *Pharmacological:* Promotes reabsorption of water by increasing the permeability of the collecting ducts in the kidney. Acts on both V_1 and V_2 receptors. Increases the smooth muscular activity of the bladder, GI tract, and uterus.
- *Clinical Effects:* Regulates water conservation. Causes vasoconstriction (pressor effect) of the splanchnic and portal vessels and, to a lesser extent, of peripheral, cerebral, pulmonary, and coronary vessels.

Indications:
- Used initially as an alternative pressor agent to epinephrine in the treatment of adult shock-refractory ventricular fibrillation/ventricular tachycardia. Current recommendations recommend early use of this drug.
- Vasodilitory shock.
- Septic shock.
- May be used as an alternative in asystole and pulseless electrical activity (PEA).

Contraindications:
- Potent peripheral vasoconstriction may provoke angina and cardiac ischemia.
- Vascular disease, especially when involving coronary arteries.
- Angina pectoris.

Adverse Reactions:
- *CV:* PVCs, CAD, CHF, may provoke cardiac ischemia and angina pectoris, severe vasoconstriction.
- *Respiratory:* Bronchoconstriction.
- *CNS:* Tremors, migraine, vertigo, seizures, coma.
- *GI:* Diarrhea, abdominal cramps, nausea, vomiting.
- *Renal:* Nephritis.
- *Other:* Increased risk of hyponatremia and water intoxication; use caution during lactation; local tissue necrosis if extravasation occurs.

Notes on Administration

Incompatibilities/Drug Interactions:
- Carbamazepine, chlorpropamide, or clofibrate may increase the antiduiretic effects of this drug.

Vasopressin Infusion

Adult Dosage

- *GI Hemorrhage:* Initial dose 0.1 to 0.4 unit/minute IV.
- *Esophageal Varices:* Initial dose 0.2 to 0.4 unit/minute IV. The maximum recommended dose is 1.0 to 2.0 units/minute.

Pediatric Dosage

- The safety and efficacy of this infusion for use in children have not been established.

Route of Administration:

- Intravenous infusion.

Onset of Action:

- Immediate.

VERAPAMIL HCl

Generic Name: Verapamil HCl.

Trade Names: Calan, Isoptin.

Class: Calcium channel blocker (Class IV).

Standard Supply: 5.0 mg/2.0 ml.

Mechanism of Action:

- Causes coronary artery vasodilation.
- Causes peripheral vasodilation.
- Causes vascular dilation.
- Decreases the rate of ventricular response associated with atrial fibrillation and atrial flutter.
- Inhibits reentry during PSVT.
- Reduces myocardial oxygen demand.
- Selectively inhibits slow calcium channels in cardiac tissue.
- Slows conduction through the AV node.

Indications:

- Narrow-complex PSVT refractory to administration of adenosine.
- Atrial fibrillation with rapid ventricular response.
- Atrial flutter with rapid ventricular response.

Contraindications:

- Hypotension.
- Cardiogenic shock.
- Wide complex tachycardia.
- Ventricular tachycardia.
- WPW syndrome.
- Sick-sinus syndrome.
- Beta-blocker medications.

Adverse Reactions:

- Bradycardia.
- Hypotension.
- Headache.
- Dizziness.
- Heart block.
- Congestive heart failure with pulmonary edema.
- Nausea and vomiting.
- Asystole.

Notes on Administration

Route of Administration:

- Slow IVP (over 1–2 minutes).

Onset of Action:

- 1–10 minutes.

Drug Interactions:

- Beta-blocker medications.
- Calcium chloride may be administered to prevent hypotensive effects in the management of a calciumchannel blocker overdose.
- Grapefruit juice increases by 50 percent the bioavailabiity by of calcium taken orally.

Adult Dosage:

- 2.5–5.0 mg slow IVP.
- Repeat in 15–30 minutes: 5.0–10 mg IVP up to a maximum of 20 mg.

Summary

This compilation of medication profiles is for quick reference only. It does not replace knowledge of specific drug inserts, protocols, and physician medical direction.

List of Abbreviations

ECG

(+)	positive (as with deflections)
(−)	negative (as with deflections)
A-fib	atrial fibrillation
ACS	acute coronary syndrome
AIVR	accelerated idioventricular rhythm
AJR	accelerated junctional rhythm
AV	atrioventricular
AVNR	AV nodal reentry
CLBBB	complete left bundle branch block
ICLBBB	incomplete left bundle branch block
ICRBBB	incomplete right bundle branch block
IVR	idioventricular rhythm
LAD	left axis deviation
LAH	left anterior hemiblock
LBBB	left bundle branch block
LGL	Lown-Ganong-Levine (syndrome)
LPH	left posterior hemiblock, aka left posterior fascicular
M/F	multiformed (as with PVCs)
NSTEMI	No ST elevation myocardial infarction
P′	P prime indicates atrial depolarization from other than SA node
PAC	premature atrial complex
PAT	paroxysmal atrial tachycardia
PJC	premature junctional complex
PR	PR interval (intrinsic)
PSVT	paroxysmal supraventricular tachycardia
PVC	premature ventricular complex
RAD	right axis deviation
RBBB	right bundle branch block
SA	sinoatrial node, aka sinus node
SC	subcutaneous, aka SQ (SC is preferred)
STEMI	ST elevation myocardial infarction
SVT	supraventricular tachycardia
TdP	Torsades de Pointes
U/F	uniform (as with PVCs)
UTD	unable to determine
VAT	ventricular activation time
VF	ventricular fibrillation
VT	ventricular tachycardia
WPW	Wolff-Parkinson-White (syndrome)

Anatomy and Physiology

ATP	adenosine triphosphate
Ca++	calcium (electrolyte)
CABG	coronary artery bypass graft
CFX	circumflex (coronary artery)
GI	gastrointestinal
K+	potassium (electrolyte)
LAD	left anterior descending (coronary artery)
LAE	left atrial enlargement
LAF	left anterior fascicle
LCA	left coronary artery
LPF	left posterior fascicle
LVH	left ventricular hypertrophy
MI	myocardial infarction
Na+	sodium (electrolyte)
RAE	right atrial enlargement
RCA	right coronary artery
RVH	right ventricular hypertrophy
SA node	sinus node

Clinical Applications

? allergies	Ask for any history of allergy, topical, oral, medication, dyes.
? medical history	Accumulate a full and focused history of the patient's past medical conditions, current illness, and allergies.
? meds	Question names of medications prescribed, borrowed, over-the-counter, and illegal—especially sexual enhancement meds—prior to considering nitroglycerin.
? vital signs	Ask for or assess blood pressure, pulse, respirations, temperature, skin, color temperature, and hydration. Includes pulse oximetry and blood glucose monitoring.
AAA	abdominal aortic aneurysm
ABCs	assessment of airway, breathing, and circulation
ACS	acute coronary syndrome; a group signs and symptoms that represent coronary occlusion
ALOC	altered level of consciousness
ALS	advanced life support
AMI	acute myocardial infarction
ASAP	as soon as possible
ATV	automatic transport ventilator
AWMI	anterior wall myocardial infarction
BLS	basic life support
BP	blood pressure
BVM	bag-valve-mask (ventilation device)
CC	chief complaint
CCU	coronary care unit
CHF	congestive heart failure
COPD	chronic obstructive pulmonary disease, aka COLD (chronic obstructive lung disease)
CPAP	continuous positive airway pressure
CPR	cardiopulmonary resuscitation
CV	cardioversion
Defib	defibrillation
Epi	epinephrine
ET	endotracheal intubation
g	gram; a unit of measurement, usually noted as lowercase *g*.
H/H	hypotension/hypoperfusion
HPI	history of present illness
Hx	history

IABP	intra-aortic balloon pump, aka intra-aortic counter-pulsation device
IM	intramuscular
IO	intraosseous
IV	intravenous
IVP	IV push; rapid intravenous push (as in injection; immediate; usually no timed delay); followed by 20 cc flush of NS (aka IVP preceded by medication name, concentration, and dosage)
IWMI	inferior wall myocardial infarction
LR	lactated Ringer's (IV solution)
LOC	level of consciousness
LWMI	lateral wall myocardial infraction (left)
mg	milligram; a unit of measurement, usually noted as lowercase *mg*.
NS	normal saline
NTG	nitroglycerin
O_2	oxygen
PE	pulmonary embolus
PEA	pulseless electrical activity
PEEP	positive end expiratory pressure
PMH	past medical history
PMI	point of maximum impulse
PPV	positive pressure ventilation
PRN	*pro re nata* (Latin—as the occasion arises; when necessary)
PTCA	percutaneous transluminal coronary angioplasty
qd	every day
qh	every hour
qhs	every night (bedtime)
RVMI	right ventricular myocardial infarction
SL	sublingual
SOB	shortness-of-breath or short-of-breath
SQ	subcutaneous
s/s	signs and symptoms
sync CV	synchronized cardioversion
TAR	traumatic aortic rupture
tPA	tissue plasminogen activator
USA	unstable angina

Pacemaker

FTC	failure to capture
FTS	failure to sense
TCP	transcutaneous pacing
RR	interval between two intrinsic ventricular complexes
RV	interval between the intrinsic QRS to the paced ventricular complex; the pacing interval
VV	interval between two ventricular paced complexes

Glossary

A

Aberrancy: QRS distortion that occurs with abnormal impulse transmission; often used when referring to a PAC or SVT with abnormal ventricular conduction; the QRS complex, instead of being narrow, is wide and distorted.

Absolute refractory period: Period of time in which cells cannot respond to a stimulus.

Accelerated idioventricular rhythm (AIVR): When a ventricular escape rhythm accelerates to greater than 40 bpm. AIVR may also be defined as an ectopic rhythm with 3 or more consecutive premature ventricular beats and a rate faster than the normal ventricular intrinsic escape rate of 20–40 bpm but slower than VT.

Accelerated junctional rhythm: When the junctional rate accelerates to greater than 60 bpm.

Accessory pathway (AP): Abnormal conduction pathway between an atrium and a ventricle. An extra bundle composed of ventricular tissue that exists outside the normal specialized conduction tissue.

Action potential: Describes the electrolyte exchanges that occur across the cell membrane of the heart during depolarization and repolarization.

Acute coronary syndrome (ACS): Group of signs and symptoms associated with myocardial ischemia and injury in compromised, and hopefully salvageable, tissue.

Advanced AV block: More than one QRS complex is missing, usually without a warning such as progressive prolongation of PR intervals.

Agida: Phrase meaning "heartburn." The spelling *acida* is also used, from the Italian *acido* (heartburn or stomach acid).

Akinesis: Lack of motion in the muscle wall of the heart.

Anorexia nervosa: Psychiatric illness that describes an eating disorder characterized by an obsessive fear of gaining weight. These patients have been known to practice voluntary starvation and excessive exercise and often use diet aids and diuretics.

Antidromic: Use of an accessory pathway in an antegrade fashion and the AV node in a retrograde direction.

Arrhythmia: Abnormalities in heart rate or rhythm.

Asystole: No cardiac electrical activity, hence no contractions of the myocardium, therefore no cardiac output or blood flow.

Atrial fibrillation: Chaotic and erratic depolarization state within the atria that results in irregular ventricular response.

Atrial flutter: Macroreentrant tachyarrhythmia resulting from an atrial ectopic arising outside the sinus node that travels in a clockwise or counterclockwise direction, in a circular fashion usually within the right atrium. Creates flutter waves.

Atrial kick: Atrial systole; the contraction of the atrium immediately before ventricular systole to increase the efficiency of ventricular function. Atrial kick contributes 6–30 percent of cardiac output.

Atrial tachycardia: Premature atrial beat that sends an impulse along an abnormal electrical path to the ventricles often at a rate range between 160 and 200 bpm. The rhythm is usually rigidly regular.

Augmented leads: Leads that are automatically set to increase in size by 50 percent without any change in the configuration of the electrodes by the machine's property; include leads aVL (augmented vector left), aVR (augmented vector right, and aVF (augmented vector foot).

Automaticity: Property of cardiac muscles that describes the ability of a cell to spontaneously generate an impulse without being externally stimulated. Cells that possess automaticity at a predictable rate serve as pacemakers.

AV dissociation: Condition where the atria and ventricles are independent. The atria usually are under the control of the sinus node and the ventricles are under the control of an escape junctional or ventricular mechanism.

AV nodal: Relating to the atrioventricular node (in origin).

AV node: The atrioventricular node (abbreviated *AV node*) is an area of specialized tissue between the atria and the ventricles of the heart, specifically located on the right side of the partition that divides the atria, near the bottom of the right atrium.

Axis: Direct path between two electrodes or between an electrode and the reference point; the direction of flow of depolarization.

B

Bifascicular block: Right bundle branch block that occurs concomitantly with left anterior fascicular block.

Bigeminy: When every other beat is an ectopic beat. For example, sinus→PAC→sinus→PAC, sinus→PJC→sinus→PJC, or sinus→PVC→sinus→PVC.

Biphasic: Having positive and negative components.

Bipolar leads: Leads that comprise one positive and one negative electrode; leads I, II, and III.

Bradycardia: Heart rate less than 60 bpm.

Brugada's sign: Overt ECG signs seen in the right precordial leads that warn of risk for sudden cardiac death.

Brugada syndrome: Group of signs and symptoms associated with the risk of sudden cardiac death. Implicated in genetic structural disorder within the heart.

Bundle branch block: Conduction disorder in one or more of the bundle branches.

Bypass tracts: An extra connection between the atria and ventricles.

C

Cardiac access: Mean direction of the wave of ventricular depolarization.

Cardiac output: Amount of blood ejected during ventricular systole in a given period of time, usually 1 minute. Stroke volume (the amount of blood ejected by the left ventricle) multiplied by the heart rate is the cardiac output.

Cardiac resynchronization therapy (CRT): Is a treatment for selected patients with heart failure-induced conduction disturbances and ventricular dyssynchrony. CRT is designed to reduce symptoms and improve cardiac function by restoring the mechanical sequence of ventricular activation and contraction.

Chest pain: Subjective term described as a physical hurt or disorder in the area of the chest.

Climacteric: Period in a man's life corresponding to menopause.

Compensatory pause: Distance from the previous normal beat to the next normal beat following the PVC is the same as two normal RR intervals.

Complete AV block: Independent beating of the atria and ventricles due to complete refractoriness in the AV junction, at the level of the AV node or infranodal.

Conductivity: Property of cardiac muscle that describes the ability to transmit an impulse from cell to cell.

Contiguous: Two or more leads that look at the same anatomical area of the heart.

Contractility: Property of cardiac muscle that describes the ability of the heart to react to electrical conduction with an organized mechanical response.

Cyanosis: Physical sign characterized by blue mucous membranes, lips, nail beds, and skin.

D

Delta wave: Initial slurring of the QRS complex. A premature upstroke to the QRS complex due to activity of an atrioventricular bypass tract. This is seen in preexcitation states such as the Wolff-Parkinson-White pattern. As a result, the PR interval is shortened. It does not have to be seen in all leads.

Depolarization: Electrical activation of myocardial cells due to the spread of an electrical impulse.

Digitalis effect: Negative scooping or slurring of the ST segment seen in patients on a digitalis preparation; not to be interpreted as digitalis toxicity.

Diphasic: Having two phases a wave form with positive and negative components within the same duration of time as a normally configured wave form.

Dyskinesia: Paradoxical bulging of the heart wall during ventricular systole.

Dyspnea: Difficulty in breathing.

Dyssynchrony: Delayed ventricular activation and contraction.

E

Early transition: Increase from negative to positive QRS complexes before V_3.

Ectopy: Cells that possess automaticity in competition with pacemakers.

End-diastolic (PVC): When a PVC occurs at the end or just after a sinus P wave.

Endocarditis: Inflammation of the endocardium.

Endocardium: Innermost layer of tissue that lines the heart and part of the heart valves.

Epicardium: Innermost of the two layers of the pericardium; continuous with the outer covering of the ventricles. Also called the visceral pericardium.

Erythema: Redness of the skin as a result of a widening of the small blood vessels near its surface. Causes include fever and inflammation.

Escape rhythm: Development of alternate pacemakers to stimulate the heart when there is sinus node slowing or arrest. The atria, AV junction, or ventricles may be the site of a single escape complex or a sustained escape rhythm.

Excitability: Property of cardiac muscles that describes the capacity of a cell to respond to a stimulus.

F

Fascicles: Bundles of fibers; left anterior and left posterior fascicles extend from the left main bundle branch.

Fascicular block: Disruption in conduction within one or more of the extensions of the bundle branches.

Fibrillation: Chaotic activity due to multiple ectopic foci.

Fibrinolysis: Process wherein a fibrin clot, the product of coagulation, is broken down. Its main enzyme, plasmin, cuts the fibrin mesh at various places, leading to the production of circulating fragments that are cleared by other proteases or by the kidney and liver.

First-degree AV block: Delay in AV conduction reflected in a consistently prolonged PR interval greater than 0.20 second.

Fixed atherosclerosis obstruction: Localized accumulations of lipid-containing material (atheromas) within or beneath the intimal surfaces of blood vessels.

Focal atrial tachycardia: Where an atrial ectopic rises from a localized area in the atria conducts through to the ventricles and causes a rapid ventricular response.

Frontal plane: In anatomy, an imaginary plane that divides the body into anterior (ventral) and posterior (dorsal) halves along the longitudinal (left-right) axis.

Frontal plane leads: Leads that visualize current flow that is right, left, inferior, and posterior; the limb leads.

Fusion beat: Abnormal QRS complex that occurs when the ventricles are activated partly by a sinus impulse, and partly by the PVC.

H

Heart rate: The number of contractions or how fast the heart beats per minute (bpm).

Hemiblock: Fascicular block. Can be left anterior or left posterior. It is best to specify the affected fascicle.

Horizontal plane: Plane perpendicular to the chest and frontal plane.

Horizontal plane leads: Leads that visualize current flow that is right, left, anterior, or posterior; the precordial leads.

Hypercalcemia: Condition in which there is an excessive amount of calcium in the blood; serum levels greater than 2.46 mEq/L (ionized). Also reported as greater than 10.4 mg/dL.

Hyperkalemia: Condition in which there is an excessive amount of potassium in the blood; serum levels greater than 6.0 mEq/L.

Hypermagesemia: Condition in which there is an excess amount of magnesium in the blood; serum levels greater than 2.4 mEq/L.

Hypernatremia: Condition is which there is an excess of sodium in the blood; serum levels greater than 147 mEq/L.

Hyperpnea: When increased breathing is required to meet demand, as during and following exercise or when the body lacks oxygen (hypoxia); for instance, in high altitude or as a result of anemia. Hyperpnea may also occur as a result of sepsis, and is usually a sign of the beginning of refractory sepsis. *Hyperpnea* is *not* synonymous with *tachypnea*. Tachypnea differs from hyperpnea in that tachypnea is rapid, shallow breaths, whereas hyperpnea is deep breaths.

Hypertrophy: Condition in which there is an increase in left ventricular muscle mass as a result of increased workload on the heart.

Hypocalcemia: Condition in which there is abnormally low levels of calcium in the blood; serum levels less than 2.24 mEq/L (ionized). Also reported as less than than 8.8 mg/dL.

Hypokalemia: Condition in which there is abnormally low levels of potassium in the blood; serum levels less than 3.0 mEq/L.

Hypomagnesemia: Condition in which there is abnormally low levels of magnesium in the blood; serum levels less than 1.6 mEq/L.

Hyponatremia: Condition in which there is abnormally low levels of sodium in the blood; serum levels less than 135 mEq/L.

Hypoperfusion: Diminished flow of oxygenated blood through an organ or organs.

I

Idiojunctional rhythm: Heart rhythm from the junction of the atrioventricular (AV) node and the bundle of His conducting an impulse to the ventricles but without retrograde conduction to the atria.

Idiopathic: Arising spontaneously for no reason or from an obscure or unknown cause.

Idioventricular rhythm (IVR): Heart rhythm from impulses propagated by an independent focus within the ventricles, with a rate of 20 to 40 bpm.

Infarction: Necrosis to heart muscle; usually the result of occlusion of a coronary artery.

Infranodal: Below the AV node.

Injury: Damage to tissue; may be reversible.

Internodal: Within the node; the median bundle of the heart's conductive system that leads to the AV node. This bundle was named *Wenckebach's bundle*, and is one of four internodal pathways, the others being the posterior internodal tract (Thorel's pathway), and the two branches of the anterior internodal tract (Bachmann's bundle plus a descending branch). Also known as intranodal bypass tract.

Interpolated PVC: When a PVC occurs between two consecutive sinus QRS complexes. Also described as being sandwiched in between two sinus QRS complexes.

Intranodal bypass tract: See *internodal*.

Intrinsicoid deflection: Deflection made during the time from the beginning of the initial inscription of the QRS to the point where the impulse arrives under a particular electrode of a lead; used to measure ventricular activation time.

Ischemia: Absolute or relative shortage of the blood supply to an organ (i.e., a shortage of oxygen, glucose, and other blood-borne fuels). Deficiency in perfusion of oxygenated blood.

Isoelectric line: Flat ECG line found between wave forms or cycles; for example, between the T wave and the next wave.

J

James fibers: Atrio-His bundle connections thought to be the basis for the short PR interval syndrome. These fibers should be distinguished from the controversial internodal tracts of the atrium. Also known as James tracts.

J point: The point where the QRS ends and meets up with the ST segment.

Junctional (AV) tachycardia: Cardiac rhythm usually originating at the junction of the atrioventricular (AV) node and the AV bundle at heart rates greater than 100 bpm. Junctional tachycardia is regular.

Junctional escape beat: When a junctional-induced QRS occurs after a pause in the underlying rhythm as seen in ECG.

Junctional rhythm: When the role of pacemaker is sustained by the bundle of His.

K

Kent bundle: Bundle of modified cardiac muscle fibers that begins at the AV node as the trunk of the AV bundle and passes through the right AV fibrous ring to the membranous part of the intraventricular septum where the trunk divides into two branches; the right and the left crus of the AV bundle. The two crura ramify in the subendocardium of their respective ventricles.

L

Lack of R-wave progression: Loss of R waves in the precordial leads when anterior forces are lost.

Late transition: Increase from negative to positive QRS complexes after V_3.

LBBB: Left bundle branch block.

Left axis deviation: When the flow of depolarization is superior and toward the left of normal.

Left ventricular strain pattern: On ECG, ST depression and T-wave inversion in left lateral precordial leads.

Lown-Ganong-Levine (LGL) syndrome: Accessory pathway that connects the atria directly to the bund of His. This accessory pathway does not share the rate-slowing properties of the AV node and may conduct electrical activity at a significantly higher rate than the AV node.

Low voltage: Lower than normal amplitude (less than 5 mm) for a given wave form at normal standard calibration.

M

Mahaim's fibers: Portions of the electrical conduction system of the heart that connect somewhere into the interventricular septum.

Mobitz, Woldemar (1889–1951): Early-twentieth-century German internist who analyzed arrhythmias by graphing the relationship of changing atrial rates and premature beats to AV conduction. Through an astute mathematical approach, he was able to classify second-degree AV block into two types: Mobitz Type I (also known as Wenckebach) and Mobitz Type II.

Monophorphic: QRS complexes of the same morphology and amplitude.

Multifocal atrial tachycardia (MAT): Multiple, different atrial foci that depolarize the atria at different and rapid rates.

Multiform: QRS complexes of different morphology and amplitude.

Myocardial cells: Bulk of the heart's muscle; the contractile units of the heart.

Myocarditis: Inflammation of the myocardium.

Myocardium: Middle muscular layer of the heart, composed of spontaneously contracting cardiac muscle fibers that are arranged in elongated, circular, and spiral cells and provide the heart's contractile force. The myocardium is the thickest layer of the heart.

N

Nadir T waves: Symmetrical, negative T waves, greater than 5 mm in depth. Considered an acute sign with a high degree of suspicion of coronary artery deficit.

Necrosis: Deadening of tissue as a result of occlusion with no oxygenated blood being perfused.

Node: Bundle of fibers of the impulse conducting system of the heart. Examples are SA node and AV node.

Nonrefractory phase: Period of time when all cells are repolarized and ready to respond in a normal fashion.

Nontransmural (non-Q-wave): Myocardial infarction that does not involve all three layers of the heart.

Normal axis: Flow of electrical current downward from right to left in the heart.

NSAIDs: Nonsteroidal anti-inflammatory drugs.

O

Orthodromic: Proceeding or conducting in a normal direction.

P

Pacemaker: A cell or group of cells that generates an impulse at a predictable rate of speed.

Pairs (couplets): Two uniform PVCs occurring in succession.

Palpitation: Irregular or unusually rapid beating of the heart, either because of a medical condition or because of exertion, fear, or anxiety (usually used in the plural).

Paroxysm: Abrupt start or stop.

Paroxysmal atrial fibrillation: An episode of atrial fibrillation that begins abruptly but is self-terminating, converting within minutes, hours, or even a few days.

Paroxysmal atrial tachycardia (PAT): An atrial ectopic focus that suddenly develops a rapid rate of depolarization, thus creating a persistent tachycardia. The hallmark is the sudden onset and sudden stop; that is; it appears *and* disappears suddenly. Recurrences may the same or longer or shorter durations.

Perfusion: Distribution of blood to organs and tissues to supply nutrients and oxygen.

Pericardial effusion: Condition in which there is abnormal accumulation of fluid within the pericardial sac.

Pericarditis: Inflammation of the pericardium.

Pericardium: Fibroserous sac enclosing the heart and the roots of the great vessels.

Permanent atrial fibrillation: An episode that lasts longer than a week and where cardioversion could not be attempted, or, if cardioversion was attempted, was not successful.

Persistent atrial fibrillation: An episode of atrial fibrillation that lasts several days or weeks.

Polarity: The direction of a vector, such as the P wave or QRS complex. Can be of either positive or negative wave form as it is measured from the baseline.

P mitrale: Notched abnormal P waves.

Polymorphic: In ventricular tachycardia. QRS complexes are of varying morphology and polarity.

Poor R-wave progression: Change of amplitude in the R wave. The R wave does not increase in size as the anterior forces diminish and the positive electrode gets closer to the current flow.

Positive ST segment coving: ST segment elevations that are convex or curved in appearance as a result of myocardial injury.

P prime (P'): P wave that is generated from other than a sinus impulse.

P pulmonale: Peaked abnormal P waves.

Precordial concordance: All QRS complexes in the precordial leads are negative in polarity. Typical of ventricular tachycardia.

Precordial leads: Leads in which the exploring electrode is on the chest overlying the heart or in its vicinity.

Precordium: Area of the anterior chest overlying the surface of the heart, V_1–V_6.

Premature atrial complex (PAC): An ectopic atrial focus that propagates an impulse before the next normal sinus beat.

Premature junctional complex (PJC): Discharge of a junctional ectopic focus that causes earlier than normal retrograde atrial depolarization. Represented on the ECG by a negative (−) P'; can occur before, during, or after the QRS complex.

PR interval: Period of time from the beginning of atrial depolarization (P wave) to ventricular activation (the QRS).

Protease: Any enzyme that conducts proteolysis; that is, that begins protein catabolism by hydrolysis of the peptide bonds that link amino acids together in the polypeptide chain, which form a molecule of protein.

Pulseless electrical activity (PEA): Where the ECG of a patient in cardiac arrest continues to display a normal identifiable rhythm but the patient is unresponsive and does not have a palpable pulse.

Purkinje fibers: Fibers that work with the SA node and AV junction to control heart rate. Purkinje fibers also have the ability of automaticity and can generate their own action potentials, but at a slower rate than SA node and other atrial ectopic foci. They can serve as the last resort when the sinus and junctional pacemakers fail.

Purkinje's system: Network of Purkinje fibers that carry the cardiac impulse from the atrioventricular node to the ventricles of the heart and cause them to contract. The impulse through the Purkinje fibers is associated with the QRS complex.

P wave: Wave form representing atrial depolarization; can be positive (+) when generated by a sinus and most atrial ectopic foci; is usually negative (−) when the atria are depolarized in a retrograde fashion from the AV junction.

Q

QRS alternans: alteration of the amplitude of the R and S waves of the QRS complex.

QRS complex: Portion of the cardiac cycle corresponding to depolarization of the ventricles; made of any combination of the Q, R, and S wave forms.

QT interval: Period from the start of the QRS complex until the end of the T wave; the time from ventricular depolarization to ventricular repolarization.

Q wave: Initial negative deflection of the QRS complex shown on the ECG. Q waves are considered pathologic when they are new to the patient, and/or greater than 0.04 second. QRS complex: That portion of the cardiac cycle corresponding to depolarization of the ventricles; made of any combination of the Q, R, and S wave forms.

R

R′: Second positive (+) R in a QRS complex.

Rate-dependent bundle branch block: Development of bundle branch block (BBB) with the change of heart rate. The heart rate at which BBB appears is known as critical heart rate.

RBBB: Right bundle branch block. Results from impaired or absence of transmission of electric impulses from the atrioventricular (AV) bundle of His to the right ventricle. The block may be complete or incomplete. Causes are a lesion in the right bundle branch or a small, focal lesion in the AV bundle. RBBB is often associated with right ventricular hypertrophy, especially in athletes and individuals under 40 years of age. In older individuals RBBB is commonly caused by coronary artery disease. A complete RBBB commonly occurs after surgical closure of a ventricular septal defect.

Reciprocal leads: Leads that are in the same plane but show a reflection or mirror image.

Reentrant atrial tachycardia: When an atrial ectopic uses a macroreentrant or microreentrant circuit through atrial and AV nodal tissue and results in a rapid, regular rate.

Reentry: Ability of an impulse to reexcite some region of the atria through which it has already passed.

Reflecting leads: Leads that are facing the affected surface of the heart.

Refractoriness: Property of cardiac muscle that describes the cell's ability to reject an impulse.

Relative refractory period: Period of time when only a strong stimulus can cause depolarization.

Repolarization: Process by which a cell, after being discharged, returns to its state of readiness.

Resonance: Decreased density usually referring to assessment of sounds. *Impaired resonance* is slightly more dense; *hyperresonance* is lowest in density; dullness is a dense sound; and *tympany* refers to very low density heard over air-filled areas.

Retrograde atrial depolarization: Conduction to and activation of the atria from an impulse inferior to atrial tissue.

Right axis deviation: When the flow of depolarization is inferior and toward the right of normal.

R-on-T: When a PVC occurs anywhere on the T wave.

RR interval: Period of time between consecutive QRS complexes.

R wave: The first positive deflection of the QRS complex shown on the ECG.

R-wave progression: Increase in amplitude of the R waves in the precordial leads. If the anterior forces are intact and as the positive electrode gets closer to the current flow, the R wave becomes taller.

S

SA node: Bundle of fibers that provides the initial impulse for the heart's conduction system. Also known as the sinoatrial node.

Second-degree AV block: Condition in which one or more sinus impulses are blocked and are unable to stimulate the ventricles.

Sensitivity and specificity: In the study of ventricular hypertrophy, refers to when the criteria are very sensitive or very specific (i.e., specificity >90 percent), which means if the criteria are met, it is very likely that ventricular hypertrophy is present.

Sinoatrial (SA) block: Disorder where the atria are unable to respond to the sinus stimulus, resulting in a missed PQRST complex; sinus cadence is usually undisturbed.

Sinus arrhythmia: Irregular changes in the beating pattern of the heart.

Sinus bradycardia: Heart rate less than 60 bpm.

Sinus rhythm: Rhythmic heart rate between 60 and 100 bpm.

Sinus (SA) arrest: Sudden failure of the SA node to initiate a timely impulse.

Sinus tachycardia: Heart rate greater than 100 bpm.

Specialized cells: Cells that make up the heart's electrical conduction system.

Stroke volume: Amount of blood ejected by the left ventricle.

ST segment: Line between the QRS and the T wave that represents early ventricular repolarization.

Supraventricular: Site above the ventricles—that is, the SA node, atria, or AV junction.

Sustained atrial tachycardia: When atrial tachycardia persists and is constant with no let-up.

S wave: Last negative deflection of the QRS complex shown on the ECG. Represents completion of ventricular depolarization. Usually less than 0.04 second in duration and less than 5 mm in depth.

Synchronized cardioversion: Delivery of electrical current to coincide with a QRS complex. Energy is delivered by way of multifunction pads at a selected amount of electric current over a predefined number of milliseconds at the optimal moment in the cardiac cycle that corresponds to the R wave of the QRS complex on the ECG. Also known as reversion shock.

T

Tachycardia: Heart rate greater than 100 bpm.

Tachypnea: Rapid, shallow breaths. *Tachypnea* is *not* synonymous with *hyperpnea*. Hyperpnea is deep, often rapid breaths.

Tenting: Assessment of skin as a sign of dehydration. Gently pinch and lift up the skin on the back of the hand to form a tent, and then quickly let it go. How it stretches is an indication of its extensibility. The faster it returns to normal, the more hydrated the patient; the slower it returns, the more likely the patient is dehydrated.

Thrombolysis: Breakdown (*lysis*) of blood clots by pharmacological means. It is colloquially referred to as *clot busting*. It works by stimulating fibrinolysis by plasmin through infusion of analogs of tissue plasminogen activator, the protein that normally activates plasmin.

Torsades de Pointes (TdP): Polymorphic ventricular tachycardia with changes in the QRS axis (twisting of the points).

Trabeculae: Muscular extensions of the myocardium. Rounded or irregular muscular columns that project from the whole of the inner surface of the ventricle.

Trending: Repeated ECG recording with comparison to allow for diagnosis and evaluation of interventions.

Trifascicular block: Condition in which a block is located in each of the three main fascicles on the bundle branch system.

Triggered activity: Tachycardias that result when low-amplitude oscillations occur at the end of the action potential.

Tripod position: Characteristic use of three points of support sitting leaning forward with hands supported on the knees, or on either side of the thighs.

T wave: Wave form corresponding to ventricular repolarization.

Type I AV block: Usually presents with patterns of progressive prolongation of the PR interval, group beating, and a missing QRS complex. Thought to be drug induced, often reversible, and with no other associated pathological findings. The first PR interval in the group is consistently the same.

Type II AV block: Often presents with bradycardia, differences in sinus and ventricular rates, and a ratio of P to QRS complexes, and frequently progresses to complete AV block because of pathological findings. The first PR interval in the group is consistently the same.

U

Uniform (PVCs): PVCs that look similar to each other in morphology and configuration, and in direction and amplitude.

Unipolar leads: Leads that measure the electrical voltages at one location relative to a zero potential, rather than relative to the voltages of another extremity; leads aVL, aVR, aVF, and V_1-V_6.

U wave: An ECG wave sometimes observed following the T wave; thought to be related to late repolarization of the ventricles.

V

Varying polarity: Direction of a vector, such as the P wave or QRS complex. Can be either positive or negative from the baseline.

Vector: Direction of force of electrical energy within the heart.

Ventricular activation time (VAT): Time from the beginning of the initial inscription of the QRS to the point where the impulse arrives under a particular electrode of a lead.

Ventricular bigeminy: When every other QRS is a ventricular ectopic that is sinus→PVC→sinus→PVC.

Ventricular fibrillation: Chaotic ventricular activity resulting in cardiac death. QRS complexes cannot be defined and the rate is immeasurable.

Ventricular flutter: Ventricular tachycardia at a rate of 250 to 350 bpm.

Ventricular septum: Wall separating the ventricles of the heart from one another. Primarily left ventricular tissue.

Ventricular trigeminy: When every third QRS is a ventricular ectopic.

W

Wenckebach, Karel Frederik (1864–1940): Dutch anatomist remembered primarily for his work in describing second-degree AV block (Mobitz Type I), later named the *Wenckebach phenomenon*. He is also credited with describing the median bundle of the heart's conductive system that leads to the AV node—*Wenckebach's bundle*—which is one of four internodal pathways. See also *internodal*.

Wide QRS complex tachycardia of uncertain origin: When an abnormally wide QRS complex generates a ventricular rate faster than 100 bpm. Can be supraventricular or ventricular in origin.

Wolff-Parkinson-White (WPW) syndrome: Syndrome of preexcitation of the ventricles of the heart due to an accessory pathway (AP) known as the *bundle of Kent*. This AP is an abnormal electrical communication from the atria to the ventricles. The use of the AP is often seen as a slurring on the upswing of the QRS complex (delta wave) and a shortened PR interval.

Pacemaker Terminology

A

Asynchronous: Pacemaker not synchronized by a shared signal. Pacer fires at a preset rate and does not recognize intrinsic wave forms. Also known as a fixed-rate pacemaker.

AV interval: Time between paced atrial and paced ventricular activity.

D

Demand: Pacemaker that has both sensing and pacing capabilities and responds within a specific timed interval.

E

Electronic capture: On ECG, the presence of a pacer spike in association to the wave form of the chamber being paced.

Escape interval: Time from the last sensed beat to the first pacer artifact (spike).

F

Failure to capture: When the pacemaker impulse does not result in a QRS complex.

Failure to sense: When the pacer does not sense an intrinsic wave form or interval and generates an impulse too soon.

Fusion: Collision of forces.

H

Hysteresis: Delay mechanism that allows a little more time for the intrinsic pacemaker to generate a natural impulse.

I

Inhibited: When a pacer has a sensing device that is preset to read and recognize intrinsic activity and thus does not pace. A characteristic of demand pacers.

Intrinsic: Belonging to the patient.

M

Mode of pacemaker response: Describes a pacemaker function, either demand or asynchronous.

O

Overdrive suppression: Electronic overdrive suppression; that is, the delivery of continuous rapid pacing used to control recurrent sustained supraventricular tachycardia, atrial fibrillation, and well as in Torsades de Pointes.

Oversensing: When activity other than intrinsic ventricular activity is sensed by the ventricular sensing channel and results in loss of output. Many signals could be responsible for the oversensing.

P

Pacemaker: Electronic devise that generates electrical current at a programmed rate and amplitude.

Pacemaker identification code: Five-letter code of the Intersociety Committee on Heart Disease (ICHD) designed to explain how a pacemaker operates.

Programmed upper rate limit (PURL): Upper rate limit at which a pacemaker will generate an impulse.

R

Rate-adaptive or physiologic: Pacemakers that are sensitive to the patient's physiologic parameters.

S

Sensitivity: Ability of the pacemaker to process the heart's intrinsic signals.

T

Threshold: Minimum amount of current required to elicit electronic and mechanical capture.

U

Undersensing: When the pacemaker does not sense intrinsic activity.

V

VA interval: Time between paced ventricular and paced atrial activity.

VV interval: Distance measured between two paced ventricular events.

References

Albert, J. S., Thygesen K., Antman, E., & Bassand, J. P. (2000). Myocardial infarction redefined—a consensus document of the joint European Society of Cardiology/American College of Cardiology Committee for the Redefinition of Myocardial Infarction. *Journal of the American College of Cardiology, 36,* 959–969.

American Heart Association. (2008). *Handbook of emergency cardiovascular care for healthcare providers.* Dallas, TX: Author.

American Heart Association. (2008). *STEMI: Rationalization for regionalization of care: An EMS and ED perspective.* Dallas, TX: Author.

American Heart Association. (2008). *STEMI provider manual.* John M. Field (Ed.). Dallas, TX: Author.

Antzelevitch, C. (2007). Genetic basis of Brugada syndrome. *Heart Rhythm: The Official Journal of the Heart Rhythm Society, 4*(6), 756–757.

Aronson, R. (1981). The hemodynamic consequences of cardiac arrhythmias. *Cardiovascular Reviews and Reports.* New York: le Jacq Publishing.

Balaji, S. (2009). Asymptomatic Wolff-Parkinson-White syndrome in children: An unnatural history? *Journal of the American College of Cardiology, 53,* 281–283.

Belhassen, B., Glick, A., & Viskin, S. (2004). Efficacy of quinidine in high-risk patients with Brugada syndrome. *Circulation, 110*(13), 1731–1737.

Berne, R. M., & Levy, M. N. (1981). *Cardiovascular physiology* (4th ed.). St. Louis, MO: C. V. Mosby.

Bode, C., & Zirlik, A. STEMI and NSTEMI: The dangerous brothers. An editorial. *European Heart Journal.* May 24, 2007.

Breithardt, G., & Seipel, L. (1976). The effect of premature atrial depolarization on sinus node automaticity in man. *Circulation, 53,* 920–925.

Brugada, J., Brugada, P., & Brugada, R. (1999, July). The syndrome of right bundle branch block ST segment elevation in V1 to V3 and sudden death—the Brugada syndrome. *Europace, 1*(3), 156–166.

Brugada, P., & Brugada, J. (1992). Right bundle branch block, persistent ST segment elevation and sudden cardiac death: A distinct clinical and electrocardiographic syndrome. A multicenter report. *Journal of the American College of Cardiology, 20*(6), 1391–1396.

Camm, A., Yap, J., Gruan, Y., & Merek, M. (2004). *Acquired long QT syndrome.* Futura, Blackwell Publi-shing. Published Online Nov. 2007.

Chou, T. C. (1996). *Left ventricular hypertrophy in electrocardiography in clinical practice: Adult and pediatric* (pp. 37–53). Philadelphia: W. B. Saunders.

Cohen, H. C., & Arbel, E. R. (1976). Tachycardias and electrical pacing. *Emergency Medical Clinics of North America, 60*(2), 343–367.

Conover, M. B. (2003). *Understanding electrocardiography* (8th ed.). St. Louis, MO: C. V. Mosby.

Elkayam, U., & Gleicher, N. (1998). *Cardiac problems in pregnancy.* New York: Wiley-Liss.

Fauchier, L., Olivier, M., Casset-Seonon, D., Babuty, D., Cosnay, P., & Fauchier, J. P. (2002). Interventricular and intraventricular dyssynchrony in idiopathic dilated cardiomyopathy: A prognostic study with Fourier phase analysis of radionuclide angioscintigraphy. *Journal of the American College of Cardiology, 40*(11), 2022–2030.

Feola, M., Ribichini, F., Gallone, G., Ganzit, G., & Gribaudo, C. (1994). Analysis of right electrocardiographic leads in 195 normal subjects. *Giornale Italiano di Cardiologia, 24*(4), 376–389.

Ferri, F. F. (2006). *Ferri's clinical advisor: Instant diagnosis and treatment* (8th ed., p. 540). St. Louis, MO: C. V. Mosby.

Goldberger, E. (1982). *Textbook of clinical cardiology.* St. Louis, MO: C. V. Mosby.

Gómez-Barrado, J. J., Turégano, S., Polo, J., and Carreras, R. (2008). *Torsades de pointes and a prolonged QT interval in the context of a very low-calorie-diet.* Sociedad Española de Cardiología/Ediciones Doyma S. L.

Hayes, D. L., & Vlietstra, R. E. (1993). Pacemaker malfunction. *Annals of Internal Medicine, 119*(8), 828–835.

Herring, N., & Paterson, D. J. (2006). ECG diagnosis of acute ischaemia and infarction: Past, present and future. Burdon Sanderson Cardiac Science Centre, Department of Physiology, Anatomy and Genetics, Oxford University. *QJM, 99*(4), 219–230.

Hess, O. M., & Carroll, J. D. (2007). Clinical assessment of heart failure. In Libby, P., Bonow, R. O., Mann, D. L., & Zipes, D. P., eds. *Braunwald's heart disease: A textbook of cardiovascular medicine.* (8th ed.). Philadelphia: Saunders Elsevier; chap 23.

Hicks Keen, J., & Saunorus Baired, M. (1998). Torsades de pointes: Success equals recognition. *St. Journal of Emergency Nursing, 21*(2): 142–144.

Hong, K., Berruezo-Sanchez, A., Poungvarin, N., Oliva, A., Vatta, M., Brugada, J., et al. (2004). Phenotypic characterization of a large European family with Brugada syndrome displaying a sudden unexpected death syndrome mutation in SCN5A. *Journal of Cardiovascular Electrophysiology, 15*(1), 64–69.

Horenstein, M. S., & Hamilton, R. M. (2008). *Atrioventricular block, second degree.* The Hospital for Sick Children and Research Institute, University of Toronto, Canada. Retrieved from the eMedicine Web site: http://emedicine.medscape.com/article/890621-overview.

Jacobsen, C. (2008). Understanding atrioventricular blocks; Part I. First-degree and second-degree atrioventricular blocks. *AACN Advanced Critical Care, 19*(4), 478–484.

Jacobsen, C. (2009). Understanding atrioventricular blocks; Part II. High-grade and third-degree atrioventricular blocks. *AACN Advanced Critical Care, 20*(1), 112–118.

James, T. N., & Sherf, L. (1968). Ultrastructure of the human atrioventricular node. *Circulation, 37*, 1049.

Katz, A. M. (2006). *Physiology of the heart* (4th ed.). Philadelphia: Lippincott Williams & Wilkins.

Klabunde, R. E. (2005). *Pulmonary capillary wedge pressure: Cardiovascular physiology concepts.* Philadelphia: Lippincott Williams & Wilkins.

Lemery, R., Kleinebenne, A., Nihoyannopoulos, P., Aber, V., Alfonso, F., & McKenna, W. J. (1990). Q waves in hypertrophic cardiomyopathy in relation to the distribution and severity of right and left ventricular hypertrophy. *Journal of the American College of Cardiology, 16*(2), 368–374.

Marriott, H. J., Nelson, W. P., & Schocken, D. D. (2007). *Concepts and cautions in electrocardiography.* Denver, CO: MedInfo, Inc.

Marriott, H. J. L., & Conover, M. B. (1998). *Advanced concepts in arrhythmias* (3rd ed.). St Louis, MO: C. V. Mosby.

Marriott, H. J. L., Schwartz, N. L., & Bix, H. H. (1962). Ventricular fusion beats. *Circulation, 26*, 880–884.

Montalescot, G., Dallongeville, J., Van Belle, E., Rouanet, C. B., Degrandsart, A., & Vicaut, E. for the OPERA Investigators. STEMI and NSTEMI: Are they so different? 1 Year outcomes in acute myocardial infarction as defined by the ESC/ACC definition (the OPERA registry). *European Heart Journal,* January 24, 2007.

Moore, L. *Amniotic Fluid Embolism.* eMedicine update, August 12, 2008.

Napolitano, C., & Priori, S. G. (2006). Brugada syndrome. *Orphanet Journal of Rare Diseases, 1*, 35.

Nelson, Gregory S.PhD; Berger, Ronald D.MD, PhD; Fetics, Barry J. MSE; Talbot, Maurice RN; Spinelli, Julio C. PhD;

Hare, Joshua M. MD; Kass, David A. MD. *Left Ventricular or Biventricular Pacing Improves Cardiac Function at Diminished Energy Cost in Patients With Dilated Cardiomyopathy and Left Bundle-Branch Block (Circulation. 2000;102:3053.)* © 2000 American Heart Association, Inc.

Novey, D. W. (1988). *Rapid access guide to the physical examination.* Yearbook Medical Publishers, Inc.

Okin, P. M., Devereux, R. B., Nieminen, M. S., Jern, S., Oikarinen, L., Viitasalo, M., et al. Relationship of the electrocardiographic strain pattern to left ventricular structure and function in hypertensive patients: The LIFE study. *Journal of the American College of Cardiology, 38*, 514–520.

Okreglicki, A. M., Hongsheng M. G., Rosero, S., Daubert, J. P., Huang, D., Budzikowski, A. S., et al. (2006). *Atrial tachycardia: Treatment & medication.* Retrieved from the eMedicine Web site: http://emedicine.medscape.com/article/151456-treatment

Olgin, J. E., & Zipes, D. P. (2007). Specific arrhythmias: Diagnosis and treatment. In Libby, P., Bonow, R. O., Mann, D. L., & Zipes, D. P., eds. *Braunwald's heart disease: A textbook of cardiovascular medicine* (8th ed., chap. 35). St. Louis, MO: W. B. Saunders.

Opie, L. H. (2004). *Heart physiology from cell to circulation* (4th ed.). Philadelphia: Lippincott Williams & Wilkins.

Pavia, S. V., & Wilkoff, B. L. (2001). Biventricular Pacing for Heart Failure. In Young, J. B., ed. *Cardiology Clinics.* (Vol. 19, No. 4) (pp. 637–651). Philadelphia: WB Saunders Co.

Prehospital thrombolytic therapy in patients with suspected acute myocardial infarction. The European Myocardial Infarction Project Group. (1993). *New England Journal of Medicine, 329*(6), 383–389.

Rosen, M. J. (2002). *Rosen's emergency medicine: Concepts and clinical practice* (5th ed., pp. 1080–1081). St. Louis, MO: C. V. Mosby.

Santinelli, V., Radinovic, A., Manguso, F., Vicedomini, G., Gulletta, S., Paglino, G., et al. (2009). The natural history of asymptomatic ventricular pre-excitation: A long-term prospective follow-up study of 184 asymptomatic children. *Journal of the American College of Cardiology, 53*, 275–280. doi:10.1016/j.jacc.2008.09.037.

Seidel, H., Ball, J. W., Dains, R. N., & Benedict, G. W. (2006). *Mosby's Guide to physical examination,* (6th ed.). St. Louis, MO: CV Mosby.

Shapiro, E. (1980). The electrocardiogram and the arrhythmias: Historical insights. In Mandel, W. J., ed. *Cardiac arrhythmias: Their mechanisms, diagnosis and management* (pp. 1–12). Philadelphia: Lippincott.

Shah, C. P., Thakur, R. K., Xie, B., & Hoon, V. K. (1998). Clinical approach to wide QRS complex tachycardias. *Emergency Medicine Clinics of North America, 16*(2), 331–360.

Silverman, M. E., Upshaw, C. B., Jr., & Lange, H. W. (2004). Woldemar Mobitz and his 1924 classification of second-degree atrioventricular block. Historical Perspective. *Circulation, 110*, 1162–1167.

Singh, V. N., & Sharma, R. K. (2006). *Accelerated idioventricular rhythm*. Retrieved from the eMedicine Web site: http://emedicine.medscape.com/article/150074-overview

Smith, R. C. (1996). *The patient's story: The integrated patient interview*. Little, Brown and Company.

Strohmer, B., Chen, P.-S., & Hwang, C. (2000). Radiofrequency ablation of focal atrial tachycardia and atrioatrial conduction from recipient to donor after orthotopic heart transplantation. *Journal of Cardiovascular Electrophysiology, 11*(10), 1165–1170.

Swartz, M. H. (1998). *Textbook of physical diagnosis: History and examination,* W. B. Saunders.

Urban, M. J., Edmondson, D. A., & Aufderheide, T. P. (2002). Prehospital 12-lead ECG diagnostic programs. *Emergency Medicine Clinics of North America, 20*(4), 725–841.

Veress, G. (1994). Hypokalemia Associated with infra-His Mobitz type second degree A-V block. *Chest, 105.,* 1616–1617.

Wagner, G. S. (1994). *Marriott's practical electrocardiography* (9th ed.). Baltimore: Williams & Wilkins.

Watanabe, H., Koopmann, T. T., Le Scouarnec S., Yang, T., Ingram, C. R., Schott, J. J., et al. (2008). Sodium channel beta1 subunit mutations associated with Brugada syndrome and cardiac conduction disease in humans. *Journal of Clinical Investigation, 118*(6), 2260–2268.

Wellens, H. J., & Conover, M. B. (2006). *The ECG in emergency decision making* (2nd ed.). Philadelphia: W. B. Saunders.

White, R. D. (1992). Prehospital 12-lead ECG. *Annals of Emergency Medicine, 21*(5), 586.

Wood, S. L., Sivarajam Froelicher, E. S., Adams Motzer, S., & Bridges, E. J. (2004). *Cardiac nursing* (5th ed.). Philadelphia: Lippincott Williams & Wilkins.

Yarlagadda, C. (2009). Pacemaker malfunction. Retrieved from the eMedicine Web site: http://emedicine.medscape.com/article/156583-overview.

Zalenski, R. J., Cook, D., & Rydman, R. (1993). Assessing the diagnostic value of an ECG containing leads V4R, V8, and V9: The 15-lead ECG. *Annals of Emergency Medicine, 22,* 786–793.

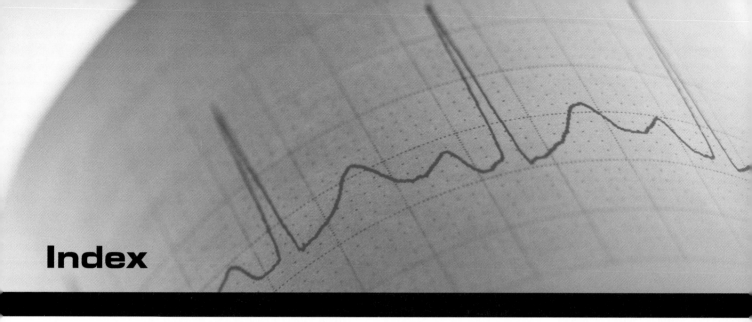

Index

A

Abbreviations, 477–479
  anatomy and physiology, 478
  clinical applications, 478–479
  ECG, 477
  electronic pacemaker, 479

ABCD survey, 425–426

Abciximab, 444–446

Aberrant ventricular conduction, 110, 114–116, 115f

Absolute refractory period, 16

Accelerated idioventricular rhythm (AIVR), 159–161, 160f

Accelerated junctional rhythm, 97–98, 98f, 101

Accessory pathway, 231, 232

Acetylcholine, 16, 121

Acetylsalicylic acid (ASA), 443–444

Action potential, 13

Acute coronary syndrome, 250, 431

Acute myocardial infarction, 274. *See also* Myocardial infarction

Acute onset, 126

Adenosine, 446–447

Advanced (high-grade) AV block, 180–183, 181f, 182f

Afterdepolarization, 113, 147, 149, 155

Akinesis, 258

Amiodarone HCl, 447–448

Amplitude, measurement of, 32

Anatomy abbreviations, 478

Anatomy of heart. *See* Cardiac function

Anorexia nervosa, 46

Anterior leads, 28

Anterior wall myocardial infarction (AWMI), 180, 184, 199, 264–265, 264f, 265t

Anterolateral wall myocardial infarction, 265–266, 267f

Anteroseptal wall myocardial infarction, 265, 266f

Antiarrhythmic medications
  abnormal QT intervals and, 46
  alterations on ECG tracing and, 48

Antidromic tachycardia, 237

Aortic valve, 4

Apical pulse, 4

Arrhythmias, 82–83
  accessory pathway physiology, 232
  concealed accessory pathway, 236
  due to abnormal conduction pathways, 231–245
  ECG rhythm identification practice, 243–245
  Lown-Ganong-Levine (LGL) syndrome, 239
  medication-induced, 48
  preexcitation, 232, 233f, 234–239, 236f

Arterial perfusion, 194

Assessment, 437–442
  of asystole, 438
  of monitor pattern, 441–442
  of narrow QRS complex assessment, 439–440
  of narrow QRS tachycardia, 438
  of pulseless electrical activity, 439
  of slow rates in hypotensive/hypoperfusing patients, 437–438
  of ventricular fibrillation, 438
  of wide complex QRS, 440–441
  of wide QRS tachycardia, 439

Asynchronous pacemakers, 293, 295

Asystole, 161–162, 161f, 430, 438

Atria, 6

Atrial bigeminy, 112, 112f

Atrial ectopy, pregnancy and, 111

Atrial fibrillation, 126–131, 127f, 129f
  causes and consequences, 128
  ECG characteristics of, 127–128
  intervention, 130

Atrial flutter, 112, 123–126, 124f, 125f
  causes and consequences, 125
  with 2:1 conduction, 123–124
  ECG characteristics of, 124–125

Atrial kick, 6

Atrial mechanisms, 107–132
atrial fibrillation, 126–131, 127f, 129f
atrial flutter, 123–126, 124f, 125f
atrial versus sinus and junctional ectopics, 130–131t
ECG rhythm identification practice, 133–140
multifocal atrial tachycardia (MAT), 116, 116f
nonconducted (blocked) PAC, 110–112, 110f, 111f
premature atrial complex (PAC), 108–112, 109f, 109t

Atrial pacemakers, 296

Atrial stretch, 111

Atrial tachycardia, 112–113, 113f, 174

Atropine sulfate, 448–449

Augmented leads, 22, 23, 23f

Augmented vector foot, 23

Augmented vector left, 23

Augmented vector right, 23

Automaticity, 14–15

Autonomic nervous system, 16

AV conduction defects, 173–186
advanced (or high-grade) AV block, 180–183, 181f, 182f
complete AV block, 184–186, 185f, 186t
ECG rhythm identification practice, 188–192
first-degree AV block, 174–176, 175f, 175t, 186t
second-degree AV block Type I, 174, 176–178, 177f, 178f, 183t, 186t
2:1 block, 180, 181f, 182

AV dissociation, 100

aVF lead, 22, 23, 28

AV interval, 288, 289, 289t, 298, 298f

AV junction, 17, 18f. See also Junctional mechanisms

aVL lead, 22, 23, 28

aVR lead, 22, 23

Axis
calculation of, 65–68, 65f–68f
defined, 22, 63
ECG rhythm identification practice, 72–76
left axis deviation, 65, 65f
Lewis circle, 69–70, 70f
normal and abnormal values, 69
normal axis, 64, 66
right axis deviation, 64, 64f

B

Bazette formula, 41

Bifascicular block, 203, 205–206

Bigeminy, 112, 112f

Bipolar leads, 22–23, 29, 291

Blocked PAC. See Nonconducted (blocked) PACs

Blood temperature pacemakers, 299

Bradycardia, 34
digitalis and, 49
narrow QRS complex, 427
sinus bradycardia, 80–82

Bradycardia-dependent branch block, 196

Brugada syndrome, 276–277

Bundle branch block, 193–194
ECG changes in, 195–203
left bundle branch block, 199, 201–203
rate-related bundle branch block, 196
right bundle branch block, 196–199, 198f

Bundle of His, 17–18

Bundle of Kent, 232, 233f, 240

Bypass tracts, 232

C

Calcium
abnormally low levels, hypocalcemia and, 51
excessive, hypercalcemia and, 50

Calcium chloride, 450

Cardiac axis. See Axis

Cardiac care guidelines (emergency). See Emergency cardiac care guidelines

Cardiac function, 1–11
cardiac muscle, 5–8
cardiac position and movement, 3–4, 4f
cardiac valves, 4–5, 5f
coronary artery perfusion, 9–11, 10f
mechanical structures of heart, 3, 3f

Cardiac output, 2

Cardiac serum enzyme markers, 272

Cardioversion
emergency, 122
synchronized, 120, 122–123, 153
unsynchronized, 156

Carotid sinus massage (CSM), 121

Catheter dislodgement, 302–303

Cerebrovascular disorder. See Stroke

Chamber enlargement, 223f
left atrial enlargement, 216
right atrial enlargement, 43, 215–216

Chest leads. See Precordial (chest) leads

Chest pain
cocaine-induced, 277
terms used to describe, 2

Chordae tendinae, 4–5

Chronic, defined, 126

Chronic obstructive pulmonary disease, 273

Cincinnati Prehospital Stroke Scale, 434

Circus-movement tachycardia, 236

Clinical applications, abbreviations for, 478

Clinical lead groups, 28–29

Coarse atrial fibrillation, 126

Coarse ventricular fibrillation, 157, 159f

Cocaine-induced chest pain and infarction, 277

Committed pacemakers, 289

Common left bundle, 193

Compensatory pause, 145–146

Complete AV block, 184–186, 185f, 186t

Complete left bundle branch block, 206, 208–209, 208t, 209f

Complexes, 38–39

Concealed conduction, 147

Conductivity, 15

Contiguous leads, 28

Continuous pacemakers, 293

Contractility, 15

Controlled atrial fibrillation, 126

Cornell voltage criteria, 221

Coronary artery disease
    left anterior descending CAD, 199
    sinus arrest and, 84

Coronary artery perfusion, 9–11, 10f, 248–249

Couplets, 148

Coving, 48

D

Deep spiral muscle groups, 7

Delta waves, 45, 232, 234, 234f, 240

Demand, 288

Demand pacemakers, 294–295, 299

Depolarization, 18. See also Axis
    atrial, P waves and, 37
    defined, 13–14
    displays, 31
    retrograde atrial depolarization, 93
    septal, 196
    ventricular, normal sequence of, 195

Diaphragmatic myocardial infarction, 261–262, 262t

Diastole, 4, 6

Diazepam, 451–452

Digitalis effect, 48–49

Digitalis toxicity, 101, 102

Diltiazem HCl, 452–454

Diphasic wave form, 22, 31

Dive reflex, 121

Dopamine, 454–455

Drug-induced changes, on ECG, 47–49

Drug use, in medical history, 48

Dual chamber pacemaker, 297–298, 301–302

Dyskinesia, 258

E

Early transition, 26

Ectopic, 108

Ectopic cells, 141

Ectopy, 15
    differentiation of atrial versus sinus and junctional
        ectopics, 130–131t
    ventricular, 142

Electrical conversion, 130

Electrical mechanical dissociation (EMD), 163

Electrocardiogram (ECG). See also Assessment; Myocardial
        perfusion deficits and ECG changes
    abbreviations, 477
    assessing dual chamber pacemaker on, 301–302
    assessing monitor pattern using multiple lead ECG, 442
    assessing the pacemaker ECG, 300–302
    drug-induced changes on, 47–49
    function of, 21
    monitoring myocardial ischemia, injury, and necrosis,
        254–261
    monitor pattern assessment, 441
    multiple lead system, 21–29
    normal ranges/variations in adult 12-lead, 423–424
    sinus mechanism configurations/proposed treatment,
        86t–87t
    standard 12-lead, 252
    ST segment monitoring, 274–276, 275f, 276t
    ventricular strain pattern, 223, 224t–225t, 225

Electrolyte imbalances
    abnormal QT intervals and, 46
    alterations in duration/amplitude of ECG wave forms
        and, 47
    ECG wave forms/complexes and, 52t–53t

Electronic capture, 300, 302

Electronic pacemakers
    abbreviations used with, 479
    asynchronous, 293, 295
    atrial, 296
    catheter dislodgement, 302–303
    catheters and electrodes, 291

Electronic pacemakers (*continued*)
    classification, 293
    components, 290–293
    demand pacemakers, 294–295
    ECG rhythm identification practice, 305–310
    failure to capture, 300
    failure to function, 299–300
    failure to sense, 300
    fusion, 292–293
    hysteresis, 295–296, 295f
    interference, 303
    malfunction of, 299–300
    pacemaker energy, 291–292
    pacemaker function, 289, 289t
    pacemaker identification code, 288
    perforation, 302
    for sinus arrest, 84
    skeletal muscle inhibition, 302–303
    temporary and permanent pacing, 293–296
    terminology, 488
    ventricular, 296–299, 296f–298f
Electrophysiologic testing, 152
Electrophysiology of heart, 13–18
    cardiac cycle phases, 14, 15f
    cardiac muscle properties, 14–16
    electrical conduction system, 9, 16–18, 17f, 18f
    nervous system control of heart, 16
Emergency cardiac care guidelines, 425–436
    acute coronary syndrome, 431
    asystole, 430
    elevated blood pressure in acute ischemic stroke, 436
    fibrinolytic criteria for AMI, 432
    fibrinolytic criteria for CVA, 435–436
    narrow QRS complex bradycardia, 427
    narrow QRS complex tachycardia, 429
    prehospital stroke criteria, 434–435
    primary ABCD survey, 425
    SAMPLE, 427
    secondary ABCD survey, 426
    suspected stroke (EMS assessment and actions), 432–434
    ventricular fibrillation and pulseless ventricular tachycardia, 429
Emergency cardioversion, 122
Emphysema, 53, 273
End-diastolic PVC, 146, 147f
Endocardium, 6
Epicardium, 6
Epinephrine, 16, 455–457
Eptifibatide, 457–458
Escape interval, 294
Escape junctional complex, 95–96, 96f
Excitability, 15

F
Failure to capture, 292, 300
Failure to function, 299–300
Failure to sense, 300, 301f
Fascicular blocks, 65, 203–206
    bifascicular block, 203, 205–206
    left anterior fascicular block, 203, 205–206
    left posterior fascicular block, 206
Fast cells, 141
Fibrinolysis, 250
Fibrinolytic criteria
    for AMI, 432
    for CVA, 435–436
Fibrinolytic-revascularization therapy, 251
Fibrous pericardium, 5–6
Fib waves, 126
Fine atrial fibrillation, 127
Fine ventricular fibrillation, 157, 159f
    asystole versus, 161
First-degree AV block, 174–176, 175f, 175t, 186t
Fixed atherosclerotic obstruction, 250
Fixed coupling, 147, 148
Fixed-rate pacemakers, 293
Flutter waves, 123
Focal atrial tachycardia, 112
Frontal plane, 22, 29
Fully committed pacemakers, 289
Furosemide, 458–459
Fusion, 290f, 292–293
Fusion beats, 151
F waves, 126

G
Global lead changes, 53

H
Handbook of Emergency Cardiovascular Care for Health Care Providers (2008), 437
Heart rate, 2
Hemiblock, 203
Hexaxial reference system, 65
High-grade (advanced) AV block, 180–183, 181f, 182f
Horizontal plane, 24
Hypercalcemia, 46, 50, 52f
Hyperkalemia, 46, 49, 49f, 258, 273

Hypertrophic cardiomyopathy (HCM), 56, 273

Hypertrophy, 217–225
  left ventricular, 218–219, 219f
  QRS changes, 219–223
  right ventricular, 215, 217–218, 217f, 218f
  ventricular strain pattern, 223, 224f–225f, 225

Hypocalcemia, 51, 51f

Hypokalemia, 50, 50f

Hypomagnesemia, 46

Hypoperfusion, 81, 86, 184

Hypothermia, 40

Hypoxia, 2

Hysteresis, 295–296, 295f

I

Idiojunctional rhythm, 100, 101f

Idiopathic PACs, 111

Idioventricular rhythm (IVR), 158–159, 160f. *See also*
  Accelerated idioventricular rhythm (AIVR)

Implantable cardioverdefibrillator (ICD), 277

Incomplete left bundle branch block, 202

Index of Lewis, 220

Infarction, 247. *See also* Myocardial infarction

Inferior leads, 28

Inferior wall myocardial infarction, 261–262, 262t, 263f

Inferoposterior wall myocardial infarction, 250

Infranodal, 178, 184

Inhibited pacemakers, 298–298

Injury, 247

Intermittent ventricular tachycardia, 152–153, 153f

Interpolated PVC, 146–147

Intersociety Committee on Heart Disease, 288

Intervals, 38

Intracranial pressure (ICP), increase in, 56, 57f, 274

Intranodal bypass tract syndrome, 239

Intraventricular conduction defects, 64
  bundle branches and arterial perfusion, 194–195, 194f
  complete left bundle branch block, 206, 208–209, 208t
  ECG changes in bundle branch block, 195–203
  ECG rhythm identification practice, 209–213
  fascicular blocks, 203–206
  normal sequence of ventricular depolarization/QRS
    vector, 195
  trifascicular block, 209

Intrinsicoid deflection, 202

Ischemia, 247

Isoelectric line, 40

Isoproterenol, 459–461

J

James, T.N., 18, 94

James fibers, 232, 239

J point, 40, 277

Junctional escape beat, 95–96, 96f, 101

Junctional mechanisms, 93–102
  accelerated junctional rhythm, 97–98
  ECG rhythm identification practice, 103–106
  escape junctional complex, 95–96
  idiojunctional rhythm, 100
  junctional rhythm, 96–97
  junctional tachycardia, 98
  origin of, 94–95
  premature junctional complex, 98–100
  summary of causes of, 100–102

Junctional pacing function, 18

Junctional rhythm, 95, 96–97, 97f

Junctional tachycardia, 98, 98f, 101

K

Kent bundles, 232, 233f, 240

L

LAD disease, 10

Lateral leads, 28

Lateral wall myocardial infarction, 268f, 268t

Leads, 21–23, 28, 291. *See also* Multiple lead system; specific lead;
  specific type of lead

Left anterior descending (LAD), 10, 248, 250

Left anterior fascicular block, 193
  myocardial infarction and, 206
  right bundle branch block and, 205–206

Left anterior hemiblock, 203, 206

Left atrial enlargement (LAE), 44

Left atrium, 3

Left axis deviation, 65, 65f, 68

Left bundle branch block, 194, 199, 201–203, 221
  incomplete, 202
  resulting from myocardial infarction, 202–203

Left circumflex artery, 248

Left coronary artery, 248

Left main branch, 193

Left main trunk, 10

Left posterior fascicular block, 193, 206, 208f

Left ventricle, 3

Left ventricular hypertrophy, 194, 218–219, 219f, 222f, 273
   axis, 221
   with left bundle branch block, 221
   with right bundle branch block, 221

Left ventricular strain, 223

Lewis circle, 69–70, 70f

Lidocaine HCl 2%, 461–462

Limb leads, 22–23, 29

Los Angeles Prehospital Stroke Screen, 434–435

Lown-Ganong-Levine (LGL) syndrome, 239

Low-voltage QRS, 51–53

M

Macrocircuits, 119

Macroreentrant tachyarrhythmia, 123

Magnesium sulfate, 462–464

Mahaim's fibers, 232

Marriott, Henry J., 26

MCL leads, 26–28

Medications. *See also* specific drug
   medication-induced ECG changes, 47–49, 52t–53t
   medication profiles, 443–476
   tachycardia and, 79
   that can cause TdP, 155

Metabolic status pacemakers, 299

Microcircuits, 118

Midazolam, 464–465

Mitral and tricuspid valves, 4

Mitral valve, 5

Mobitz I. *See* Second-degree AV block Type I

Mobitz II. *See* Second-degree AV block Type II

Mode of pacemaker response, 288

Monomorphic ventricular tachycardia, 150–152, 151f

Morphine sulfate, 465–467

Multifocal atrial tachycardia (MAT), 116, 116f

Multiform PVCs, 147, 148

Multiple lead system, 21–29
   augmented leads, 23
   clinical lead groups, 28
   hazards of improper lead placement, 28–29
   limb leads, 22–23
   MCL leads, 26–28
   monitoring posterior surface of heart, 25–26, 26f
   precordial (chest) leads, 24–25

Mural thrombus, 129

Myocardial cells, 14

Myocardial infarction
   anterior wall, 264–265, 264f, 265t
   anterolateral wall, 265–266, 267f
   anteroseptal wall, 265, 266f
   consequences of coronary artery occlusion, 250–252
   inferior wall (diaphragmatic), 261–262, 262t, 263f
   interoposterior wall, 250
   lateral wall, 266–268, 268f, 268t
   nonclassic ECG presentation of, 274
   pathophysiology of, 249–254
   posterior wall, 269, 270f, 271t
   reflecting and reciprocal leads, 252–253
   right ventricular, 269, 271–272, 271f, 272t
   and unstable angina compared, 250

Myocardial perfusion deficits and ECG changes, 247–278
   anterior wall MI, 264–265, 264f, 265t
   anterolateral wall MI, 265–266, 267f
   anteroseptal wall MI, 265, 266f
   Brugada syndrome, 276–277
   cocaine-induced chest pain and infarction, 277
   coronary artery perfusion, 248–249
   ECG indicators of, 261
   ECG rhythm identification practice, 279–285
   inferior wall MI, 261–262
   lateral wall MI, 266–268, 268f, 268t
   monitoring myocardial ischemia, injury, necrosis, 254–261
   nonclassic ECG presentation of acute MI, 274
   non-Q-wave MI, 272
   pathophysiology of MI, 249–254
   posterior wall MI, 269, 270f, 271t
   pseudo-infarction patterns, 273–274
   right ventricular MI, 269, 271–272

Myocardium, 5, 6

N

Nadir T wave, 40, 258, 259f

Narrow QRS complex, analysis of, 439–440

Narrow QRS complex bradycardia, 427

Narrow QRS complex tachycardia, 428

Narrow QRS tachycardia, 438

Necrosis, 247, 250

Nervous system, 16

Net area of the QRS. *See* Axis

New onset atrial fibrillation, 126

Nitroglycerin, 467–468

Nodal, 173

No-man's-land lead, 23

Nonconducted (blocked) PACs, 110–112, 110f, 111f

Non-Q-wave myocardial infarction, 272

Nonrefractory period, 16

Nontransmural (non-Q wave), 261, 272

Norepinephrine, 16

Northwest lead, 23

Notation, 289

NSTEMI (no ST segment elevation), 250–251

O

Orphan lead, 23

Orthodromic tachycardia, 236

Overdrive pacing, 156

Oversensing (pacemakers), 292, 300

Oxygen, 468–470

P

Pacemaker cells, 14–15. *See also* Sinus node

Pacemaker identification code, 288

Pacemakers. *See* Electronic pacemakers

PA interval, 289

Paired PVCs, 148

Papillary muscles, 5

Parasympathetic systems, 16

Paroxysmal atrial fibrillation, 126, 128

Paroxysmal atrial tachycardia (PAT), 116–117

Paroxysmal supraventricular tachycardia, 232

Paroxysmal tachycardia, 94

Partially committed pacemakers, 289

Patient assessment. *See* Assessment

Percutaneous transluminal coronary angioplasty, 250

Perforation, 302

Perfusion, 6, 9–11, 10f
ECG indicators of deficits, 261

Pericardial effusion, 54–55
low-voltage QRS and, 51

Pericardial tamponade, 55

Pericarditis, 53–55, 257

Pericardium, 4–5

Peripheral embolus, 129

Permanent atrial fibrillation, 126

Permanent pacing, 293

Persistent atrial fibrillation, 126

P mitrale, 44, 216, 216f

Pneumothorax, 273

Polymorphic ventricular tachycardia, 154–156, 154f

Poor R-wave progression, 26, 27f

Positive ST segment coving, 256

Posterior descending artery, 248

Posterior wall myocardial infarction, 269, 270f, 271t

Potassium
decreased, hypokalemia and, 50
increased, hyperkalemia and, 49

P prime (P′), 37, 94, 96, 97, 99

P pulmonale, 43, 215, 216f

PQRST complex, 54

Precordial (chest) leads, 24–25, 29

Preexcitation
defined, 232
degrees of, 234–235
ECG wave forms affected by, 232, 233f, 234–236

Pregnancy, atrial ectopy and, 111

Premature atrial complex (PAC), 37, 37f, 108–112, 109f, 109t
with aberrant ventricular conduction, 114–116, 115f
ECG characteristics of, 108–109
nonconducted (blocked), 110–112, 110f, 111f

Premature junctional complex (PJC), 98–100, 99f

Premature ventricular complex (PVC), 142–150, 143f–150f, 144t
ECG characteristics of, 143–144
end-diastolic, 146
with full compensatory pause, 145–146
interpolated, 146–147
intervention, 150
multiform, 148
narrow complex, 144–145, 145f
pairs or couplets, 148
recognizing, 142–143
R-on-T phenomenon, 150, 152f
trigeminy, 149
uniform, 147
variations in, 145–150
ventricular bigeminy, 149

Premature ventricular ectopic complex (PVC), 37, 37f

Primary ST-T wave changes, 196

PR interval, 38, 43, 44, 44f

Procainamide HCl, 470–471

Programmed upper rate limit (PURL), 298, 299

Prolapsed valve, 5

Pseudo-infarction patterns, 273–274

Pseudonormalization, 53

Pulmonary embolism, 57, 58f, 129, 273

Pulmonic circulation, 3

Pulmonic valve, 4

Pulse generator, 290, 294f

Pulseless electrical activity (PEA), 162–163, 163f, 439

P waves, 17, 37, 37f, 42f, 43. *See also* P prime (P′)
  abnormal, 43–44
  junctional-induced, 100
  sinus-induced, 78–80, 82, 83, 85

Q

QRS alternans, 236, 236f

QRS axis. *See* Axis

QRS changes, 219–223

QRS complex, 17, 27f, 38–39, 42f, 43
  abnormal, 45–46
  low-voltage, 51–53
  net area of, 63, 64f (*See also* Axis)
  PVCs and, 142–143

QRS vector, normal sequence of, 195

QT interval, 41, 41f, 43
  abnormal, 45, 48

Quadrant method, of calculating axis, 67

Q waves, 38, 260–261, 260f

R

Radiofrequency catheter ablation, 123

Ramus intermedius, 248

Rate-adaptive or physiologic pacers, 298

Rate and rhythm, calculating, 32–36, 33f, 35f, 36f

Reciprocal leads, 252–254, 253f, 254f, 263f, 267f, 268f, 275f

Reentrant atrial tachycardia, 112, 123, 131

Reentry, 118, 142, 149

Reentry tachycardia, 236

Reflecting leads, 252–254, 253f, 253t, 254f, 257f

Refractoriness, 16

Relative refractory period (RRP), 16

Repolarization, 14, 18
  early repolarization, 274

Retrograde atrial depolarization, 93

Rhythm. *See* Rate and rhythm, calculating

Right atrial enlargement (RAE), 43, 215–216

Right atrium, 3

Right axis deviation, 64, 64f, 68

Right bundle branch block, 193, 194, 196–199, 198f, 221
  acute myocardial infarction and, 199
  incomplete, 198–199
  left anterior fascicular block and, 205–206

Right coronary artery, 248

Right ventricle, 3

Right ventricular hypertrophy, 215, 217–218, 217f, 218f

Right ventricular myocardial infarction, 269, 271–272, 271f, 272t

Right ventricular strain, 225

R-on-T PVCs, 150, 152f

R prime (R′), 38

RR intervals, 35, 35f

rS complex, 45

R/S voltage criteria, 221

RV interval, 289

R wave, 38

R-wave progression, 26, 27f

S

SA node, 78, 79

Sawtooth baseline, 123

Scooping, 48

Secondary T waves, 196

Second-degree AV block Type I, 174, 176–178, 177f, 178f, 183t, 186t

Second-degree AV block Type II, 176, 178–180, 183t, 186t

Semilunar valves, 4

Sensitivity (of pacemakers), 292

Sensitivity (true positive rate), 221

Septal depolarization, 196

Septal leads, 28

Septal perforating arteries, 248

Serous pericardium, 6

Serum biomarkers, 251

Sherf, L., 18, 94

Sinoatrial block. *See* Sinus (SA) block

Sinoatrial node. *See* SA node

Sinus arrest, 83–85
  causes, 84
  intervention, 84–85

Sinus arrhythmia, 82–83

Sinus bradycardia, 80–82

Sinus exit block. *See* Sinus (SA) block

Sinus mechanisms, 77–86
  ECG rhythm identification practice, 88–92
  sinoatrial (SA) block, 85–86, 85f, 86f
  sinus arrest, 83–85, 84f
  sinus arrhythmia, 82–83, 83f
  sinus bradycardia, 80–82, 81f

sinus rhythm, 78–80, 78f
sinus tachycardia, 79–80, 79f
Sinus node
blood supply to, 9
bradycardia and tachycardia, 34
function of, 17
parasympathetic stimulation and, 16
Sinus node artery, 248
Sinus rhythm, 78
Sinus (SA) block, 85–86
Sinus tachycardia, 79–80, 174, 237
Skeletal muscle inhibition, 302–303
"Skipped beat," 111
Sleep apnea, 84
Slow cells, 141
Sodium Bicarbonate, 471–472
Sokolow-Lyon criteria, 221
Specialized cells, 14
Specificity (true negative rate), 221
$S_1Q_3T_3$ pattern, 57
STEMI (ST segment elevation), 250
Stroke
atrial fibrillation and, 129–130
elevated blood pressure in acute ischemic stroke, 436
fibrinolytic criteria for, 435–436
prehospital stroke criteria: detection dispatch delivery, 434–435
suspected stroke emergency guidelines, 432–434
Stroke volume, 2
ST segment, 40, 42f, 43
continuous monitoring of, 274–276, 275f, 276t
depression, 254–255
elevation of, 255–258, 255f–257f, 261
ST-T abnormalities, 258
Sudden unexpected death syndrome (SUDS), 276–277
Superficial muscle groups, 7
Supraventricular, 107–108
Supraventricular mechanisms, differentiating, 109
Supraventricular tachycardia (SVT), 117–123, 118f–123f, 231
causes and consequences, 120
ECG characteristics of, 119–120
intervention, 121
Sustained atrial tachycardia, 117
Sustained SVT, 117
Sustained ventricular tachycardia (sustained v-tach), 151
S wave, 38
Sympathetic systems, 16

Symptomatic patient, defined, 2
Synchronized cardioversion, 102, 120, 122–123, 153
Systemic circulation, 3
Systemic vascular resistance, 3
Systole, 4, 6–8

T
Tachycardia, 34
antidromic, 237, 238f
atrial, 112–113, 113f, 174
intermittent ventricular, 152–153, 153f
junctional, 98, 98f, 101
monomorphic ventricular, 150–152, 151f
multifocal atrial (MAT), 116, 116f
narrow QRS, 438
narrow QRS complex, 428, 438
orthodromic, 236–237
paroxysmal, 94, 232
paroxysmal atrial, 116–117
polymorphic ventricular, 154–156, 154f
sinus, 79–80, 174, 237
supraventricular (SVT), 117–123, 118f–123f, 231
ventricular, 429
Tachycardia-dependent branch block, 196
Tamponade, 55, 163
T distortion, 108
Temporary pacing, 293
Threshold, 291
Thromboembolic occlusion, 250
"Time is muscle," 254
Tirofiban, 472–474
Torsades de Pointes (TdP), 46, 56, 154–156
TP segment, 53
Transcutaneous pacemakers, 290
Transition zone, 26
Transmural infarctions, 261
Transvenous radio-frequency ablation, 242
Trending, 248, 274
Tricuspid valve, 5
Trifascicular block, 209
Trigeminy, 149
Triggered activity, 113
Triggered ventricular pacemakers, 297–298
Troponins, 251
T waves, 40–41, 41f, 42, 43
changes/abnormalities, 258–259, 259f
secondary, 196

12-lead ECG, 225, 252

Two-step method, of calculating axis, 66, 66f

2008 Handbook of Emergency Cardiovascular Care for Health Care Providers, 437

2:1 block, 180, 181f, 182

Type I AV block (second-degree), 174, 176–178, 177f, 178f, 183t, 186t

U

Uncontrolled atrial fibrillation, 126

Undersensing (pacemakers), 292

Uniform PVCs, 147

Unipolar leads, 22, 291

Unstable angina, 250–251

Unsynchronized cardioversion, 156

U waves, 41, 42–43, 42f, 43, 260
  abnormal, 46–47

V

Vagal tone, increasing, 121

Vagus, 16

Valsalva's maneuver, 121

Valve cusps, 4

Varying polarity, 154

Vascular resistance, 3

Vasopressin, 474–475

Vector, 65

Ventricles, 6–8, 7f

Ventricular aneurysm, 55, 55f, 257

Ventricular bigeminy, 149

Ventricular depolarization, normal sequence of, 195

Ventricular diastole, 4, 6, 8–9, 9f

Ventricular fibrillation, 156–158, 429
  coarse vs. fine, 157, 159f
  mistaken as TdP, 155
  patient assessment, 438

Ventricular flutter, 156

Ventricular hypertrophy, 64, 217–225
  left ventricular, 218–219, 219f
  right ventricular, 217–218, 217f, 218f

Ventricular mechanisms, 141–172
  accelerated idioventricular rhythm, 159–161, 160f
  asystole, 161–162, 161f
  ECG rhythm identification practice, 165–172
  guide to ECG analysis of, 164t
  idioventricular rhythm, 158–159, 160f
  intermittent ventricular tachycardia, 152–153, 153f
  monomorphic ventricular tachycardia, 150–152, 151f
  polymorphic ventricular tachycardia, 154–156, 154f
  premature ventricular complex (PVC), 142–150
  pulseless electrical activity, 162–163, 163f
  ventricular fibrillation, 156–158
  ventricular flutter, 156

Ventricular pacemakers, 296–299, 296f–298f
  overdrive suppression, 299
  rate-responsive, 299
  triggered ventricular pacemakers, 297–298
  ventricular demand pacemakers, 297

Ventricular strain pattern, 223, 224f–225f, 225

Ventricular systole, 4, 6–8, 9f

Ventricular tachycardia, 429

Verapamil HCl, 475–476

Visceral pericardium. See Epicardium

Voltage, measurement of, 32

V_1 through V_{6R} leads, 24–26, 28

W

Wave forms, 36–39
  abnormal, 43–47
  alterations of, 47–58
  summary, 43t

Wenckebach periodicity (Wenckebach phenomenon), 177. See also Second-degree AV block Type I

Wide QRS complex tachycardia of uncertain origin, 152–153

Wide QRS tachycardia, 439

"Widow maker," 10

Wolff-Parkinson-White syndrome, 240, 241f, 242, 273